WE

D0551903

£21.99.

Muscles, Bones and Skin

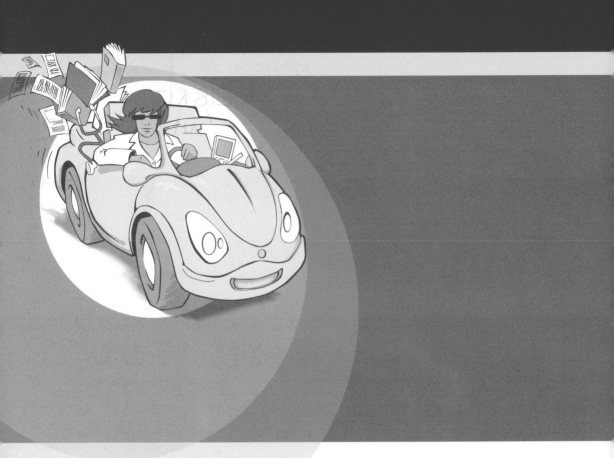

First and second edition authors:
Sona V. Biswas
Rehana Iqbal
Sîan Knight BMedSci

CRASH COURSE

Third Edition

Muscles, Bones and Skin

Series editor
Daniel Horton-Szar
BSc (Hons), MBBS (Hons), MRCGP

Northgate Medical Practice
Canterbury
Kent, UK

Faculty advisors
Andrew Joseph Gerard McDonagh
MB ChB, FRCP

Consultant Dermatologist
Sheffield Teaching Hospitals NHS
Foundation Trust & Honorary
Clinical Senior Lecturer
University of Sheffield
Sheffield, UK

Anthony Gerard Wilson
MB PhD FRCP DCH

Reader in Rheumatology
Section of Musculoskeletal
Sciences
School of Medicine & Biomedical
Sciences
Royal Hallamshire Hospital
Sheffield, UK

Judith E Ritchie

BMedSci

Medical Student, University of Sheffield Medical School
Sheffield, UK

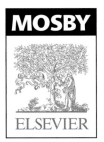

Edinburgh • London • New York • Oxford • Philadelphia • St Louis • Sydney • Toronto 2008

MOSBY
ELSEVIER

Commissioning Editor:	**Alison Taylor**
Development Editor:	**Lulu Stader**
Project Manager:	**Jess Thompson**
Page Design:	**Sarah Russell**
Cover Design:	**Stewart Larking**
Icon Illustration:	**Geo Parkin**
Illustration Management:	**Merlyn Harvey**
Illustrator:	**Marion Tasker**

© 1998, Mosby International Ltd
© 2003, Elsevier Science Ltd
© 2008, Elsevier Limited. All rights reserved.

First edition 1998
Second edition 2003
Third edition 2008

ISBN: 9780723434344

British Library Cataloguing in Publication Data
A catalogue record for this book is available from the British Library

Library of Congress Cataloging in Publication Data
A catalog record for this book is available from the Library of Congress

Note
Knowledge and best practice in this field are constantly changing. As new research and experience broaden our knowledge, changes in practice, treatment and drug therapy may become necessary or appropriate. Readers are advised to check the most current information provided (i) on procedures featured or (ii) by the manufacturer of each product to be administered, to verify the recommended dose or formula, the method and duration of administration, and contraindications. It is the responsibility of the practitioner, relying on their own experience and knowledge of the patient, to make diagnoses, to determine dosages and the best treatment for each individual patient, and to take all appropriate safety precautions. To the fullest extent of the law, neither the Publisher nor the Authors assumes any liability for any injury and/or damage to persons or property arising out or related to any use of the material contained in this book.

The Publisher

Working together to grow
libraries in developing countries

www.elsevier.com | www.bookaid.org | www.sabre.org

ELSEVIER   BOOK AID International   Sabre Foundation

ELSEVIER   your source for books,
journals and multimedia
in the health sciences

www.elsevierhealth.com

The
Publisher's
policy is to use
**paper manufactured
from sustainable forests**

Printed in China

Preface

Medicine is the scientific field that concerns the maintenance or restoration of health and requires a broad yet comprehensive scientific knowledge of the functioning of the body's systems, together with clinical knowledge of the disease processes that affect them and the treatments available. Modern medical curricula integrate these areas of knowledge, producing a requirement for a broad scope of knowledge that can appear overwhelming to students embarking on a medical education. Herein lies the distinct advantage of the Crash Course series over most conventional medical textbooks, as they deliver core systematic knowledge of health and disease in a concise yet comprehensive format. Crash Course: Muscles Bone and Skin dissects the fields of rheumatology, orthopaedics and dermatology to produce categorical chunks that are easy to digest. The glossary allows rapid reference of key terms, and the self-assessment section provides the opportunity to review your knowledge using modern formats of assessment adopted in medical schools today.

The unique format of the *Crash Course* series has made them highly popular and an essential tool for students in both preclinical and clinical stages of training, myself included, and it has been a privilege to be involved in editing and authoring this edition. I hope you find it useful and accessible, and I wish you well in all your exams and your future medical career.

Judith Ritchie

Muscles, bones and skin are big subjects with important connections to many areas of medical practice. In this book, the basic science and disease topics are integrated to meet the needs of the contemporary medical school curriculum. Using a summarizing style of text with plenty of pictures and tables, the material is presented in a format to help with rapid learning and revision.

Dr Andrew Joseph Gerard McDonagh
Faculty Advisor

Musculoskeletal abnormalities are major causes of morbidity; back, neck and soft tissue problems such as tenosynovitis are major causes of days lost from work and a major reason for attendance at primary care clinics. The inflammatory joint diseases such as rheumatoid arthritis are also relatively common, but our increasing understanding of the mediators of joint inflammation and destruction has resulted in the recent therapeutic introduction of inhibitors of proinflammatory cytokines. This book gives a comprehensive insight into the pathogenesis, clinical features and treatments of these common conditions in a user-friendly format.

Dr Anthony Gerard Wilson
Faculty Advisor

More than a decade has now passed since work began on the first editions of the *Crash Course* series, and over 4 years since the publication of the second edition. Medicine never stands still, and the work of keeping this series relevant for today's students is an ongoing process. This third edition builds on the success of the previous ones and incorporates a great deal of new and revised material, keeping the series up to date with the latest medical research and developments in pharmacology and current best practice.

As always, we listen to feedback from the thousands of students who use *Crash Course*, and have made further improvements to the layout and structure of the books. Each chapter now starts with a set of learning objectives, and the self-assessment sections have been enhanced and brought up to date with modern exam formats. We have also worked to integrate points of clinical relevance into the basic medical science material, which will not only add to the interest of the text but will reinforce the principles being described.

Despite fully revising the books, we hold fast to the principles on which we first developed the series: *Crash Course* will always bring you all the information you need to revise in compact, manageable volumes that integrate basic medical science and clinical practice. The books still maintain the balance between clarity and conciseness, and provide sufficient depth for those aiming at distinction. The authors are medical students and junior doctors who have recent experience of the exams you are now facing, and the accuracy of the material is checked by senior faculty members from across the UK.

I wish you all the best for your future careers!

Dr Daniel Horton-Szar
Series Editor

Acknowledgements

There are so many thank-yous for so many people who have kept me going this year. Thank you to everyone at Elsevier, particularly Lulu, for her support, reassurance and lovely pictures of the Scottish scenery. Thank you to everyone working with me within the Department of Surgical Oncology for being so fantastic and supportive as I juggled research and writing; to Peter and Lynda for their support, and to Cathryn and Rose who kept me laughing every evening! To Phoenix and Fox for their continuous support, endless encouragement and boundless hilarity. To Louise for 'bigging me up' at the times I've felt small. To Moe, whose love, companionship and total faith have kept me going through the early starts and the long hours. And a special thank you to my mum June, a pillar of support and faith and a wonderful friend.

Figure acknowledgements

Fig. 1.7, 4.5, 4.10, 4.18, 4.20A, 5.30, 5.31 and 5.32 redrawn with permission from P G Bullough and V J Vigorita. Orthopaedic Pathology, 3rd edition. TMIP, 1997.

Figs. 2.8B, 2.9, 2.20, 4.8A–C and 6.3 reproduced with permission from A Stevens and J Lowe. Human Histology, 2nd edition. Mosby, 1997. Fig. 2.8B also courtesy of T Gray.

Figs. 3.1, 3.9 and 5.1 reproduced with permission from R M H McMinn, P Gaddum-Rosse, R T Hutchings and B M Logan. McMinn's Functional and Clinical Anatomy. TMIP, 1995.

Figs. 4.1, 11.6 and 10.9 reproduced with permission from J A Gosling, P F Harris, J R Humpherson, I Whitmore and P L T Wilan. Human Anatomy, Color Atlas and Text, 3rd edition. TMIP, 1996.

Fig. 4.6 adapted with permission from Basic Histology, 8th edition, by L.C. Junqueira, Appleton & Lange, 1995.

Figs. 4.13, 4.21, 5.6 and 5.7 reproduced with permission from A Stevens and J Lowe. Pathology. Mosby, 1991.

Figs. 5.10, 5.11, 5.18, 5.21, 5.28 and 5.29 redrawn with permission from O Epstein, G D Perkin, D P deBono and J Cookson. Clinical Examination, 2edition, Mosby, 1997.

Colour figures in Chapter 7 reproduced with permission from G White. Levene's Color Atlas of Dermatology, 2nd edition. Mosby, 1997.

With the exception of Figs. 7.6 and 7.24 from Genera and Systemic Pathology, 3rd edition, JC Underwood, Harcourt, 2000.

Dedication

For my late father, John, whose love and blessings inspire me to achieve, and who guides me in spirit in all that I do.

Contents

Contents

Glossary

Acetylcholine   a neurotransmitter released and acting at cholinergic autonomic synapses and neuromuscular junctions

Actin   a protein that polymerizes to form myofilaments, often called thin filaments, within each sarcomere.

Action potential   an electrical signal produced by a neuron, created by a change of electrical charge across a membrane

Aponeurosis   a broad thin sheet of collagenous connective tissue through which several muscles or a group of muscles attach to bone

Chronotrope   an agent that increases (positive chronotrope) or decreases (negative chronotrope) the rate or frequency of cardiac contraction

Cross-bridge   a myosin head that projects from the surface of a thick filament and which can bind to an active site of a thin filament in the presence of calcium ions, responsible for producing contraction

Dermis   cutaneous connective tissue layer situated between the epidermis and the submucosa

DMARD   disease-modifying antirheumatic drug

Dystrophin   a protein present in skeletal and cardiac muscle that forms complexes with glycoproteins of the sarcolemma, essential for its proper functioning

Eccrine gland   cutaneous sweat glands under sympathetic nervous control independent of hair follicles. Involved in thermoregulation

EDV   end-diastolic volume: the volume of blood in the ventricle of the heart at the end of diastole

Endocardium   simple squamous epithelium lining the heart, continuous with the endothelium of the great vessels

Endomysium   a thin layer of connective tissue that surrounds each individual muscle fibre, containing the nerves, blood vessels and lymphatics that supply it

Epicardium   a connective tissue layer surrounding the outside of the heart, continuous with the pericardium

Epidermis   the epithelium covering the skin surface

Exocrine gland   a gland that releases its secretions via a duct, e.g. salivary or sweat glands

Gower's sign   when a patient must use his or her upper body in order to rise from sitting to standing. A sign of proximal muscle weakness

Hair follicle   a tubular structure containing a single hair, lined by a stratified squamous epithelium that begins at the surface of the skin and ends at the hair papilla

Hair root   a cone-shaped structure consisting of a connective tissue papilla and its overlying matrix, a layer of epithelial cells that produces the hair shaft

Hallux   big toe

Hamartoma   a benign growth composed of cells and tissues normally present in that area, growing in a disorganized manner

Hyperkeratosis   thickening and hardening of the skin

Immunofluorescence   a laboratory investigation using fluorescent microscopy to detect an antigen. Can be direct or indirect, depending on the method used

Inotrope   an agent that increases (positive inotrope) or decreases (negative inotrope) the force of a muscular contraction. Most commonly used with reference to agents that affect heart muscle

Insensible perspiration   water loss by evaporation across the epithelium of the skin or the alveolar surfaces of the lungs

Isometric contraction   muscular contraction producing tension but no movement

Isotonic   muscular contraction producing movement, but with equal tension throughout the movement

Keratolytic   a topical substance used to soften and promote epidermal peeling in certain conditions, e.g. warts

Myofibril   organized collections of myofilaments within muscle cells

Myofilaments   fine protein filaments of a muscle composed primarily of the proteins actin (thin filaments) and myosin (thick filaments)

Motor unit   term describing a single motor neuron and the muscle fibres that neuron innervates

Myosin   a protein that forms myofilaments that utilize ATP molecules to interact with actin myofilaments in order to produce contraction

NSAID   non-steroidal anti-inflammatory drug

Pacemaker cells   cells of the sinoatrial node that set the pace of cardiac contraction

Pacinian corpuscle   a cutaneous receptor sensitive to vibration

Parasympathetic division   division of the autonomic nervous system, responsible for activities that conserve energy and lower the metabolic rate

Parasympathomimetic   drugs that mimic the actions of parasympathetic stimulation

Parathyroid glands   four small glands embedded in the posterior surface of the thyroid, responsible for parathyroid hormone secretion

Parathyroid hormone   a hormone secreted by the parathyroid gland when plasma calcium levels fall below the normal range, causing increased osteoclast activity, increased intestinal calcium uptake, and decreased calcium ion loss at the kidneys

Pericardium   the fibrous sac that surrounds the heart and whose inner, serous lining is continuous with the epicardium

Perimysium   the connective tissue sheath that covers a bundle of muscle fibres, dividing them into fasciculi

Sarcolemma   the cell membrane of a muscle fibre

Sarcomere   the contractile unit of striated myofibrils composed of thick (myosin) and thin (actin) filaments interacting with each other

Sarcoplasmic reticulum   specialized form of endoplasmic reticulum in muscle fibres. Important in storage and release of calcium during the process of contraction

Sensible perspiration   water loss due to sweat gland secretion

Subluxation   an incomplete or partial dislocation of a joint

Subungual hyperkeratosis   excessive proliferation of the nail bed and hyonychium, which can lead to the nail separating from the underlying nail bed

Subungual haematoma   an accumulation of blood under the nail to produce a solid swelling or haematoma

Sympathetic nervous system   division of the autonomic nervous system responsible for 'fight or flight' reactions, mobilizing energy in times of stress

Sympathomimetic   drugs that mimic the actions of sympathetic stimulation

Syncytium   cells that act together as a functional unit. Where this occurs in the heart it is called cardiac syncytium

Tendon   inelastic flexible cord composed of closely compacted collagen fibres that attach muscle to bone

Topical   application directly to the skin

Valgus   angulation away from the midline of the body

Varus   angulation inwards towards the midline of the body

BASIC MEDICAL SCIENCE OF MUSCLES, BONES AND SKIN

Musculoskeletal system— an overview

Objectives

By the end of this chapter you will be able to:
- Explain the components of the musculoskeletal system
- Discuss the general functions of the musculoskeletal system
- Describe the stimulation of skeletal, cardiac and smooth muscle
- List the general functions of the skin
- Name the three layers of the skin
- Define connective tissue and outline its functions and classification
- Describe the components of connective tissue.

OVERVIEW OF THE MUSCULOSKELETAL SYSTEM

Introduction

The musculoskeletal system comprises muscles, bones and joints. It makes up most of the body's mass and performs several essential functions, including:

- The maintenance of body shape
- The support and protection of soft tissue structures
- Movement
- Breathing
- The storage of calcium and phosphate in bone.

Connective tissue

Most of the musculoskeletal system is made up of connective tissue such as bone and cartilage. Connective tissue comprises specialized cells embedded in an extracellular matrix of collagen, elastin and structural proteoglycans. In bone, this matrix is mineralized and rigid.

Muscle

There are three types of muscle: skeletal, cardiac and smooth (Fig. 1.1), each having a characteristic histological structure (Fig. 1.2).

- Skeletal muscle—striated voluntary muscle controlled by the nervous system. Most muscle in the body is of this type
- Cardiac muscle—striated muscle of the heart

- Smooth muscle—non-striated involuntary muscle controlled by a variety of chemical mediators. Smooth muscle is important in the function of most visceral tissues, e.g. blood vessels, the gastrointestinal and reproductive tracts.

Energy stored in tissues as adenosine triphosphate (ATP) is converted by muscle tissue into mechanical energy. This produces movement or tension.

The contraction of muscle requires stimulation. The type of stimulation varies: for example, skeletal muscle is activated by motor neurons, cardiac muscle initiates its own contractions, and smooth muscle is activated by a variety of chemical mediators. Stimulation of muscle causes protein filaments, called actin and myosin, within its cells to interact and produce a contractile force.

The skeleton

The skeleton consists of bone, cartilage and fibrous ligaments. A joint is the site at which bones are attached to each other. The range of movement at the joint, and whether a joint is rigid or flexible, depends on the joint structure.

Bone

Bone is rigid and forms most of the skeleton. It functions as a supportive framework for the musculoskeletal system, and the bony sites for muscle attachment provide the mechanical basis for

Fig. 1.1 Properties of the three different muscle types

	Skeletal	Cardiac	Smooth
histological appearance	cross-striated, multinucleated muscle fibres	cross-striated, single-nucleated muscle fibres containing intracellular discs	non-striated, spindle cells with a single nucleus
site	skeletal covering	muscular component of the heart	found in wall of blood vessel, airways and walls of hollow organs
cell size	50–60 μm in diameter, up to 10 cm long	15 μm in diameter, 100 μm long	2–10 μm in diameter, 20–400 μm long
control	voluntary/reflex; controlled by somatic nervous system	self-regulated by pacemaker cells; heart rate can be altered by autonomic nervous system	involuntary control or regulation by inherent contraction initiation (visceral smooth muscle)
nature of contraction	rapid contraction and relaxation	spontaneous and rhythmical contraction	slow and sustained contraction
function	voluntary movement of skeleton and posture maintenance	contractions pump blood around the body	related to the structure, e.g. regulation of blood-vessel diameter, hair erection, etc.

locomotion. Other functions of bone include mineral storage in the matrix and formation of blood cells (haemopoiesis) within the marrow.

Cartilage

Cartilage is a resilient tissue that provides semirigid support in some parts of the skeleton. Cartilage is also a component of some types of joint. Most bone is formed within a cartilaginous template during development.

Ligaments, tendons and aponeuroses

Ligaments, tendons and aponeuroses are fibrous tissues that connect the various components of the musculoskeletal system.

- Ligaments are flexible bands that connect bones or cartilage together, strengthening and stabilizing joints
- Tendons are connections between muscle and bone that transmit the force of contraction during movement

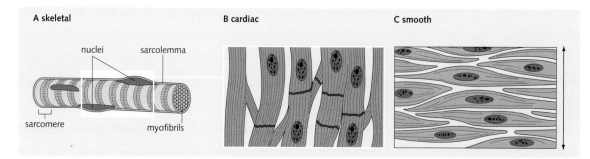

Fig. 1.2 The appearance of muscle fibres. (A) Skeletal muscle; (B) cardiac muscle; (C) smooth muscle.

- An aponeurosis may be considered as a broad, sheet-like tendon into which more than one muscle can insert.

A sprain occurs when the ligaments supporting a joint are overstretched, which can occur, for instance, during sports. It causes swelling, pain and erythema of the area. Ice should be applied to the site of the sprain, the joint should be elevated and the patient should rest. Mild compression may also help.

Joints

Joints are composite structures between bones. They may also include cartilage and fibrous connective tissue. There are several types of joint. The strength of a joint and the range of movement it allows depend upon its position and configuration.

Control of the musculoskeletal system

The musculoskeletal system is controlled by the nervous system to produce coordinated movements and locomotion. There are a number of elements to this control. These include:

- Afferent neurons providing feedback from stretch receptors in muscles and tendons, and sensory nerve endings in joints and skin, synapsing at the level of the spinal cord, allowing coordination of movement
- Efferent motor neurons, which activate groups of muscle fibres to produce contraction
- Neural pathways within the spinal cord, which coordinate the action of related muscle groups (agonist–antagonist pairs, for example) and also initiate repetitive actions, such as walking ('central pattern generator').

Spinal neuronal pathways form reflex pathways called spinal arc reflexes. These allow movements to be initiated relatively rapidly when required, such as retracting the hand from a hot object.

For further information about central control of movement and locomotion, refer to *Crash course: nervous system, 2nd edn.*

SKIN

Structure

The skin is composed of three layers: an outer protective epidermis, an inner connective tissue dermis, and a fatty subcutaneous layer (see Fig. 1.3). It is characterized by a tough keratinized surface, which protects underlying tissues from the external environment.

The thickness of skin varies, depending on its location on the body and the amount of daily trauma it is subjected to. The epidermis is usually around 0.1 mm thick, but increases to between 0.8 and 1.4 mm in places such as the soles of the feet and the palms of the hands, where it undergoes repeated trauma. The dermis also follows this pattern, ranging from 0.6 mm thick on the eyelids to 3 mm on the palms and soles. The subcutaneous layer (subcutis) of the skin is much thicker than the upper layers and has a different thickness distribution: it is thickest on the abdomen, where it reaches depths of 3 cm.

Functions

In addition to its obvious role of barrier protection, skin performs many functions, including thermo-regulation, mechanical chemical and immuno-logical protection, synthesis of vitamin D and various hormones, and the perception of touch, temperature and pain sensation.

Skin derivatives

There are many derivatives of skin, including hair, nails, sebaceous glands and sweat glands, which will also be discussed in this book. These structures are so named because they have developed from cells derived from the epidermis. They perform important functions in the protection and homoeostasis of the skin.

Pathology

Because of the skin's exposure to the external environment, it is open to damage caused by infection and infestation. These will be covered later in the book (Chapter 7), as will clinical presentations caused by a range of pathologies, including inflammation, tumours, genetic disorders, systemic disease and drug-induced disorders.

CONNECTIVE TISSUE

Definition

Connective tissue is a term that describes a variety of tissue types that ultimately provide support to all other tissues and organs in the body. It comprises different types of support cells embedded in an extracellular matrix, which is composed of ground substance and fibres that the support cells secrete. It may come as a surprise to learn that red blood cells and white blood cells, such as macrophages and leukocytes, are classed as a type of connective tissue (see Fig. 1.5) Connective tissue is characterized by a high ratio of cells to matrix.

Origins

Connective tissue is derived from the embryonic mesenchyme, which itself originates from the embryonic mesoderm (Fig. 1.4).

Functions

Connective tissue performs several functions. These include:

- Mediating the exchange of nutrients and metabolic products between tissues and the circulatory system
- Mechanical support and muscle attachment
- Packaging, as connective tissue encloses and lies between other specialized tissues
- A metabolic role, in particular allowing fat storage in adipose tissue
- Insulation
- Defence and repair; some cells are involved in the immune response.

Classification

Connective tissue is classified according to its function, location, structure and properties (Fig. 1.5). Connective tissue proper refers to

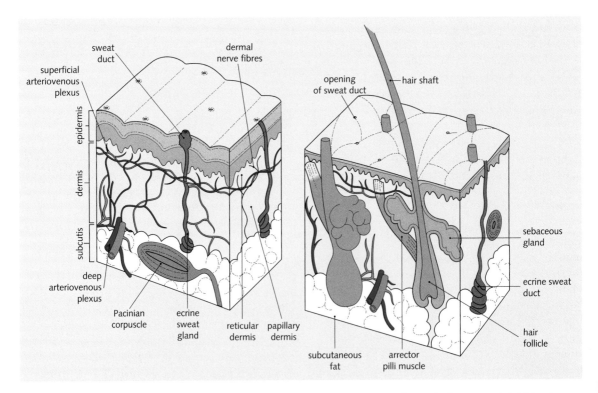

Fig. 1.3 The structure of the skin. (Adapted with permission from Gawkrodger DJ. Dermatology: an illustrated colour text. 2nd ed. Edinburgh: Churchill Livingstone, 1997.)

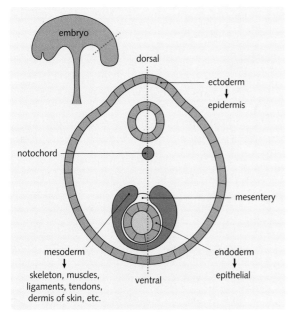

Fig. 1.4 The three primitive embryonic layers and their derivative structures.(Adapted with permission from Gawkrodger DJ. Dermatology: an illustrated colour text, 2nd edn. Edinburgh: Churchill Livingstone, 1997.)

connective tissue that contains many types of fibre and cells supported within a thick, rich extracellular matrix.

Components

The three main components of connective tissue are cells, fibres, and extracellular matrix.

Cells

Connective tissue comprises several cell types, each of which performs a certain function (Fig. 1.6).

Fibres

Collagen

Collagen is the main fibre found in the extracellular matrix of connective tissue. Collagen is formed from tropocollagen, a substance synthesized by matrix-secreting cells, predominantly fibroblasts. Tropocollagen is released into the extracellular matrix, where it is modified and arranged into fibres with other tropocollagen molecules to form collagen microfibrils. These microfibrils cluster to form bundles, or fibres, that are the basis of the polypeptide chains.

Most of the body's collagen comprises three helical polypeptide chains (Fig. 1.7). Differences in

these chains result in at least 15 types of collagen molecule, each with a particular function. They are classified into different families according to their morphological structure. Over 90% of the body's collagen is type I collagen (Fig. 1.8).

Elastin

Elastin is a component of elastic fibres. Elastic fibres are found in the skin, lung and blood vessels. They are thinner than collagen and are arranged in random sheets.

Elastin is produced from fibrillin and proelastin, a substance synthesized by matrix-secreting cells, most commonly fibroblasts. Proelastin becomes modified to elastin by the cell's Golgi apparatus, when it is released into the extracellular matrix.

Extracellular matrix

Extracellular matrix (ECM), or ground substance, surrounds the connective tissue and contains the supporting cells. The major material component of the ECM surrounding connective tissue fibres and their supporting cells is glycosaminoglycans (GAGs), protein chains bound to branched polysaccharides which, with the exception of hyaluronic acid, bond covalently to form proteoglycans. This way they can form different fibres such as fibronectin and laminin. Some structural proteoglycans are found on the surface of cells, where their functions include cell–cell recognition and migration.

> As a person ages the physiological breakdown of the skin's elastin is not replaced at the same rate. This results in wrinkles and fine lines developing. The process is accelerated by increased exposure to sunlight and is termed photoageing. It is also accelerated by smoking.

Structural proteoglycans can also function as cell adhesion molecules, facilitating communication between cells and their surrounding environment and subsequently regulating a large number of cell functions, including proliferation, gene expression, apoptosis and differentiation. Current research is under way focusing on methods of modifying the actions of these adhesion molecules, and whether this may provide possible ways in which to treat illnesses such as cancer.

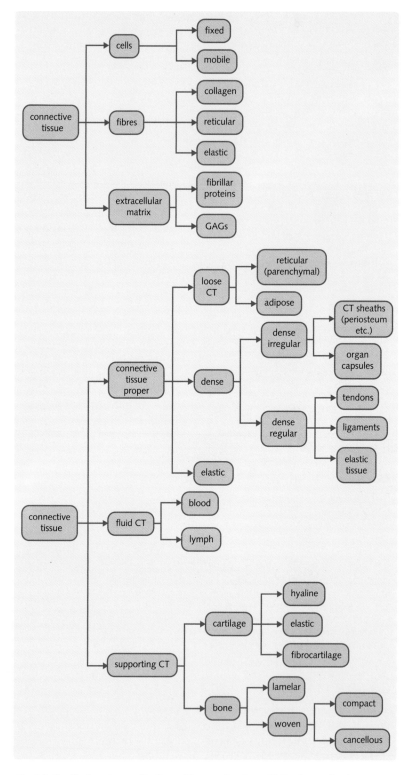

Fig. 1.5 Classification of connective tissue. CT, connective tissue; GAGs, glycosaminoglycans.

Fig. 1.6 Connective tissue cell types and their functions

	Cell type	Functions
fixed cells	fibroblasts, chondroblasts, osteoblasts, osteoclasts	synthesis and maintenance of matrix
	adipocytes	fat metabolism
	mast cells	release of histamine
	mesenchymal cells	mature cell precursors
transient cells	white blood cells	immune response
	melanocytes	pigmentation

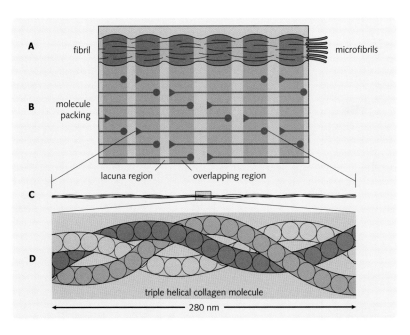

Fig. 1.7 Microstructure of the collagen fibril showing the triple helix of polypeptide (α) chains.

Fig. 1.8 Functions of collagen types

Type	Location	Functions
I	skin, tendon, ligaments, bone, fascia and organ capsules (accounts for 90% of body collagen)	provides variable mechanical support (loose or dense)
II	hyaline and elastic cartilage, notochord, and intervertebral discs	provides shape and resistance to pressure
III	connective tissue of organs (liver, lymphoid organs, etc.), blood vessels, and fetal skin	forms reticular networks
IV	basement membrane of epithelial and endothelial cells	provides support and a filtration barrier
V	basement membrane of smooth and skeletal muscle cells	provides support (other functions poorly understood)

Skeletal muscle

Objectives

By the end of this chapter you should be able to:

- Discuss the different arrangements of muscle fibres and groups and understand their effects on function
- Define the terminology associated with the structure and functions of skeletal muscle
- Understand the structure and function of the different components and subcomponents of voluntary muscle
- Know the ionic composition of the intracellular fluid and extracellular fluid in muscle fibres
- Explain the ionic basis of an action potential and the mechanisms that govern its initiation and propagation
- Understand the function of the neuromuscular junction
- Describe the mechanism of muscle contraction
- Outline the concepts that govern muscle biomechanics
- Be familiar with common pathologies that affect skeletal muscle presynaptically, postsynaptically, and at the synaptic cleft.

Muscle is a tissue made up of functionally contractile cells. These cells are capable of producing movement or tension. Other examples of contractile cells include myoepithelial cells (see p. 57) and myofibroblasts, found in connective tissue.

Three types of muscle tissue are found in the human body: skeletal, cardiac and smooth. Cardiac and smooth muscle will be discussed in more detail in Chapter 3.

Skeletal muscle

The alternative names for skeletal muscle are striated (from its histological appearance) or voluntary (from the mechanism by which contraction is controlled).

Function

Skeletal muscle has a fundamental role in voluntary movement of the skeleton and the maintenance of posture. It is also involved in the movement of the tongue, the globe of the eye and even the middle ear.

Sites

The majority of muscle found within the body is skeletal (Fig. 2.1). It is found in the limbs, thorax, abdominal wall, pelvis and face.

Control

Contraction of skeletal muscle tends to be either voluntary or reflex, and is controlled by the somatic nervous system.

Histological appearance

Skeletal muscle cells are long and thin, and are often referred to as muscle fibres. The cells are multinucleated, with the nuclei lying just inside the cell membrane (sarcolemma). The cell's contractile apparatus, termed myofibrils, runs in parallel along the length of the cell and gives the cell a characteristic striated appearance when viewed in longitudinal section.

Cell size

Skeletal muscle cells are 50–60 μm in diameter (range 10–100 μm) and up to 10 cm long.

Nature of contraction

Transient stimulation of a muscle causes rapid contraction and relaxation, producing a twitch. The nature of the stimulus is important because muscle must be stimulated rapidly and repetitively to produce the sustained contractions that are necessary for movement.

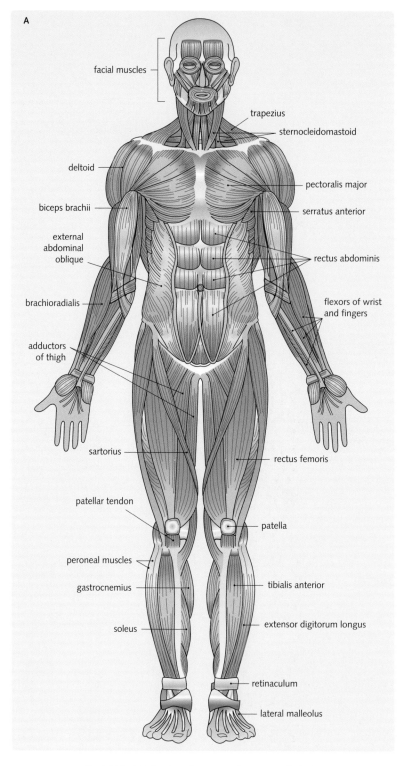

Fig. 2.1 (A) Anterior view of major muscle groups in the body.

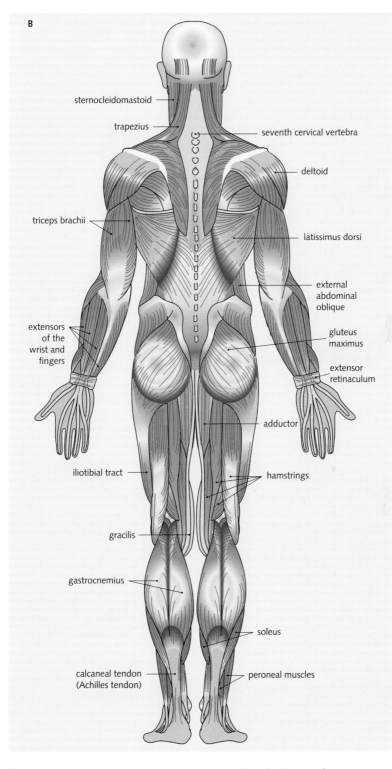

Fig. 2.1 cont'd (B) Posterior view of major muscle groups in the body. (Courtesy of Dr K.M. Backhouse.)

Muscle atrophy is the wasting of a muscle, resulting in reduced mass, size and strength. Causes of muscle atrophy include disuse due to prolonged immobility, poor circulation, poor nerve supply, or disease intrinsic to the muscle itself.

Skeletal and multi-unit smooth muscle may be referred to as neurogenic muscle, i.e. muscle in which contraction arises as a result of nerve stimulation.

Cardiac muscle may be referred to as myogenic muscle, i.e. they require no nerve stimulation for contraction that arises from within the muscle owing to the presence of pacemaker cells.

SKELETAL MUSCLE CONTRACTION

The contraction generated by a muscle depends on:

- The length of the muscle fibres
- The volume/number of muscle fibres
- The rate at which fibre length changes.

The greater the length of a muscle's fibres, the greater the range of movement it produces, whereas the bulkier the muscle, the greater the force it will generate. This can be illustrated by the following example. A long, narrow muscle will allow a greater degree of shortening, but because of its narrow cross-section it cannot generate much force of contraction. By contrast, the shorter muscle cannot contract over any great length but, because its cross-section incorporates many muscle fibres, it generates a large force of contraction.

Wasting of the body's skeletal muscle occurs in cachexia. Cachexia is also characterized by loss of weight, fatigue, weakness and anorexia. It is a group of signs and symptoms caused by a range of underlying conditions, important examples being cancer, infectious diseases such as tuberculosis, and autoimmune diseases such as SLE.

Muscle fibres assume a variety of arrangements, depending on the type of contraction the muscle will produce (Fig. 2.2). For example, a multipennate arrangement results in a large number of short fibres attached to a single tendon, and the force of contraction is great and concentrated on the tendon.

Muscle groups are arranged in pairs, which consist of:

- A functional group in which one muscle—the prime mover—is the main participant. Other muscles, termed synergists, help the prime mover to perform a movement. For example, flexion at the elbow joint is due to the action of biceps, with the help of brachialis, brachioradialis and the forearm flexor muscles
- An antagonistic group in which muscles oppose the movement of the functional group, e.g. triceps, assisted by anconeus, antagonizes the action of biceps by causing extension at the elbow (Fig. 2.3). As the force of contraction of the functional muscle(s) increases, there is coordinated relaxation of the antagonistic group.

A muscle can belong to more than one group, e.g. latissimus dorsi is involved in both adduction and extension of the shoulder joint.

Each end of a muscle is usually attached to bone. The origin, or head, is the site from which the movement originates and at which there is little movement when the muscle performs its main action (Fig. 2.3). The attachment site, distant from the origin, is commonly referred to as the site of insertion, or enthesis.

Tendons can become damaged by overuse of the muscles they attach to bone. An example of this is Achilles tendonitis, with inflammation, irritation and swelling of the Achilles tendon, which attaches the gastrocnemius and soleus to the heel. This commonly occurs through sporting activities in younger patients. However, the Achilles tendon can be also affected by some types of arthritis in older patients.

The terms proximal and distal attachment may be more appropriate terms to use as, depending on the movement, the origin (proximal attachment) may be more mobile than the insertion (distal attachment).

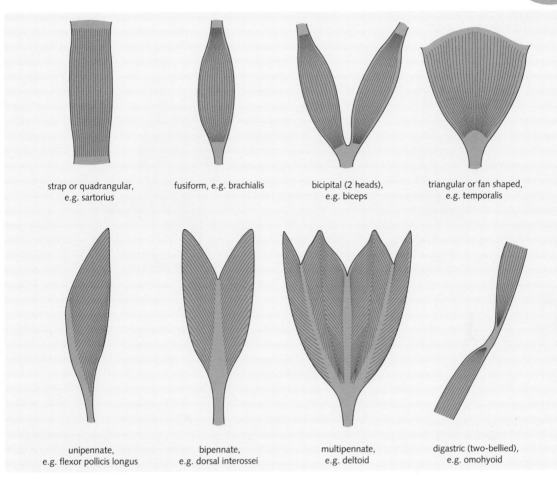

strap or quadrangular, e.g. sartorius

fusiform, e.g. brachialis

bicipital (2 heads), e.g. biceps

triangular or fan shaped, e.g. temporalis

unipennate, e.g. flexor pollicis longus

bipennate, e.g. dorsal interossei

multipennate, e.g. deltoid

digastric (two-bellied), e.g. omohyoid

Fig. 2.2 Fibre configurations and shapes of muscles in the human body

Most skeletal muscles are attached to bone by a band of fibrous connective tissue called a tendon, an inelastic, flexible cord consisting of closely packed collagen fibres. Some muscles or groups of muscles have a wide area through which they attach to bone. These muscles attach through a broader form of tendon termed an aponeurosis, a thin sheet of fibrous connective tissue. One example is the muscle groups of the anterior abdominal wall.

Not all skeletal muscle is attached to bone. For instance, the tongue has neither bony proximal nor bony distal attachments. In addition, sphincters (rings of skeletal muscle), such as the external urethral sphincter that controls the passage of urine from the bladder to the urethra, do not attach to bone.

A sesamoid bone is a small bone found within the tendons of certain muscles, e.g. the patella, and some bones in the hand and foot.

Microstructure of skeletal muscle

Arrangement of muscle tissue

Whole muscle consists of fibres arranged in parallel in bundles called fasciculi. Although skeletal muscle fibres are long, they do not extend the whole length of the muscle but are organized as overlapping bundles. This arrangement enables the force of a contraction to be transmitted throughout the muscle. Skeletal muscle fibres are arranged in parallel within a fasciculus (Fig. 2.5).

Connective tissue surrounds the individual muscle fibres (endomysium) and fasciculi (perimysium), in addition to the dense connective tissue coat surrounding the whole muscle (Fig. 2.4).

Skeletal muscle has a rich blood supply. The blood vessels and nerves divide and extend throughout the perimysium (the collagen connective tissue that surrounds fasciculi).

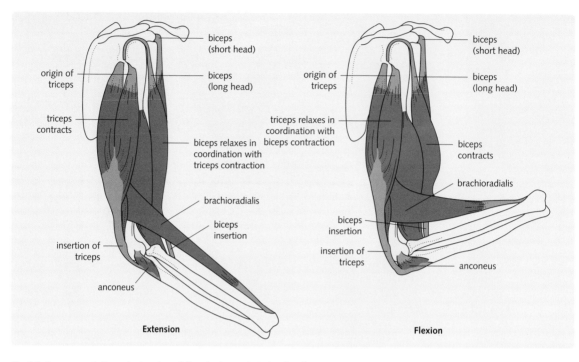

Fig. 2.3 Arrangement of muscles in antagonistic pairs demonstrated at the elbow joint.

Fig. 2.4 Cross-section of whole muscle showing the arrangement of muscles into fasciculi and fibres surrounded by connective tissue.

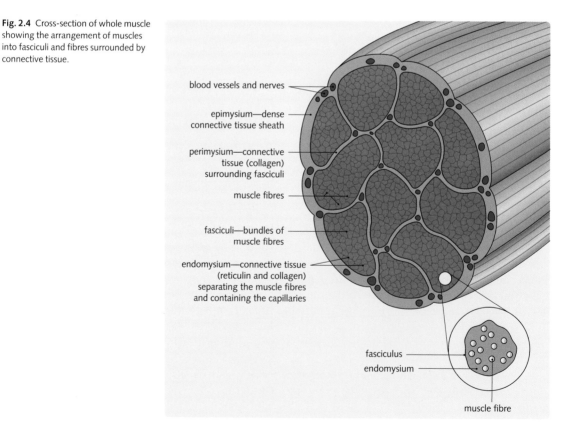

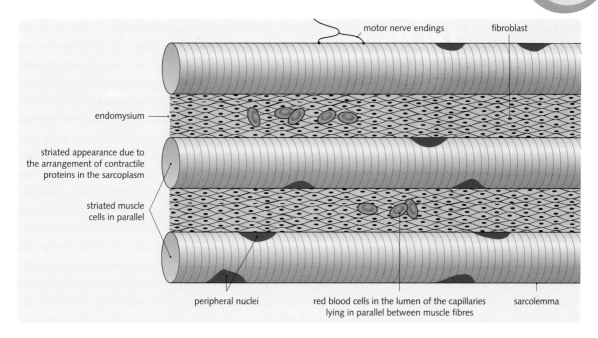

Fig. 2.5 Longitudinal section showing the arrangement of skeletal muscle fibres within a fasciculus.

The size of a fasciculus is suggestive of function. Smaller fasciculi are found in muscles involved in fine movement.

Microenvironment of skeletal muscle

Skeletal muscle fibres can be divided into three types, I, IIa and IIb, following a classification based on the speed and force of contraction and resistance to fatigue (Fig. 2.6). All three types are widely distributed throughout a muscle. The properties of the different types of muscle fibre are considered in more detail in Figure 2.23.

Sarcomere

Muscle fibres, or myofibres, are cells that contain myofibrils. Myofibrils consist of myofilaments arranged in contractile units called sarcomeres. Two types of myofilament occur:

- Thick filaments, composed mainly of myosin protein
- Thin filaments, composed mainly of actin protein.

It is the organization of these myofilaments that leads to the striated appearance of skeletal muscle when viewed in longitudinal section (Figs 2.7 and 2.8).

Fibre type	Colour	Speed and force of twitch	Resistance to fatigue
I	red (because of myoglobin)	slow, only 10% of force of type IIb	high (fatigue resistant)
IIa	intermediate	fast, but force and speed less than type IIb	intermediate (fatigue resistant)
IIb	white	fast and high force	low (fatigues after repeated stimulation), fast fatiguable

Fig. 2.6 Classification of different types of skeletal muscle fibres

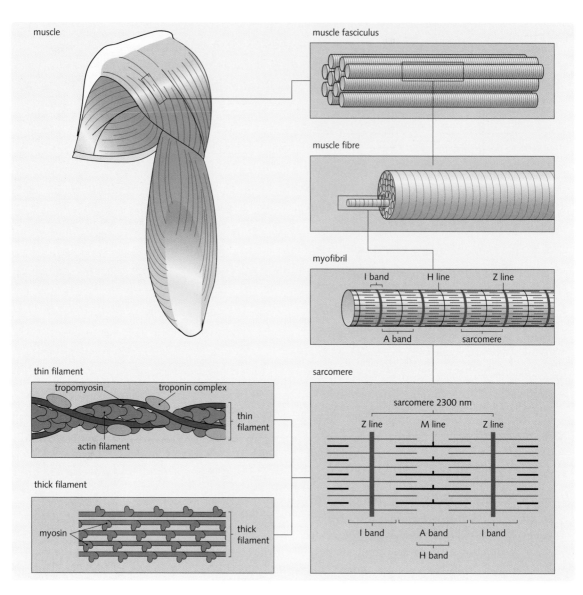

Fig. 2.7 Organization of skeletal muscle.

Cellular structure of muscle fibre

A muscle fibre is a specialized cell (Fig. 2.9) that contains:

- A cell membrane (the sarcolemma)
- Cytoplasm (the sarcoplasm)
- An endoplasmic reticulum (the sarcoplasmic reticulum).

The sarcolemma surrounds the sarcoplasm, intracellular organelles and the sarcoplasmic reticulum of the muscle fibre. In each muscle fibre cell, multiple peripheral nuclei, glycogen granules and mitochondria lie in the sarcoplasm between the myofibrils (Fig. 2.9).

The cells also contain T-tubules— channels that extend from the sarcolemma of the muscle fibre and surround each one at the junction of the A and I bands, the AI junction T-tubules ensure that all sarcomere contractions are synchronized.

Sarcoplasmic reticulum runs longitudinally along myofibrils and wraps around groups of myofibrils. In regions of T-tubules, the sarcoplasmic reticulum forms terminal cisternae.

Triads are important structures within the muscle. They consist of a T-tubule with sarcoplasmic reticulum on either side. Depolarization is transmitted through the T-tubule, causing release of calcium ions (Ca^{2+})

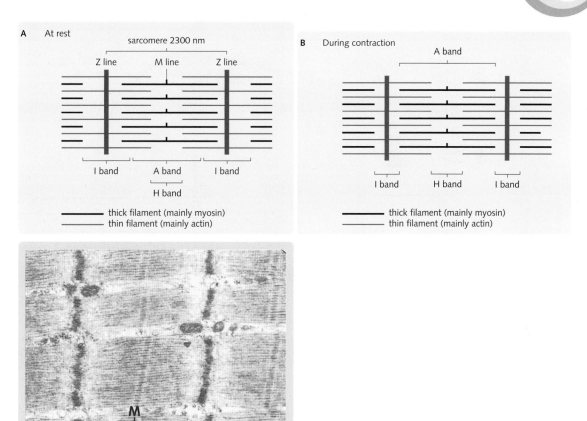

Fig. 2.8 Arrangement of contractile proteins in the sarcomere at rest and during contraction. At rest (A), the H and I bands represent areas in which the thick and thin filaments do not overlap. The Z line anchors the actin filaments and the M line anchors the myosin filaments. During contraction (B) the Z lines 'slide' closer together, causing shortening of muscle. The A band remains constant in width but the I and H bands shorten. In (C), the pattern of actin and myosin filaments is clearly demonstrated on the electron microscope image (M, M line; Z, Z line.) (Electron micrograph courtesy of Dr T Gray.)

into the sarcoplasm. Ca^{2+} in the sarcoplasm triggers muscular contraction.

Satellite cells are small, spindle-shaped cells, visible only by electron microscopy, that lie between the sarcolemma and the basal lamina in adult skeletal muscle. Where muscle damage occurs but the basal lamina remains intact, satellite cells proliferate to form myoblasts. Myoblasts fuse to form myotubules, a structure around which myofibrils assemble. New muscle fibres subsequently form in which the nuclei are centrally, rather than peripherally, placed.

If the basal lamina becomes damaged, fibroblasts are activated to repair the tissues, resulting in scar formation and a reduction in function.

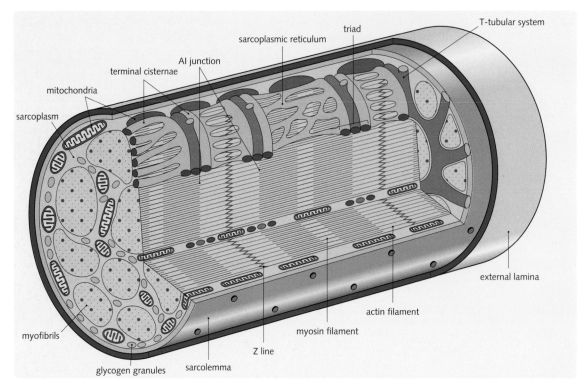

Fig. 2.9 Components of muscle fibre.

CELLULAR PHYSIOLOGY OF SKELETAL MUSCLE

Ion balance and the resting membrane potential in muscle cells

There are differences in the ionic composition of the intracellular fluid (ICF) and extracellular fluid (ECF) of muscle cells (Fig. 2.10). These differences are due to:

- The selective permeability of the cell membrane to K^+ and Cl^-
- Large intracellular anions (A^-) impermeable to the cell membrane, products of amino acid metabolism, the presence of which cause Cl^- export to the extracellular compartment and import of K^+ into the intracellular compartment.
- Relative cell membrane impermeability to Na^+.

The resulting differences in ionic distributions and permeabilities contribute to the production of the resting membrane potential.

Resting membrane potential

The resting membrane potential (RMP) is the difference in voltage between the inside and the outside of the cell at rest, with the charge being positive on the outside and negative on the inside.

Fig. 2.10 Distribution of ions in the ICF and ECF of muscle cells

Ion	ICF (mmol/L)	ECF (mmol/L)
Na^+	12	145
K^+	155	4
H^+	13×10^{-5}	3.8×10^{-5}
Ca^{2+}	8	1.5
Cl^-	3.8	12.0
HCO_3^-	8	27
A^-	155	0

A, Organic impermeant anions. (Adapted with permission from Ganong WF. Review of medical physiology, 17th edn. Appleton & Lange, 1995.)

It normally has a value of −90 mV in muscle cells. This separation of charge across the cell membrane creates the potential to do work (Fig. 2.11). The concentration gradient favours K$^+$ efflux, whereas an electrostatic gradient favours K$^+$ influx.

The main ion responsible for the RMP is K$^+$. The equilibrium potential of K$^+$ (E$_K$) is the voltage required to achieve equilibrium and therefore stop K$^+$ diffusion across the sarcolemma; this is approximately −95 mV. The RMP and the E$_K$ are very close, which suggests that the cell membrane is mainly permeable to K$^+$. The relatively small difference is due to other factors, namely:

- A small amount of Na$^+$ leaking from ECF to ICF
- Diffusion of Cl$^-$

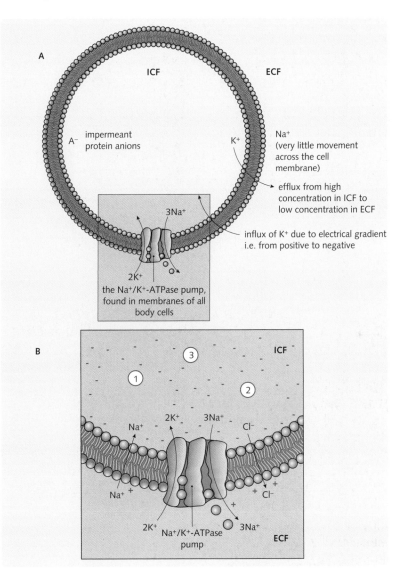

Fig. 2.11 Factors involved in the determination and maintenance of the resting membrane potential (RMP). K$^+$ is the key player. (A) The Na pump is found in membranes of all body cells. The mechanism of action is as follows: removal of three Na$^+$ and entry of two K$^+$, expending one ATP molecule; phosphorylation of the protein subunits produces a conformational change and binding of Na$^+$; dephosphorylation results in binding of K$^+$ and reversion of the protein to its original shape. The cycle is repeated 100 times per second. Other contributors to RMP are shown in (B).
1. There is a passive leakage of a small amount of Na$^+$ from ECF to ICF along a concentration gradient.
2. Passive movement of Cl$^-$ from ICF to ECF along an electrical gradient.
3. Presence of impermeant protein anions (A$^-$)
(Note that the bulk of the solution is electrochemically neutral. The excess ions close to the cell membrane are a small proportion. However, they are significant enough to cause movements across the cell membrane.) ICF, intracellular fluid; ECF, extracellular fluid.

- The presence of ions (A^-) that are impermeable to the cell membrane
- The activities of the Na^+/K^+ pump.

Na^+/K^+-ATPase pump

The Na^+/K^+-ATPase pump is found in the membranes of every cell in the body (Fig. 2.11). It transports three Na^+ molecules out of the cell and two K^+ molecules into the cell in an energy-dependent process, in a cycle of approximately 100 times a second, expending one ATP molecule each time. In doing so, the pump:

- Maintains cell water content and volume
- Cotransports and countertransports other solutes at the same time, e.g. Cl^-
- Contributes to the RMP (by maintaining an electrostatic gradient).

Electrochemical equilibrium

Electrochemical equilibrium of K^+ is achieved when the forces acting in both directions are equal, so that there is no net movement of K^+.

Equilibrium potential

The equilibrium potential (E) of a particular ion across a cell membrane can be calculated using the Nernst equation. This potential level equates to the potential that prevents net diffusion of the particular ion, determined by the ratio of concentrations of the ion on both sides of the cell membrane. The greater the ratio, the greater the Nernst potential required to prevent diffusion. (Where this potential is negative, it denotes a greater distribution of negative charge inside the cell relative to that outside the cell for that ion).

Nernst equation:

$$E = E^0 - \frac{RT}{NF} \ln \frac{{}^aRed}{{}^aOx}$$

(E^0 = formal electrode potential; R = universal gas constant; T = temperature (kelvins); ^{a} = chemical activities of reduced and oxidized side; F = charge per mole of electrons (Faraday constant); n = number of electrons transferred in an oxidization or reduction reaction; Red = concentration of reduced species/oxidizing agent; Ox = oxidized species (reducing agent). Therefore:

$$E_{ion} = \pm 61 \frac{\ln[ion]_{ECF}}{\ln[ion]_{ICF}}$$

Effects of Na^+ and K^+ channels on the membrane potential

The electrical nature of a stimulus applied to the skeletal muscle cell can alter the resting membrane potential. This creates a potential difference across the membrane that activates an important class of ion channels found in the membrane, known as voltage-gated ion channels. These play a crucial role in generating the means by which information is transmitted through the nervous system to initiate muscle cell contraction. The area immediately surrounding the channels undergoes depolarization, followed by hyperpolarization.

Depolarization

The potential difference across the cell membrane will activate nearby voltage-gated Na^+ channels, causing an Na^+ influx and the membrane potential to become less negative than the RMP.

Hyperpolarization

The Na^+ channels then close and K^+ channels open. The resulting K^+ efflux overcompensates for the voltage change that occurred in depolarization. This results in a membrane potential that is more negative than the RMP.

A cell membrane can be depolarized to any particular voltage, depending on the strength of the stimulus. However, when depolarization occurs beyond a certain 'critical' level or threshold, the cell is able to 'fire' a signal called an action potential.

Action potential

An action potential (AP) is a transient depolarization of the cell membrane beyond the 'threshold potential' followed by hyperpolarization before returning to the normal RMP (Fig. 2.12). When there is slow depolarization of a cell in response to a stimulus, an AP is generated at the threshold potential via the triggering of voltage-gated ion channels. It is an important means of transmitting information through the nervous system to excitable cells and initiating the contraction of muscle cells. The size and duration of the AP within different cell types are variable. Understanding initiation and propagation of APs to muscles is important to understand the pathophysiology of many conditions that interrupt muscle innervation.

Initiation of the action potential

APs are usually initiated:

- At synapses—specialized junctions between cells

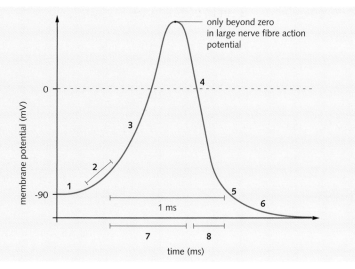

Fig. 2.12 Phases of the action potential (AP). (1) Resting membrane potential; (2) initial slow depolarization of cell in response to stimulus; (3) opening of voltage-gated Na^+ channels when threshold is reached; (4) repolarization, i.e. opening of voltage-gated K^+ channels; (5) return to resting membrane potential (−90 mV); (6) hyperpolarization due to 'excessive' K^+ efflux; (7) absolute refractory period (AP may not be initiated); (8) relative refractory period (greater stimulus than normal to initiate the AP).

- By the passage of current from one cell to another via gap junctions.

Either of these stimuli activates a slow depolarization of the cell membrane, which reaches the critical threshold level and thus generates an AP. The all-or-none law states that once an AP has been initiated, the size is constant for a given type of cell and will not be affected by altering the strength of the stimulus.

Ionic basis of the action potential

Movements of both Na^+ and K^+ across the cell membrane are important (Fig. 2.13). At rest, the voltage-activated Na^+ and K^+ channels are closed, although, as you will recall, K^+ moves along a concentration gradient through the cell membrane, maintaining the RMP.

The depolarization that produces an action potential can be broken down into two phases, early and late.

Early phase of depolarization

During the early phase of depolarization, the fast gate (m-gate) of a voltage-gated Na^+ channel opens and the slow gate (h-gate) starts to close. As the slow gate takes longer to close, there is an influx of Na^+. This results in the activation of more Na^+ channels via a feedback mechanism.

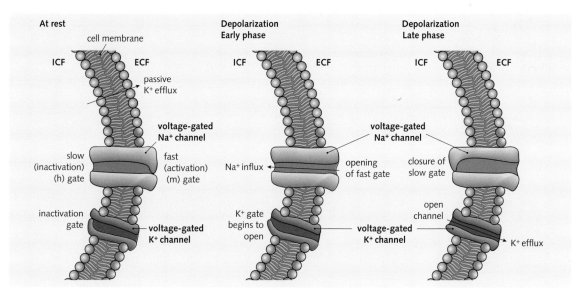

Fig. 2.13 Changes in voltage-activated channels during an action potential derived from studies using the voltage clamp and selective channel blockers. ICF, intracellular fluid; ECF, extracellular fluid.

The voltage-activated K+ channel starts to open slowly.

Late phase of depolarization

During the late phase of depolarization, the slow gate of a voltage-gated Na+ channel is closed and there is no more influx of Na+. The slow gate reopens when RMP is reached, i.e. when the fast gate is closed.

The K+ channel is open and remains so until RMP is restored. Closure of the K+ channel is slow, meaning that hyperpolarization may occur following an AP.

Propagation of the action potential

An AP occurring at any one site on the cell membrane causes voltage changes in the adjacent parts of the membrane, allowing the AP to propagate in both directions. These changes can be explained by the local circuit theory (Fig. 2.14).

Saltatory conduction

Saltatory conduction occurs in myelinated nerve fibres (Fig. 2.15). The local circuit theory still applies, but the current can leave the axon only at nodes of Ranvier. This results in a greater conduction velocity because the current density at the nodes is greater, and so depolarization is more rapid.

The circuit of current can travel a number of internodal lengths and still be able to depolarize a node to threshold. This produces a large safety factor.

Conduction velocity

In nerves, the conduction velocity (CV) ranges from 100 m/s to less than 1 m/s. Factors affecting conduction velocity are:

- Fibre diameter, i.e. myelin sheath, large nerve fibres: increasing the fibre diameter increases the conduction velocity
- Temperature: increasing temperature increases the conduction velocity. However, above 40 °C the conduction velocity decreases until there is 'heat block'

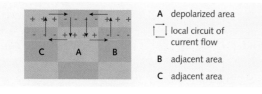

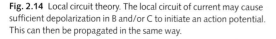

A depolarized area

local circuit of current flow

B adjacent area

C adjacent area

Fig. 2.14 Local circuit theory. The local circuit of current may cause sufficient depolarization in B and/or C to initiate an action potential. This can then be propagated in the same way.

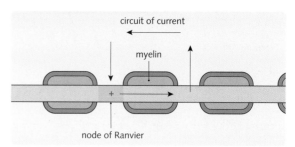

Fig. 2.15 Saltatory conduction in myelinated nerve fibres. The current is only able to leave at the nodes of Ranvier. In this way, the circuit of current can be thought of as 'jumping' from node to node, allowing a greater speed of conduction.

- Strength of local circuits: stronger local circuits result in a greater conduction velocity.

The synapse

The junction at which nerve cells communicate with each other is called a synapse. Synapses can be electrical, i.e. direct transmission of current from presynaptic cell to target cell through ion channels, or chemical, i.e. release of a chemical that binds to protein receptors on the target cell membrane, causing direct or indirect opening of ion channels (Fig. 2.16).

Transmission of a signal at a chemical synapse involves:

- An AP propagated at the presynaptic nerve terminal
- Depolarization of the nerve terminal
- Voltage-activated Ca²⁺ channels open, causing an influx of Ca^{2+}
- Vesicles in the active zone fusing with the presynaptic membrane, releasing neurotransmitter by exocytosis
- The neurotransmitter binding to protein receptors in the postsynaptic membrane
- Changes in the postsynaptic membrane, leading to depolarization or hyperpolarization of the target cell.

Electrical synapses correspond to gap junctions between certain cells (e.g. neurons, cardiac muscle cells, smooth muscle cells, epithelial cells). Transmission of a signal at an electrical synapse involves:

- Depolarization of the presynaptic membrane
- Direct flow of current through gap junction ion channels to target cell
- Depolarization of the target cell.

Fig. 2.16 Comparison of electrical and chemical synapses

Property	Electrical	Chemical
site	nerves, heart, smooth muscle, liver, epithelium	most of synapses in body, including skeletal muscle and brain
structures seen at synapse	gap junctions	presynaptic vesicles and mitochondria, postsynaptic receptors
mechanism of transmission	ionic current	chemical messenger
cytoplasmic continuity between presynaptic and postsynaptic cell	yes	no
synaptic cleft	3.5 nm	20–40 nm
nature of transmission	rapid, usually excitatory effect on target cell	synaptic delay 1–5 ms, excitatory or inhibitory effect on target cell
plasticity	no	yes
amplification of signal	no	yes

Adapted with permission from Guyton AC. Human physiology and mechanisms of disease, 5th edn. St Louis, MO: WB Saunders, 1991.

Local anaesthetics

Local anaesthetics are drugs used to provide temporary relief of pain. They are weak bases. In tissue fluid they are present in ionized and non-ionized forms, the proportions of which depend on the pH of the tissue and the pK_a (acid dissociation constant) of the drug. It is the non-ionized base that diffuses through the nerve to reach the internal side of the axoplasm, where it ionizes. It then enters the Na^+ channels on the membrane from inside the axon when the channels are open, producing a blockade.

The more common local anaesthetics include lidocaine, bupivacaine, prilocaine, benzocaine and cocaine.

Vasoconstrictors such as epinephrine (adrenaline) are often administered with local anaesthetics. The constricted blood vessels prevent too much local anaesthetic diffusing away from the relevant site, resulting in a longer duration of action and less chance of systemic toxicity. However, the vasoconstrictors are never used in sites with small blood vessels (e.g. fingers, ears), owing to the risk of tissue ischaemia resulting from vasospasm.

Mechanism of action Local anaesthetics block Na^+ channels to prevent depolarization and propagation of APs. The un-ionized form crosses the cell membrane and 10% ionizes in the cytoplasm. This ionized form then blocks open Na^+ channels from within. Nerve fibres with a small diameter are more easily blocked, hence local anaesthetics can prevent the sensation of pain without affecting touch.

Use dependency The more a nerve is stimulated the greater the block achieved, as the Na+ channels are blocked when open.

Adverse effects Local anaesthetics can affect the cardiovascular system by causing hypotension or cardiac arrest, or the central nervous system (CNS) by causing restlessness, sleepiness, convulsions and respiratory depression. Anaphylaxis can also occur.

Neuromuscular junction

Structure of the neuromuscular junction

At the neuromuscular junction (NMJ; Fig. 2.17) each muscle fibre is innervated by one motor nerve. The axon of each motor neuron divides into many branches as it enters the muscle, each branch forming an NMJ with a single muscle fibre. Each muscle fibre has only one NMJ.

The nerve terminal invaginates into the muscle fibre near its midpoint to form a depression in the muscle membrane, termed the synaptic trough (gutter). However, the nerve terminal does not cross the muscle membrane.

The space between the nerve terminal and the muscle membrane is called the synaptic cleft. It is occupied by connective tissue and ECF.

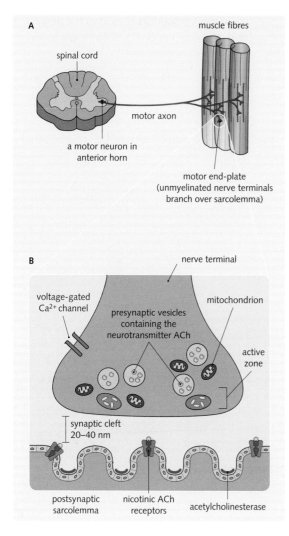

Fig. 2.17 Diagram demonstrating (A) the motor endplate and (B) the structure of the neuromuscular junction at a chemical synapse. ACh, acetylcholine.

Presynaptic nerve terminal

Vesicles

At the presynaptic nerve terminal, acetylcholine (ACh) is synthesized in the cytoplasm from choline and acetyl CoA and then stored in vesicles (about 10 000 molecules per vesicle) with an ATP molecule. At rest, 85% of ACh is stored in the vesicles and 15% is present in the cytoplasm.

Mitochondria

Numerous mitochondria are present to provide energy for the active process of choline uptake and the synthesis of ACh.

Active zones

Active zones are specialized regions of the presynaptic membrane. They are sites of neurotransmitter release and are positioned so that they lie opposite a junctional fold in the postsynaptic membrane.

Voltage-activated Ca^{2+} channels

Voltage-activated Ca^{2+} channels are believed to be adjacent to active zones. The channels open in response to an AP. The associated influx of Ca^{2+} causes the vesicles to move to the active zone.

Although the overall intracellular concentration of Ca^{2+} is relatively low, remember that there is a high concentration of Ca^{2+} in the sarcoplasmic reticulum.

Postsynaptic membrane

Motor endplate

The motor endplate is a specialized region of the muscle fibre membrane where the terminal branches of the motor nerve communicate with the muscle fibre.

Junctional folds

Junctional folds are folds in the motor endplate upon which nicotinic ACh receptors (nicAChR) are located. These folds increase the surface area upon which the transmitter can act.

Basal lamina

The basal lamina is connective tissue lying between the nerve terminal and muscle fibre membrane. Large quantities of the enzyme acetylcholinesterase are found here, particularly at the bases of the junctional folds.

Nicotinic acetylcholine receptor

This receptor (the nicAChR) consists of five protein subunits (2α, 1β, 1γ and 1δ). The binding of two ACh molecules (one to each of the two α subunits) induces a conformational change and the receptor channel opens. The channel is permeable to both K^+ and Na^+. However, concentration gradients favour Na^+ influx.

When a nerve AP arrives at the NMJ, a sequence of events takes place lasting 10–15 ms. This sequence is numbered to correspond to Figure 2.18, as follows:

1. The AP arrives at the nerve terminal.
2. The voltage-activated Ca^{2+} channels open, allowing Ca^{2+} influx.

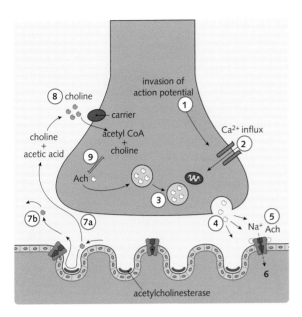

Fig. 2.18 Events at the neuromuscular junction upon the arrival of a nerve action potential. Refer to text for an explanation of the sequence (which occurs in 10–15 ms). ACh, acetylcholine.

3. Ca²⁺ influx attracts presynaptic vesicles to the active zones.
4. Vesicles fuse to the presynaptic membrane and release ACh in 'packets' by the process of exocytosis.
5. ACh diffuses across the synaptic cleft to bind to nicAChR on the junctional folds, altering the membrane's permeability to produce an influx of Na^+.
6. Na^+ influx generates an action potential at the motor endplate called an endplate potential (epp). The epp depolarizes adjacent regions of the muscle membrane. Upon reaching threshold, an AP occurs in the muscle fibre.
7. Rapid removal of ACh from the synaptic trough terminates the Na^+ influx and the activation of the receptors. The majority is removed by the action of acetylcholinesterase, which hydrolyses ACh to choline and acetic acid (7a). A small amount tends to diffuse out of the trough (7b), and this is broken down by pseudocholinesterase in the plasma.
8. Uptake of choline into nerve terminals is the rate-limiting step of ACh synthesis. This is an active process requiring the hydrolysis of ATP, and involves a high-affinity—low-capacity mechanism, which is responsible for 90% of the uptake, as well as a low-affinity—high-capacity mechanism.
9. Recycled choline reacts with acetyl CoA (which is formed in the mitochondria and transported into

the cytoplasm), reproducing ACh in the nerve terminal. The enzyme choline acetyltransferase catalyses the reaction. The vesicular membrane is also recycled by endocytosis from the nerve terminal membrane. ACh is again stored in vesicles in the nerve terminal.

Comparing the action potential in skeletal muscle and nerve

The ionic basis of the AP in skeletal muscle is the same as that of the AP in nerves. However, there are certain important differences between the two:

- The RMP in skeletal muscle is fairly constant between −80 and −90 mV, whereas the RMP in nerve varies from −40 mV in small nerves to −90 mV in large nerves
- An AP travels through skeletal muscle at a speed of 3–5 m/s and can last between 1 and 5 ms, whereas the AP in nerve can travel from less than 1 m/s up to 100 m/s, depending on a number of factors, lasting less than 1 m/s.
- The AP spreads through a skeletal muscle via the T-tubule system, whereas in nerve cells, depolarization of the membrane is sufficient.

Drugs acting at the neuromuscular junction

Drugs acting presynaptically

Hemicholinium acts presynaptically at the NMJ by blocking the uptake of choline, which results in a slow depletion of ACh in the nerve terminal. Hemicholinium-3 is sometimes used as a research tool in animal and in-vitro experiments.

Botulinum toxin acts by inhibiting ACh release at the presynaptic membrane. The aminoglycoside antibiotic group can also inhibit ACh release here, which can result in the uncommon side effect of neuromuscular blockade.

Of the seven serotypes of botulinum toxin that have been identified, serotype A is used to treat a variety of conditions. Widely known under its trade name of Botox, it can be used to treat conditions causing muscular contractions, such as strabismus and blepharospasm, as well as those producing excessive glandular secretions, such as hyperhidrosis. It is also used for cosmetic reduction of facial wrinkles that occur due to relaxation of the underlying muscles.

Drugs enhancing transmission

Anticholinesterases enhance transmission at the NMJ by increasing the time that ACh is present in the synaptic cleft.

Mechanism of action Anticholinesterases inhibit acetylcholinesterase. There are three main types of anticholinesterase:

- Short-acting (up to 15 min) drugs such as edrophonium (these bind reversibly to the active site of the enzyme)
- Intermediate-acting drugs, e.g. pyridostigmine and neostigmine (these bind covalently to the enzyme)
- Long-acting drugs, e.g. organophosphorus compounds (these form strong covalent bonds with the active site; they are often referred to as irreversible, as the enzyme is inactivated for a long period of time; they have no clinical use, but are used in chemical weapons).

Indications Edrophonium assists in the diagnosis of myasthenia gravis. An intravenous injection leads to short-term improvement in muscle strength. Treatment involves the use of intermediate-acting anticholinesterases. Anticholinesterases reverse competitive neuromuscular block after surgery.

Adverse effects Side effects of anticholinesterases include paradoxical depolarizing neuromuscular block; convulsions, coma and respiratory arrest if a lipid-soluble anticholinesterase (e.g. physostigmine) is used; symptoms associated with the parasympathetic nervous system, as ACh is the neurotransmitter acting on muscarinic receptors.

Drugs acting postsynaptically

Neuromuscular-blocking drugs are either competitive or depolarizing.

Competitive drugs

Tubocurarine and gallamine are examples of competitive neuromuscular-blocking drugs.

Mechanism of action Neuromuscular-blocking drugs compete with ACh for binding sites on the ACh receptor in the postsynaptic membrane. There is no opening of the ion channel when they bind, therefore AP generation in muscle is less likely. Their action is reversed by anticholinesterases and enhanced by general anaesthetics.

Indications Neuromuscular-blocking drugs are used during surgery to relax skeletal muscles, and prior to electroconvulsive therapy.

Adverse effects Side effects of neuromuscular-blocking drugs include a decrease in blood pressure owing to blockage of autonomic nicotinic receptors, and anaphylaxis.

Depolarizing drugs

Suxamethonium is an example of a depolarizing drug.

Mechanism of action Depolarizing drugs are agonists of nicotinic acetylcholine receptors and block transmission by producing prolonged membrane depolarization and desensitization of the receptors. Their action is potentiated by anticholinesterases.

Indications Depolarizing drugs are used in surgery to relax skeletal muscles, and for electroconvulsive therapy. Although competitive blockers are more widely used, depolarizing drugs tend to be used for brief procedures.

Adverse effects As initial stimulation occurs before blockage, asynchronous muscle fibre twitches may result in muscle pains following the use of depolarizing drugs. Other side effects include bradycardia due to action on muscarinic receptors.

Excitation–contraction coupling

Excitation–contraction coupling refers to the events that occur once the AP has been initiated in the sarcolemma, including the resulting contraction and relaxation of the muscle.

Initiation of an action potential in muscle fibre

The endplate potential (epp) results from a single neuronal AP and is usually greater in amplitude than that required to initiate an AP in muscle fibre. For this reason the NMJ is said to have a very high 'safety factor' for activation to occur.

Propagation of an action potential into muscle fibre via T-tubules

An AP is propagated into muscle fibre via the T-tubules in a sequence of events (the following numbers refer to Fig. 2.19):

1. Bidirectional propagation of the AP occurs along the sarcolemma. This causes excitation of muscle fibre along its whole length, so that all sarcomeres contract simultaneously.
2. The AP is then propagated into the muscle fibre via the T-tubules. There are two T-tubules per sarcomere; these encircle the myofibril at the AI junction. T-tubules communicate with the extracellular space.
3. The sarcoplasmic reticulum on both sides of the T-tubule communicates with the T-tubule via junctional feet. Depolarization of the

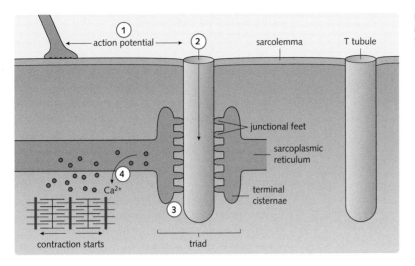

Fig. 2.19 Sarcoplasmic release of intracellular Ca^{2+}. The numbers refer to the text.

T-tubule results in a signal from the T-tubule to the sarcoplasmic reticulum terminal cisternae.

4. Ca^{2+} channels then open in the sarcoplasmic reticulum and Ca^{2+} moves along a concentration gradient into the sarcoplasm around the myofibrils.

Muscle contraction

Two types of molecule—thick and thin filaments—are involved in muscle contraction (Fig. 2.20). Their ability to interact and create the contraction depends on accessory proteins, a group of structural proteins that align the two molecules, allowing them to associate in the right place at the right time. Examples of these accessory proteins include tropomyosin and α-actinin (see p. 30).

Thick filament

Myosin is the main component of the thick filament. It is a much larger protein than actin. It consists of a tail, a neck and a head region. The head region possesses ATPase activity and can attach to specific binding sites on the actin molecule. The neck region is flexible, a property that is necessary for attachment and detachment to the actin filament. The tail region provides strength during contraction.

Thin filament

The thin filament is an intricate arrangement of actin, tropomyosin and troponin molecules intertwined with each other.

Actin is the main component of the thin filament. It is capable of binding the five following proteins.

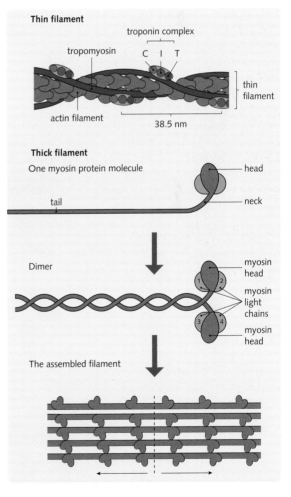

Fig. 2.20 Different arrangement of contractile proteins in thin filament (actin) and thick (myosin) filament.

Tropomyosin is a structural (accessory) protein found bound to actin filaments. Each tropomyosin is bound to seven actin filaments. Tropomyosin 'covers' the myosin-binding sites on the actin filament, thereby preventing a myosin–actin interaction.

Troponin is a protein that consists of a complex of three subunits:

- T, which binds one tropomyosin
- C, which has a high affinity for Ca^{2+}
- I, which has a high affinity for actin (hence the attachment of tropomyosin to actin).

The binding of Ca^{2+} causes a change in shape and movement of the associated tropomyosin. This uncovers the myosin-attachment site on actin.

α-Actinin is a structural protein that is found in the Z line. Two actin filaments bind by their tails to one molecule, and its role is to anchor them to the Z line and keep them in place.

Mechanism of contraction

Huxley's cross-bridge cycle

Huxley's cross-bridge cycle demonstrates the shortening of the sarcomere caused by the sliding of the actin filaments. The numbers correspond to those in Figure 2.21, as follows:

1. In the resting state, the myosin-binding sites on the actin molecule are covered by tropomyosin.
2. An increase in intracellular Ca^{2+} results in the binding of Ca^{2+} to troponin C. The binding of Ca^{2+} causes a conformational change in the troponin complex, resulting in movement of the tropomyosin and uncovering of the myosin-binding sites.
3. The myosin head attaches to an actin molecule and releases the phosphate group.
4. This attachment causes the myosin head to tilt towards its tail, thereby pulling the actin filament in that direction. Tilting of the head causes release of adenosine diphosphate (ADP).
5. A molecule of ATP binds to the myosin head. This causes detachment of the head from the actin.
6. The ATPase action of the myosin head cleaves ATP, resulting in a myosin head with attached ADP and phosphate. The energy derived from this process causes straightening (or 'untilting') of the head, preparing it for reattachment.

Fig. 2.21 Interaction of myosin heads with thin filaments during contraction. The numbers refer to the text.

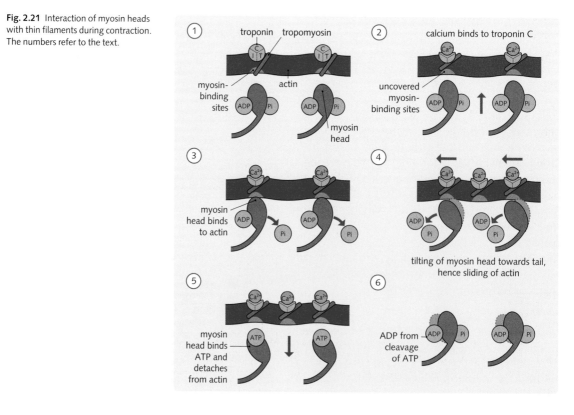

The whole process is repeated. In this way the myosin head 'walks' along the actin filament. This is the basis of the 'sliding filament' theory.

Relaxation of muscle

Relaxation of muscle is Ca^{2+} dependent. Upon repolarization of the muscle fibre, Ca^{2+} is actively pumped back out of the cell and into the sarcoplasmic reticulum. The intracellular Ca^{2+} concentration drops, causing calcium molecules to detach from troponin, and the active sites quickly become recovered by tropomyosin, preventing further association with myosin.

Bioenergetics of muscle contraction

Muscle contraction results in energy expenditure during:

- Interaction of actin and myosin filaments during contraction through the ATPase activity of the myosin head
- Pumping of Ca^{2+} from the sarcoplasm back into the sarcoplasmic reticulum after contraction
- Restoration of the intracellular ionic environment after muscle contraction, because of the actions of the Na^+/K^+-ATPase pump.

Sources of energy

Short term

Sarcoplasm ATP molecules are present in sarcoplasm. These would be expended within the first 2 seconds of contraction if they were not replaced.

Creatine phosphate At rest, the skeletal muscle produces more ATP than it requires and converts this energy into high-energy phosphate bonds to creatine, a molecule formed from fragments of amino acids, storing the energy in the form of creatine phosphate. It can be used to phosphorylate ADP to ATP by the enzyme creatine phosphokinase at a time when this energy is required. It is produced and stored in the Z line.

Myokinase The enzyme myokinase catalyses the transfer of a phosphate group from one ADP molecule to another to form ATP and the byproduct AMP.

Intermediate term

Anaerobic glycolysis This causes the breakdown of glucose to lactate and pyruvate, with the release of energy, which is used to convert ADP to ATP. ATP is generated at double the rate of oxidative phosphorylation. See *Crash Course: Metabolism and Nutrition* for more detail.

Anaerobic glycolysis is predominant in type II muscle fibres, which have few mitochondria but many glycogen granules. This is an intermediate-term source of energy only, as lactate and pyruvate accumulate in the cell.

Long term

Oxidative phosphorylation This is an aerobic process in which ATP is liberated from fats, carbohydrates and protein. See Crash Course: Metabolism and Nutrition for more information.

Energy can be provided for longer periods (a few hours) than with glycolysis.

Type I muscle fibres are suited to oxidative phosphorylation as they have numerous mitochondria and lipid droplets.

> Creatine kinase (also known as CK and creatine phosphokinase) is one of the enzymes released by damage to or lysis of muscle cells, and elevated levels can often be detected in blood tests soon after damage has occurred. Elevated CK levels can arise as a result of rhabdomyolysis, myocardial infarction, myositis, myocarditis and malignant hyperthermia.

Myofibre cytoskeleton

The cytoskeleton of the muscle fibre is essential to the mechanical stability and function of muscle. The proteins present in the myofibre cytoskeleton are dystrophin and bridging glycoproteins. This cytoskeleton forms an important link between the inside of the cell and the extracellular matrix. The extracellular matrix supports the muscle fibre, reducing the likelihood of tearing on contraction.

The intracellular actin filaments are linked to dystrophin, which in turn is linked to a number of glycoprotein complexes that bridge the surface of the sarcolemma to the cell surface. These glycoproteins link to a laminin component of the basement membrane (Fig. 2.22). This association allows force generated by the muscle to be transferred to the extracellular matrix in the external lamina.

Some of these linking proteins can be genetically absent or defective, resulting in an increased chance of the muscle fibres tearing on contraction. Affected individuals develop one of the forms of muscular dystrophy, such as Duchenne muscular dystrophy.

Fig. 2.22 Components of the myofibre cytoskeleton and their linkage with the extracellular matrix.

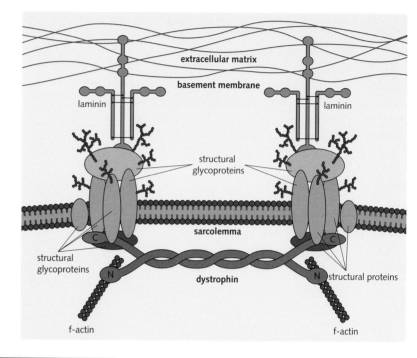

FUNCTIONS OF SKELETAL MUSCLE

Motor unit

The term 'motor unit' refers to the motor neuron and all the muscle fibres innervated by it. Each motor neuron may innervate many muscle fibres, but a single muscle fibre receives input from only one motor neuron. The muscle fibres innervated by a single motor neuron are spread out within the muscle, rather than simply being clumped together. However, the muscle fibres within a motor unit are of the same type and contract simultaneously.

The number of muscle fibres innervated by a motor neuron is known as the innervation ratio. A smaller number of muscle fibres per motor neuron is present in muscles involved in fine, precise movements, e.g. ocular muscles, whereas a larger number is seen in muscles involved in gross movements, e.g. maintaining posture.

There are three different types of motor unit (Fig. 2.23):

- Slow, resistant to fatigue
- Fast, resistant to fatigue
- Fast, fatiguable.

Orderly recruitment

Small motor neurons innervate slow muscle fibres (type I), whereas fast muscle fibres (types IIa and IIb) are innervated by larger motor neurons. This is referred to as the size principle.

Smaller motor neurons require a smaller excitatory input for activation. During reflex or voluntary movement for a given excitatory input, it is the slow units that are activated first. This results in an orderly recruitment of muscle fibres, with activation of slow units first, followed by fast fatigue-resistant units, and finally fast fatiguable units. This is important *in vivo* as it allows movement to be graded by altering the level of excitatory input rather than having to select different fibre types.

Many healthy people experience episodes of eyelid twitching from time to time. This uncontrollable, repetitive twitch is called a blepharospasm, with episodes lasting on and off for a few days. It can be triggered by fatigue, stress and caffeine. Uncommonly, it is associated with blurred vision and photosensitivity. Severe blepharospasm is rare, and small botulinum injections can temporarily stop spasms in these cases.

Effects of denervation and reinnervation on motor units

Denervation of a motor unit results in atrophy of the muscle fibres within that unit. There may also be fibrillations on the electromyogram, shown as fine,

Fig. 2.23 Properties of different motor unit types

Property	Motor unit type		
	slow, resistant to fatigue	fast, non-fatiguable	fast, fatiguable
fibre diameter	small (type I)	intermediate (type IIa)	large (type IIb)
force of contraction	low	intermediate	high
myosin–ATPase activity (indicates rate of ATP hydrolysis and therefore speed of twitch)	low	low	high
source of energy	oxidative phosphorylation	oxidative phosphorylation and some anaerobic glycolysis	anaerobic glycolysis
glycogen content	low	intermediate	high
mitochondria	many	many	few
capillaries	many	many	few
function	fine movement and maintenance of posture	sustained activity	brief strong contractions, e.g. jumping

irregular contractions of individual fibres, and an increase in sensitivity to circulating ACh.

Clinically, the signs of a lower motor neuron lesion are seen, which include decreased muscle tone and power, diminished reflexes and muscle wasting. Some of the muscle fibres are replaced by fibrous and fatty tissue. However, this fibrous tissue shortens and contractures may form.

Muscle mechanics

Length–tension relationship

The force or tension a muscle fibre generates depends on the number of cross-bridge interactions, therefore ultimately it depends on the length of the sarcomere (Fig. 2.28). There is an optimum range of lengths at which the force generated is at its maximum (Fig. 2.28). This can be explained by the sliding filament theory: if a sarcomere is overstretched, the overlap between actin and myosin is reduced and there are fewer actin–myosin interactions and less force.

Alternatively, if the sarcomere is maximally shortened, the ends of the thin filaments can overlap and disrupt actin–myosin interactions. The myosin heads are also unable to pivot, and so essentially no tension can be produced. Therefore, muscle fibres contract to produce the optimal amount of force

when the sarcomeres are within a narrow range of resting lengths (Fig. 2.28).

Isometric contraction

Isometric (iso = same, metric = length) contraction occurs in muscle with a constant length. An example of isometric contraction is a person holding a weighty plastic bag of shopping while remaining stationary, e.g. when waiting for the bus.

Isometric tests can be used to compare force against duration of contraction of different muscles (Figs. 2.24 and 2.25).

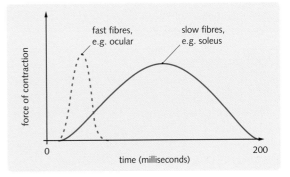

Fig. 2.24 Duration of contraction in different muscles demonstrated by isometric tests.

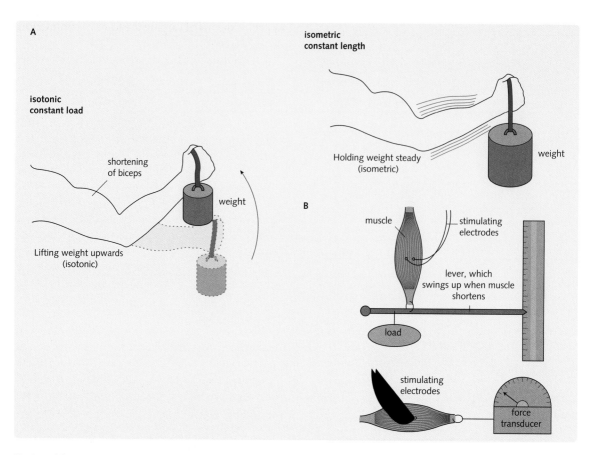

Fig. 2.25 (A) Measurement of isotonic and isometric contractions. (Modified from Guyton AC. Physiology and mechanisms of disease, 8th edn. St Louis, MO: WB Saunders, 1992.) (B) Situations involving isotonic and isometric contractions. (Adapted with permission from Ganong WF. Review of medical physiology, 17th edn. Norwalk, CN: Appleton Lange, 1995.)

Isotonic contraction

Isotonic (iso = same, tonic = tone or weight) contraction occurs in muscle with a constant tension. The length of the muscle changes while maintaining constant tension. An example of isotonic contraction is a bodybuilder lifting a free weight, actively contracting the biceps to lift the weight towards him or her.

Isotonic tests can be used to compare the speed of shortening of different muscle types (Fig. 2.25).

Producing tension

The amount of tension one muscle fibre can produce depends entirely on the number of actin–myosin interactions in its sarcomeres. Every action potential in skeletal muscle results in a similar amount of Ca^{2+} release in the muscle fibre. So, unlike myocardium, the strength of contraction in skeletal muscle is not dependent on the sarcoplasmic Ca^{2+} concentration, as each AP results in sufficient Ca^{2+} release to produce

the maximum response (Fig. 2.26). In response to the increased Ca^{2+} concentration, all myosin heads within the zone of (actin–myosin) overlap interact with the actin (thin) filaments. Therefore, even at its initial resting length, the muscle fibre is either 'on' and actively producing tension, or 'off' and relaxed, with no intermediate state. This is known as the all-or-none principle.

The amount of tension a whole skeletal muscle fibre can produce is determined primarily by:

- The frequency of stimulation to the muscle
- The number of muscle fibres stimulated.

Frequency of muscle stimulation

A single stimulus will consistently produce a maximal response resulting in one contraction, which, when it occurs singularly, is termed a *twitch*. The duration of the twitch varies according to the type of muscle in which it is generated. For example, a twitch in an eye

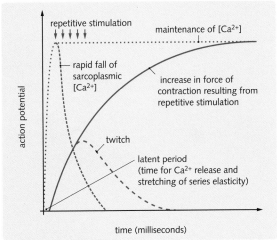

Fig. 2.26 Relationship of sarcoplasmic [Ca^{2+}] to force of contraction in skeletal muscle. Repeat stimulation results in maintenance of intracellular [Ca^{2+}]. Series elasticity refers to the inherent elasticity of muscle tissue, including its non-contractile C/T matrix. The latent period can be thought of as 'taking up the slack' before contraction of the tissue begins. In repetitive stimulation the elastic elements remain stretched, improving muscle efficiency. (Adapted with permission from Berne RM, Levy MN. Physiology, 3rd edn. Chicago: Mosby Year Book, 1993.)

muscle can be as brief as 7.5 ms, whereas in the soleus muscle it can last 100 ms.

The more stimulations applied to a muscle, the greater the number of contractions produced, and so with repetitive stimulations the muscle fibres have less time to relax in between. Increasing the frequency of stimulation allows the force of each contraction to add up, or summate. Summation of twitches is an important means of varying the force of contraction (Fig. 2.27).

When a muscle fibre receives a second stimulus before the relaxation phase of the previous twitch has ended, the second resulting contraction is more powerful than the preceding one. This concept is termed *wave summation* (or summation of twitches). As the frequency of stimulation is increased, the muscle fibre begins to produce a stronger and more sustained contraction, a waveform called unfused (incomplete) tetanus.

Fused (complete) tetanus occurs where there is no muscle relaxation between each stimulus, resulting in fusion of consecutive twitches and a smooth, sustained contraction.

Tetany is spasm, twitching of the skeletal muscle due to low levels of extracellular Ca^{2+}. A decrease in extracellular Ca^{2+} lowers the threshold for activation of muscle and nerve cells.

There are physiological limits to the amount of tension that can summate with each stimulation. For instance, if you were to examine the electrical activity of the muscle using an electromyogram, where each successive stimulation repeatedly coincides with the end of the relaxation phase of the previous twitch, the following contraction will develop a slightly higher tension than the previous one in a step-like manner, but only for the first 30–50 stimulations. Thereafter, it maintains a quarter of the maximum tension that would be produced if complete tetanus were produced. This effect is termed *treppe* (German

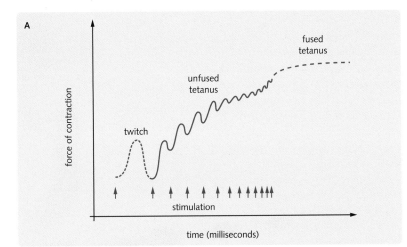

Fig. 2.27 Summation of twitches. As the time between each twitch decreases, the force of the contraction increases, showing the modulating effect of stimulation frequency. (Adapted with permission from Kapit W. Physiology colouring book. London: HarperCollins, 1987.)

(Continued)

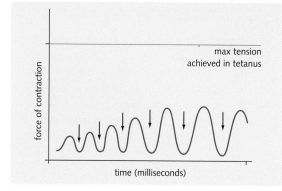

Fig. 2.27 cont'd

for 'stairs'). It is believed to be due to a gradual rise in cytoplasmic Ca^{2+} concentration, as the Ca^{2+} ion pumps in the sarcoplasmic reticulum are unable to eliminate all the Ca^{2+} before the next stimulation.

Number of fibres stimulated

The total force exerted by an active skeletal muscle depends on how many muscle fibres are activated. As a movement is initiated, the motor neurons to the muscles required are stimulated. The greater the number of active motor units, the greater the muscular tension that is produced. This concept is termed *recruitment*.

However, to ensure that the muscle is not exhausted of energy supplies, muscles undergoing sustained contraction do not activate all motor units at once. They are activated on a rotating basis, allowing some to recover while others are working. This mechanism is called *asynchronous motor unit summation*.

Muscle tone

Even when it is not contracting, a muscle at rest will always have some active motor units, so as to produce some background tension within the muscle; this is called muscle tone. Muscle tone is important to maintain body posture and stabilize the position of bones and joints in relation to one another. Muscle tone is constantly monitored by specialized intrafusal fibres found within the muscle spindles contained in every muscle fibre, and they feed back to the CNS, allowing modification where it is required. The motor response to such information is commonly known as a reflex.

Force–velocity relationship

The force–velocity relationship is found by stimulating a muscle under isotonic conditions and measuring the speed of shortening with different loads. The speed of shortening is decreased with increasing loads (Fig. 2.29A). There is an inverse relationship between the amount of resistance and the speed of contraction.

Speed of shortening varies with different fibre types. This occurs because of the existence of myosin isoforms. In fast fibres, myosin ATPase activity is rapid and therefore cross-bridge cycling and shortening of muscle fibres is more rapid (Fig. 2.29B).

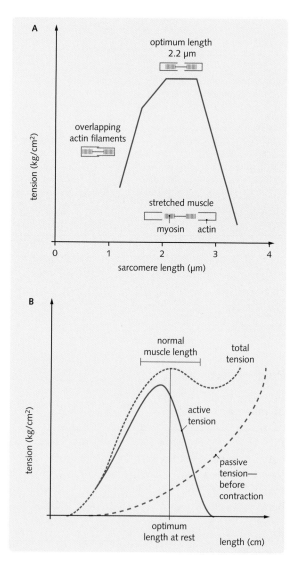

Fig. 2.28 (A) Effect of sarcomere length on the active tension developed by an individual muscle fibre upon contraction. (B) Effect of muscle length on tension. Increasing the passive tension initially increases the total tension. Further increases in passive tension lead to a decrease in active tension.

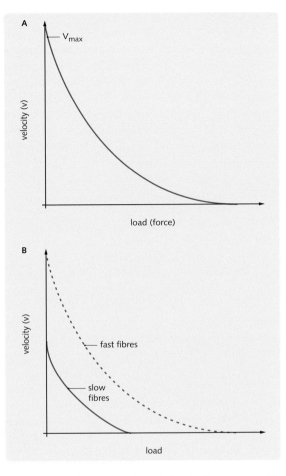

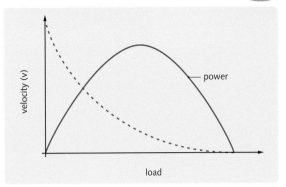

Fig. 2.30 Maximal power results from a balance between speed of shortening and load.

Fig. 2.29 Graphs showing that (A) speed of contraction decreases with increasing load, with maximum velocity occurring with zero load; and (B) maximum speed of contraction in fast-twitch fibres is greater than that in slow-twitch fibres.

Power curves

Power = velocity × load (Fig. 2.30). The power of muscle contraction is influenced by the speed of shortening (velocity) and the load. Although increasing the load would seem to favour the equation, this is not the case, because increasing the load would decrease the speed of shortening. Hence maximal power is actually achieved by a balance between the load and the speed of shortening.

Muscle plasticity

Muscle plasticity refers to adaptive changes in the characteristics of a muscle fibre that occur to match function. Factors that may be altered include muscle-fibre diameter, length, strength and vascular supply.

The fibre types may also be altered, but to a lesser extent as these are determined by the motor neuron by which they are innervated.

Fast fibres are interconvertible, i.e. fast glycolytic fibres may be converted to fast oxidative, and vice versa. Slow and fast fibres are not interconvertible.

Effect of exercise on muscle

An increase in muscle mass occurs as a result of either hypertrophy or hyperplasia.

Hypertrophy of muscle is an increase in the *size* of individual muscle fibres, resulting in an increase in the force of contraction. This is caused by regular contraction of the muscle at maximal force.

Hyperplasia of muscle is defined as an increase in the *number* of muscle cells. It occurs to a lesser extent than hypertrophy. It occurs when large fibres divide lengthwise.

Regular, sensible levels of exercise training increase the activity and sensitivity of muscle spindles, which subsequently produces an increase in muscle tone. Increased tone speeds up the recruitment process during voluntary contraction, as more motor units are already active at rest so there are fewer to activate on stimulation. In addition, exercise has the aesthetic advantage of giving muscle a firmer, more defined appearance.

A lack of exercise causes muscle atrophy. This is a decrease in muscle fibre size resulting from lack of stimulation.

Although muscle characteristics are the same in both men and women, men generally have more muscle mass than women because muscle size is increased by stimulation from the male sex hormone testosterone.

Relationship of muscle characteristics to function

Sprinters have a greater number of fast fibres, as they require rapid, large-force contractions, whereas marathon runners have a greater number of slow muscle fibres, as they require sustained, low-force contractions. The number of slow muscle fibres is largely genetically determined. Training may enhance the effect of these muscle fibres by increasing their size and vascular supply.

Individual skeletal muscle fibres may be regarded as a syncytium, as each fibre is made up of a number of myoblasts that have fused. However, skeletal muscle fibres contract independently of each other, and therefore skeletal muscle is not referred to as a syncytium.

DISORDERS OF SKELETAL MUSCLE

Disorders of the neuromuscular junction

Disorders of the NMJ can be classified into two types: presynaptic or postsynaptic. Both present with muscle weakness.

Disorders of the NMJ are not diseases of the muscle but rather disorders of function, hence atrophy tends to be a late feature.

Presynaptic abnormalities

Botulism
Aetiology Botulinum toxin is a neurotoxin produced by the bacterium *Clostridium botulinum*, a Gram-positive, spore-forming anaerobe that is found in soil and seafood products worldwide. It can germinate, grow and produce toxin where foods are not preserved properly, such as in home-preserved vegetables and food products and lightly preserved canned meats and fish. Toxin is destroyed by normal cooking at above 85 °C for 5 minutes.

Pathogenesis There are three modes of acquisition for botulism, the most common being the consumption of contaminated food products. Wound botulism is rare, and results from systemic spread of toxin produced from spore germination in the anaerobic conditions in wounds, and is associated with trauma, surgery and intravenous (IV) drug use. Infantile botulism results from C. *botulinum* colonization of an immature intestinal flora.

There are seven types of botulism, categorized from A to G, with A, B and E being common causes of human botulism.

Once in the bloodstream, the toxin blocks the uptake of choline at the presynaptic membrane of peripheral cholinergic synapses, including the NMJ and those muscles innervated by cranial and spinal nerves. It is internalized into the nerve terminal, where it mediates breakdown of the ACh exocytosis apparatus, irreversibly blocking ACh release.

Clinical features Botulism is a paralytic disease, and signs and symptoms depend on the muscles that become paralysed. When it is acquired from food, symptoms and signs usually appear within 12–36 hours of consumption, whereas it can take up to 2 weeks with wound botulism. Characteristic early symptoms and signs include marked fatigue, vertigo, weakness, followed by blurred vision, dry mouth, and difficulty in swallowing or speaking. Botulism causes symmetrical descending paralysis, particularly of the face and respiratory muscles. Symptoms and signs of infantile botulism include constipation, loss of appetite, weakness, and loss of head control.

Diagnosis The diagnosis of botulism is clinical and is confirmed by detection of the endotoxin in food or faeces.

Management Botulism is managed by administration of antitoxin and supportive care, including intensive respiratory support. Antibiotics may also be required.

Prognosis Most patients recover if given prompt treatment, but there is an associated mortality of 5–10% of cases.

Lambert–Eaton myasthenic syndrome
The Lambert–Eaton myasthenic syndrome is a non-metastatic complication of malignancy that involves the development of antibodies against voltage-gated Ca^{2+} channels in the presynaptic membrane, resulting in impaired ACh vesicle release.

Lambert–Eaton myasthenic syndrome is associated with malignancy, most commonly small-cell lung carcinoma, affecting approximately 3% of sufferers in the USA.

Patients with Lambert–Eaton myasthenic syndrome present with progressive weakness and fatiguability that interferes with everyday activities and quality of life. It affects both sexes equally, but is more common in older patients. Death is usually due to the underlying malignancy.

Postsynaptic abnormalities

Myasthenia gravis

Epidemiology Myasthenia gravis occurs most commonly in the third decade and has a male : female ratio of 1 : 2.

Aetiology The cause of myasthenia gravis is unknown. It is a rare autoimmune disease that affects peripheral nerves, with the development of antibodies against postsynaptic nicotinic ACh receptors at the neuromuscular junction (Fig. 2.31).

Pathology In 90% of patients there are IgG antibodies to the ACh receptor in the postsynaptic membrane. These bind and block the receptor binding sites and ultimately destroy the receptor.

Clinical features The main symptoms of myasthenia gravis are muscle weakness and progressively reduced muscle strength with use of the muscle and recovery on rest.

The ocular, bulbar and cranial muscles are most commonly affected. Symptoms and signs manifest when the number of receptors are reduced to around 30% of the normal amount. Symptoms and signs include ptosis and diplopia. There is generalized muscular weakness and the patient may be in respiratory distress. Symptoms are worse on exercise. Muscle bulk is maintained until late in the disease.

Myasthenia gravis generally follows a course of intermittent remission and relapse.

Other autoimmune diseases, e.g. rheumatoid arthritis and systemic lupus erythematosus (SLE), can be associated with myasthenia gravis. About 75% of sufferers have a degree of thymus gland abnormality.

Owing to a difference in the antigenicity of the nicotinic receptors in the different types of muscle, cardiac and smooth muscle are not affected.

Neonatal myasthenia may be seen in the newborn babies of mothers with the disease. The baby presents with poor limb movements and poor feeding. These symptoms last a few weeks until the maternal antibodies decrease.

Diagnosis About 90% of patients with myasthenia gravis have circulating anti-ACh receptor antibodies. Diagnosis is based on the edrophonium (Tensilon) test (Fig. 2.32). This involves giving an injection of edrophonium, a short-acting anticholinesterase. As anticholinesterase drugs inhibit the enzyme acetylcholinesterase (which hydrolyses ACh, thereby terminating the activation of ACh receptors on the muscle fibre), ACh is present in the synaptic cleft for longer and there is a greater probability that it will bind to the ACh receptor. In this way, muscle

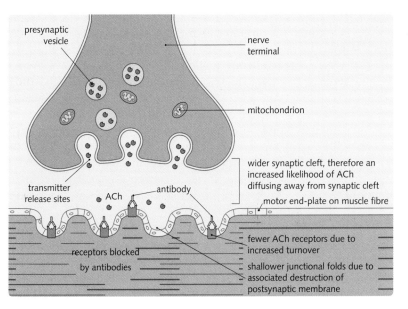

Fig. 2.31 Features of the neuromuscular junction in myasthenia gravis.

presynaptic vesicle

nerve terminal

mitochondrion

transmitter release sites

ACh   antibody

wider synaptic cleft, therefore an increased likelihood of ACh diffusing away from synaptic cleft

motor end-plate on muscle fibre

receptors blocked by antibodies

fewer ACh receptors due to increased turnover

shallower junctional folds due to associated destruction of postsynaptic membrane

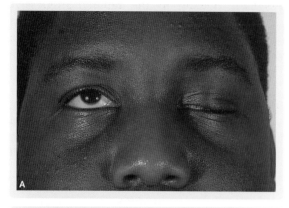

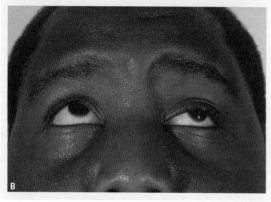

Fig. 2.32 The Tensilon test. (A) Muscle weakness caused by repeated facial movements. (B) There is rapid improvement after administration of edrophonium, a short-acting anticholinesterase. (Courtesy of Dr GD Perkin.)

contraction can take place sufficiently for the patient to regain normal muscle strength temporarily. Screening for thymoma should be considered in those diagnosed with myasthenia gravis.

An electromyogram (EMG) shows a decreased response to stimulation.

Management Management of myasthenia gravis is by the administration of long-lasting anticholinesterases, such as pyridostigmine, the dose being tailored to the patient's response. Long-lasting anticholinesterases prolong the presence of ACh in the synaptic cleft, thereby increasing the likelihood of ACh binding to a receptor.

In patients with an associated thymoma, thymectomy is needed.

Immunosuppressants such as prednisolone or azathioprine are commonly used to suppress autoimmunity and progression of the disease.

Prognosis The course of myasthenia gravis is variable, with patients experiencing varying degrees of morbidity depending on the severity of their weakness and the degree to which it interferes with day-to-day activities. Because of muscle weakness patients are at higher risk of suffering aspiration, pneumonia and falls, and some may experience side effects from their medication. In the modern medical era, patients can expect a near-normal life expectancy. Death may result from aspiration pneumonia.

> Lower motor neuron signs can easily be remembered using the adage 'everything goes down'—there is decreased tone, decreased or absent reflexes, muscle atrophy and weakness, and fasciculations.

Inherited myopathies
Muscular dystrophies
The muscular dystrophies are a group of genetic and inherited diseases involving progressive skeletal muscle degeneration and weakness.

X-linked dystrophies
In over a third of cases, the mutation occurs in the affected boy and there is no relevant family history. In over half of cases, the mother is a carrier for the mutated gene. The majority of female carriers are unaffected by the disease, but a small minority ('manifesting carriers') develop a mild degree of muscle weakness themselves.

Duchenne muscular dystrophy
Epidemiology Duchenne muscular dystrophy (DMD) is the most common form of muscular dystrophy, occurring in 1 in 4000 live male births.
Aetiology DMD is an X-linked recessive disorder. It is caused by mutation of the gene for dystrophin protein, the second largest mammalian gene.
Pathology In DMD, a mutation occurs on the short arm of the X chromosome, the site (Xp21) coding for dystrophin protein. The lack of dystrophin protein results in impaired anchorage of muscle fibres to the extracellular matrix, making the fibres more susceptible to tearing upon repeated contraction. Damaged fibres allow an influx of Ca^{2+}, leading to irreversible cell death.
Clinical features Symptoms of DMD usually appear before 6 years of age. Early symptoms include progressive weakness of muscles of the legs and pelvis, eventually involving the arms, neck and other areas. Signs include loss of muscle mass (atrophy),

with initial enlargement of the calf muscles. These muscles are eventually replaced by fat and connective tissue (a process called pseudohypertrophy). Sufferers develop a waddling gait and Gower's sign owing to the proximal myopathy (Fig. 2.33).

Diagnosis   The average age at diagnosis of DMD is 5 years.

Diagnosis is based on a raised serum creatinine phosphokinase. Muscle biopsy also reveals necrosed muscle fibres surrounded by fibrous tissue and fat (Fig. 2.34). The muscle fibres are variable in diameter, owing to the body's attempt at regeneration.

Complications   These include marked scoliosis of the chest and back, frequent falls and progressive difficulty in walking, intellectual impairment (30%), muscle contractures in the legs due to fibrosis of damaged muscle fibres, and cardiomyopathy.

Management   There is no cure for DMD. Treatment is supportive and is aimed at controlling symptoms, maintaining the use of the muscles and maintaining maximum quality of life.

Identification of female carriers is possible and genetic counselling should be offered.

Prognosis   Owing to the rapidly progressive disability caused by the disease, most patients are wheelchair bound by their teens. Death usually occurs by 25 years of age, typically due to disorders arising from failure of the respiratory muscles.

Becker's muscular dystrophy

Becker's muscular dystrophy is an X-linked disorder and a related variant of DMD. It is less common, occurring in 3–6 per 100 000 male births. Although both Becker's and DMD relate to dystrophin production, they differ in that dystrophin production is absent or grossly abnormal in DMD, whereas in Becker's insufficient dystrophin is produced, with consequent instability of the muscle cell membrane.

Becker's shows similar clinical features and complications to DMD, although progression of the disease is slower. Again there is no known cure and management is supportive.

In males, symptoms usually appear by 11 years of age, the patient becoming unable to walk at around 25. Death usually occurs in the 40s.

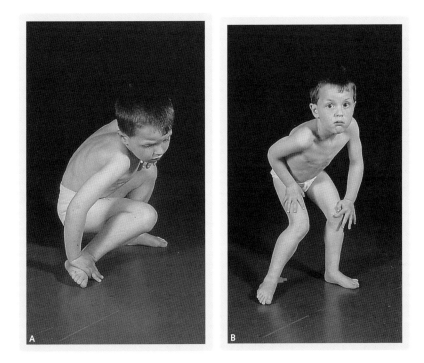

Fig. 2.33 Gower's sign, showing the difficulty encountered in standing from the prone position in patients with Duchenne muscular dystrophy. (A) This child needs to turn prone to rise, then uses his hands to climb up on his knees. (B) Once at knee level, the hands are released and the arms and trunk are swung sideways and upwards to reach an upright position. Note the hypertrophied calves (due to deposition of fat and fibrous tissue). (Courtesy of Dr T Lissauer and Dr G Clayden.)

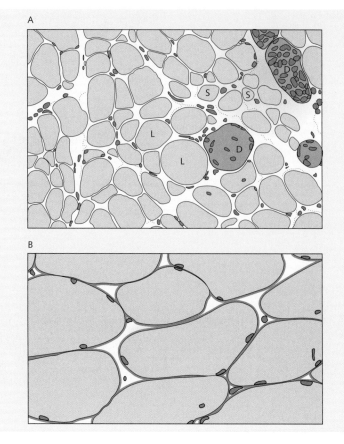

Fig. 2.34 (A) A micrograph of a frozen section of skeletal muscle of a child with Duchenne muscular dystrophy. Note the marked variation in fibre size, large (L) abnormally small (S) and dead fibres (D) being removed by phagocytic cells. (B) Normal skeletal muscle stained by immunocytochemistry which demonstrates the localization of dystrophin in the sarcolemma. In Duchenne muscular dystrophy this is absent.

Of the inherited myopathies, Duchenne muscular dystrophy is a common topic in exams.

Autosomal dystrophies

Limb girdle dystrophy

There are several different forms of limb girdle dystrophy, autosomal recessive dystrophies in which there are mutations of the genes encoding components of the muscle fibre and its contractile apparatus, resulting in the muscles being unable to produce the proteins required for them to function properly. It tends to present in childhood or young adult life, with onset of symptoms usually occurring between the ages of 10 and 30 years. It is characterized by a symmetrical, proximal and slowly progressive weakness of the muscles of the pelvic and shoulder girdle, with distal muscles not being affected until late in the disease (Fig. 2.35).

Clinical features are muscle weakness, myoglobinuria, myotonia, cardiomyopathy and elevated serum CK. Pseudohypertrophy of the calves is less common than in Duchenne muscular dystrophy.

Muscle biopsy shows findings similar to those of Duchenne muscular dystrophy. Treatment is primarily supportive.

Prognosis involves a variable degree of disability. Disability is more progressive where the disease manifests in childhood. It is not a fatal disease, but morbidity and mortality occur where the heart and lung muscles become affected.

Facioscapulohumeral dystrophy

Facioscapulohumeral dystrophy is an autosomal dominant disorder. The onset of the condition is anywhere between 10 and 70 years of age, most

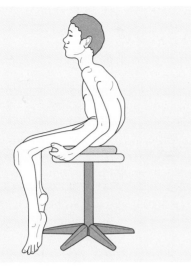

Fig. 2.35 Severe limb girdle dystrophy demonstrating proximal muscle wasting and kyphosis.

commonly producing face and shoulder girdle weakness. Winging of the scapulae is characteristic. Pseudohypertrophy is rare.

Muscle biopsy shows findings similar to those of Duchenne muscular dystrophy.

Individuals show a mild degree of disability.

Myotonic disorders

Myotonic disorders are a group of conditions in which there is a delay in muscle relaxation after voluntary contraction.

Myotonic dystrophy

Epidemiology Myotonic dystrophy occurs in 1 in 8000 people.

Aetiology Myotonic dystrophy is an autosomal dominant disorder. Genetic causes have been identified for three forms of myotonic dystrophy: DM1 (Steinert's disease), DM2 (proximal myotonic myopathy), and congenital myotonic dystrophy, each varying in severity and prognosis.

Pathology In affected families the disease can display the phenomenon of anticipation, with onset occurring at progressively lower ages and an increase in severity of disease in successive generations.

Clinical features Myotonic dystrophy commonly presents in the 20s or 30s, with life expectancy typically to the sixth decade. Characteristic features are myotonia, muscle wasting and weakness initially developing in the limbs, characteristic facies, and cranial muscle involvement (Fig. 2.36). Muscles involved with involuntary processes, such as

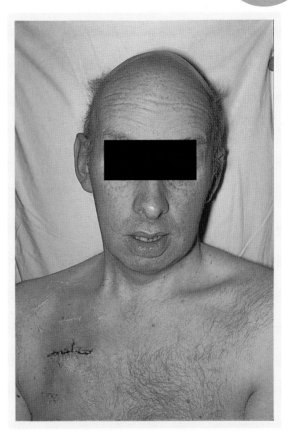

Fig. 2.36 Typical 'monk-like' appearance seen in an adult with myotonic dystrophy. Note the facial weakness, atrophy of temporal and sternocleidomastoid muscles, and frontal baldness. (Courtesy of Dr GD Perkin.)

breathing, and muscles surrounding internal organs may also be affected by the disease. Cognitive defects may also be present.

Other associated findings include cataracts, frontal balding, cardiac conduction abnormalities, gonadal atrophy and glucose intolerance.

There is a high rate of complications with the use of general anaesthesia in patients with myotonic dystrophy, including cardiac arrhythmias and postoperative respiratory problems, necessitating intensive monitoring before, during and after any surgery.

Diagnosis The diagnosis of myotonic dystrophy is mainly clinical, although an electromyogram (EMG) is characteristic. A muscle biopsy can also show dystrophic changes.

Management There is no cure for this condition. Management is supportive and involves treating the clinical manifestations, in order to maximize the patient's quality of life.

Prognosis   Death is usually due to cardiomyopathy or involvement of the respiratory muscles.

Metabolic myopathies

The metabolic myopathies are a heterogeneous group of conditions in which there are abnormalities in muscle energy metabolism.

Primary metabolic myopathies

Glycogen storage disorders   Glycogen storage disorders are caused by genetic abnormalities of glycolytic enzymes inherited in an autosomal recessive manner. The degree of muscle involvement is variable between the major types of primary metabolic myopathy.

Symptoms arise as a result of the decreased availability of energy from glycolysis, which is due to an impaired ability to mobilize glucose from glycogen.

Glycogen storage disorder type V (McArdle's syndrome) is an autosomal recessive disorder in which there is a deficiency of skeletal muscle myophosphorylase. Symptoms include temporary weakness and muscle cramps on exercise. There is an associated myoglobinuria. There is no rise in venous lactate during exercise, which aids diagnosis by enzyme analysis of muscle tissue. Life expectancy is not affected. Patients are advised to avoid exercise.

Lipid disorders   In the lipid disorders the availability of energy to muscle is reduced owing to abnormalities in fatty acid metabolism. Patients usually present with hypotonia in infancy, or muscle weakness and cramps later.

Symptoms are worse with prolonged exercise or fasting.

Mitochondrial disorders   The mitochondrial disorders are inherited. These are more commonly abnormalities of either the mitochondrial genome (more commonly) or the nuclear genome.

The age of onset is variable. The muscle weakness (particularly of the extraocular muscles) may be isolated or associated with neurological and metabolic disturbances.

Muscle biopsy shows abnormal mitochondria with crystalline inclusions.

Mitochondrial myopathy may develop in patients on long-term zidovudine therapy, i.e. patients infected with HIV.

Secondary metabolic myopathies

Myopathic symptoms can occur as a result of a whole range of electrolyte disturbances, e.g. Ca^{2+}, Mg^{2+}, K^+ etc.

Endocrine disorders are examples of secondary metabolic myopathies that are acquired.

Periodic paralyses

The periodic paralyses are a rare group of disorders characterized by repeated attacks of muscle weakness. There are three types: hypokalaemic, hyperkalaemic and normokalaemic.

Hypokalaemic periodic paralysis   This is an autosomal dominant condition that presents in adolescence and is remitting in the late 30s.

Attacks often occur after strenuous exercise or a heavy carbohydrate meal. During an attack the serum potassium concentration is low (2.5–3.5 mmol/L): attacks are terminated by the administration of intravenous potassium chloride.

Diuretic therapy and thyrotoxicosis must be excluded as possible causes of the myopathy.

Hyperkalaemic periodic paralysis   This is an autosomal dominant condition. It presents in childhood and is remitting in the 20s.

Attacks may occur after strenuous exercise and are terminated by intravenous calcium gluconate. During an attack the serum potassium concentration is high (6–7 mmol/L). Attacks are shorter than those associated with hypokalaemia.

Normokalaemic periodic paralysis   This is a very rare condition. The attacks respond to sodium.

Acquired myopathies

Idiopathic inflammatory myopathies

The idiopathic inflammatory myopathies are uncommon disorders and have a male: female ratio of 1:2. Most people with idiopathic inflammatory myopathy present in middle age.

Polymyositis

Polymyositis is the most common inflammatory myopathy. It usually affects those over 20 years of age and rarely affects children, with the peak age of onset being between 45 and 60 years of age.

Aetiology   The cause of polymyositis is not known, although it may be autoimmune, involving stimulation of T cells by a muscle antigen, resulting in a destruction of muscle fibres. A viral cause (Coxsackie virus) has been suggested.

Polymyositis can occur as a non-metastatic complication of malignancy, as more than 10% of patients have an underlying malignancy that presents later, e.g. carcinoma of the breast, bronchus or gastrointestinal tract. In this instance the male: female ratio is reversed.

Pathology   In polymyositis there is inflammation and destruction of both type I and type II muscle fibres because of the action of cytotoxic T lymphocytes. Histologically there is fibre necrosis, muscle atrophy and evidence of fibre regeneration.

Clinical features   The condition develops over 3–6 months. There is progressive, symmetrical, proximal muscle weakness, with muscle tenderness and wasting. A symmetrical non-erosive arthritis affects the knees, wrists and hands. Patients develop morning stiffness, and complain of fatigue, fever, anorexia and arthralgia. Distal muscle weakness is rare and implies advanced disease. The respiratory and heart muscles may also be affected. Dysphagia and dysarthria are other features.

Polymyositis can be associated with other connective tissue diseases, such as systemic lupus erythematosus (SLE), rheumatoid arthritis and Sjögren's syndrome. Features typical of connective tissue diseases may be present, e.g. Raynaud's phenomenon, in which there is intermittent vasospasm of arterioles in the hands and feet in response to cold and emotional stimuli. It is usually painful and the affected part of the body changes colour from pale to blue to red.

Diagnosis   Diagnosis is clinical:

- Muscle enzymes such as serum creatine phosphokinase are frequently markedly elevated.
- Characteristic abnormalities on EMG and muscle biopsy are evident.

Antinuclear antibodies (Jo-1) and rheumatoid factor may also be present, and can be of prognostic value.

Management   Management aims to minimize the immunological response and slow the progression of the disease using immunosuppressive drugs and corticosteroids. Physiotherapy aims to prevent disuse atrophy of muscles. Symptomatic therapy is used to reduce pain.

Underlying malignancy must be excluded.

Prognosis   The course of polymyositis is variable.

Death can result from aspiration pneumonia and respiratory or heart failure.

Dermatomyositis

Dermatomyositis shares many most features of polymyositis but with characteristic cutaneous pathology. However, unlike polymyositis, dermatomyositis can affect children, with a peak age of onset of 5 years. The peak age of onset of adult disease is 50 years. The cause is unknown, although associations have been made with HLA types such as DR5 and abnormal T-cell activity. It can also be drug induced, and infections such as Coxsackie virus have also been suggested.

Clinical features   The initial presentation is commonly with skin disease. In fact, 40% of sufferers only develop cutaneous features of the disease and have no musculoskeletal involvement. Muscle disease can present at the same time, or months to years later. Cutaneous features include:

- A characteristic purple heliotrope rash, typically on the eyelids, although it may spread to other sites
- An erythematous rash on the face, scalp, shoulders and hands
- Nailfold telangiectasia.

Management   Management is the same as for polymyositis (see Chapter 7). Patients with skin disease should be advised to minimize their exposure to light and to use sun protection.

Inclusion-body myositis

Inclusion-body myositis affects mainly the elderly and is clinically similar to polymyositis. It is a progressive disorder and immunosuppressive therapy is not effective.

Electron microscopy demonstrates the presence of filamentous inclusions in the muscle fibres.

Endocrine myopathies (or secondary metabolic myopathies)

Corticosteroid-induced myopathy

Corticosteroid-induced myopathy is caused by an excess of corticosteroid, e.g. in Cushing's syndrome or in people on steroid therapy.

The myopathy is proximal, i.e. it affects the upper parts of the arms and legs.

There is a raised creatine kinase concentration, and muscle biopsy reveals selective atrophy of type II muscle fibres.

Thyroid disease

Thyrotoxicosis may be associated with a proximal myopathy.

Hypothyroidism may result in a proximal myopathy, and affected individuals may experience muscle stiffness.

Osteomalacia

All causes of osteomalacia (e.g. vitamin D deficiency, liver failure, liver-enzyme-inducing drugs) may result in a proximal myopathy.

Toxic myopathies

Toxic myopathies are caused by excessive intake of alcohol or drugs.

Alcohol abuse

In toxic myopathy caused by excess alcohol, two patterns are seen:

- Subacute proximal myopathy (which may be reversed in the early stages); this is seen in chronic alcoholics. Selective atrophy of type II muscle fibres occurs.
- Acute myopathy associated with severe muscle pain due to acute alcohol excess; myoglobinuria may also occur.

Drug-induced myopathies

Agents that may cause a subacute proximal myopathy include cholesterol-lowering agents (e.g. benzofibrate), as well as chloroquine, penicillamine and lithium. Patients may respond to cessation of the drug.

Viral myalgias

The viral myalgias are muscle weaknesses associated with a viral illness, usually respiratory.

Chronic fatigue syndrome is a disorder in which the patient presents with debilitating fatigue, muscular pain with associated pain on movement, and mental fogginess. The cause is unknown and other associated symptoms include poor concentration, insomnia and depression. Professional opinions differ and have led to a degree of controversy as to whether this is a psychological or a skeletal muscle disorder.

Cardiac and smooth muscle

3

Objectives

By the end of this chapter you should be able to:
- Understand the initiation and propagation of the cardiac action potential (AP)
- Describe the ionic basis of the AP in the sinoatrial node compared to that in the Purkinje cells
- Discuss the differences in contraction between cardiac and skeletal muscle
- Explain the effect of the autonomic nervous system on heart rate
- Describe how smooth muscle cells are arranged
- Describe the arrangement of myofilaments in smooth muscle
- Describe the mechanisms involved in changing intracellular calcium levels
- Describe how smooth muscle contraction differs from skeletal muscle contraction and the effect of this
- Outline the functions of smooth muscle in the body.

CARDIAC MUSCLE

Structural organization of muscle in the heart

The heart has three layers: inner (endocardium), middle (myocardium) and outer (pericardium) (Fig. 3.1).

Endocardium

The inner layer, or endocardium, is made up of endothelial cells that respond to pressure changes, stretch, and a variety of circulatory substances.

Myocardium

The middle layer, or myocardium, consists of the cardiac muscle responsible for generating the force to pump blood around the body. It is thicker in the ventricles, the thickest layer being found in the left ventricle.

Pericardium

The outer layer, or pericardium, consists of two layers: the innermost epicardium (visceral pericardium), which is intimately related to the myocardium; and the pericardium (parietal pericardium), which forms the outermost layer of the heart. The two layers are separated by a potential space called the pericardial

cavity, into which secreted pericardial fluid lubricates the two layers during contraction.

Microstructure of cardiac muscle

Cardiac muscle cells are relatively small, about 15 μm wide and 100 μm long.

The arrangement of actin and myosin in cardiac muscle is similar to that in skeletal muscle. However, unlike skeletal muscle, cardiac myocytes are mononuclear, with a centrally placed nucleus. They are shorter than skeletal muscle cells and lack support cells (e.g. satellite cells), which leaves them unable to regenerate if they are damaged.

Myocytes are directly related to one another by low-resistance anchoring junctions called intercalated discs (Fig. 3.2). These anchor the cells to one another, anchor the actin filaments to each end of the cell to facilitate contraction, and facilitate the passage of membrane excitation, allowing rapid propagation of action potentials (APs) from cell to cell.

Cellular physiology of cardiac muscle

Initiation of the cardiac action potential

Under normal circumstances, the AP is initiated in the sinoatrial (SA) node, which is located in the right atrium under the crista terminalis. Under normal

Fig. 3.1 Macroscopic organization of the heart.

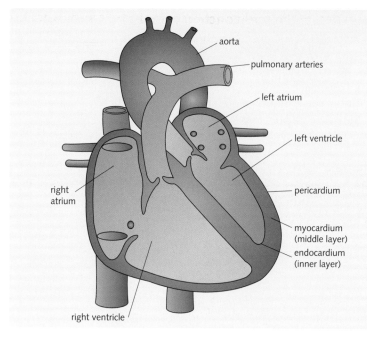

aorta

pulmonary arteries

left atrium

left ventricle

pericardium

myocardium (middle layer)

endocardium (inner layer)

right atrium

right ventricle

Fig. 3.2 Microscopic structure of cardiac muscle. Note that there are far fewer mitochondria in cardiac muscle than in skeletal muscle.

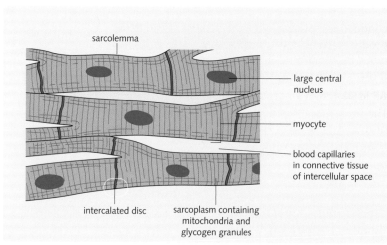

sarcolemma

large central nucleus

myocyte

blood capillaries in connective tissue of intercellular space

intercalated disc

sarcoplasm containing mitochondria and glycogen granules

conditions, the SA node functions as the heart's pacemaker. APs are generated at a greater rate in SA node pacemaker cells than in pacemaker tissue elsewhere in the heart, a property that allows the node to initiate depolarization, determining and controlling the heart rate for the whole heart. This property is called automaticity, so the SA node sets the rhythm for the heart overall.

In addition, tissue in the AV node, bundle of His and Purkinje fibres is often referred to as a latent pacemaker, as it has the potential to function as pacemaker tissue and can take over if the normal pacemaker fails.

In some heart disorders, the sinoatrial node loses its ability to initiate myocardial contractility, in which case a patient may require a pacemaker. This is a battery-operated device implanted subcutaneously that has a pulse generator producing electrical impulses conducted by electrodes to stimulate the heart to contract. Pacemakers are usually programmed to produce impulses 'on demand', i.e. when the heart misses a beat, helping to regulate the rate of contraction within a programmed threshold. They usually last 7–15 years before needing replacement.

Propagation of the cardiac action potential

Propagation occurs rapidly owing to the presence of gap junctions between adjacent cardiac myocytes. The AP is propagated from the SA node to the atrioventricular (AV) node, situated in the interatrial septum near the opening of the coronary sinus, through which the coronary veins drain into the right atrium. From there it passes to the bundle of His (AV bundle), through the fibrous ring at the atrioventricular junction into the interventricular septum, where it divides into the left and right bundle branches. These bundles break up into Purkinje fibres, from which the travelling AP facilitates contraction of papillary muscles just before it facilitates simultaneous contraction of both ventricles, from the apex up towards the base (Fig. 3.3).

Conduction is slow in the AV node, resulting in a delay of 0.1s before excitation of the ventricles that facilitates contraction of the atria before the ventricles, thereby allowing emptying of the atria.

Ionic basis

The action potential produced in the myocytes of the conducting system is different in nature from those produced in contractile myocytes. However, both types of AP last about 300 ms, much longer than those of nerve cells (3 ms).

AP in SA and AV nodes

The resting membrane potential (RMP) of the cells of the SA node is unstable and the inward current is carried by Na^+ and K^+. However, the K^+ outward current is reduced, resulting in the RMP rising to threshold more easily and more frequently than in other myocytes. Ultimately, this results in an increased number of APs and increased firing. The threshold drifts from −55 mV (lower than the RMP of ventricular and atrial myocytes) to −40 mV.

The conducting AP also looks different from that of contractile myocytes (Fig. 3.4A). Most notably, the upstroke is slow, because it is mediated by Ca^{2+} current.

AP in contractile myocytes

Unlike the SA node, the upstroke of the AP is mediated by fast Na^+ channels, resulting in a fast upstroke (Fig. 3.4B). Ca^{2+} channels are opened, producing a plateau phase that is further prolonged by the action of Ca^{2+}/Na^+ exchangers unique to cardiac cells. K^+ channels open in the late phase, producing repolarization.

The plateau phase of the AP makes the myocyte refractory for the duration of the twitch, preventing tetany from occurring in the heart. This is essential, as cardiac muscle in tetany would be incapable of pumping blood.

Excitation–contraction coupling

Excitation–contraction coupling of cardiac muscle is essentially the same as in skeletal muscle. It involves:

• Spread of the AP over the myocyte membrane
• Influx of Ca^{2+}
• Contraction, owing to the formation of cross-bridges and sliding of filaments.

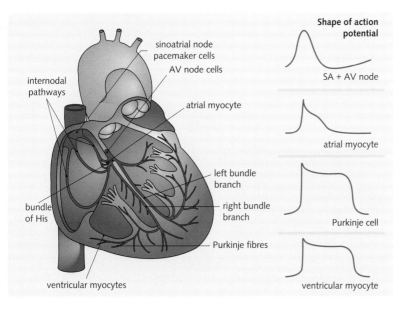

Fig. 3.3 Conducting system of the heart showing the location of the different types of myocyte and the action potentials associated with them. AV, atrioventricular; SA, sinoatrial.

Shape of action potential

SA + AV node

atrial myocyte

Purkinje cell

ventricular myocyte

sinoatrial node pacemaker cells
AV node cells
internodal pathways
atrial myocyte
left bundle branch
right bundle branch
bundle of His
Purkinje fibres
ventricular myocytes

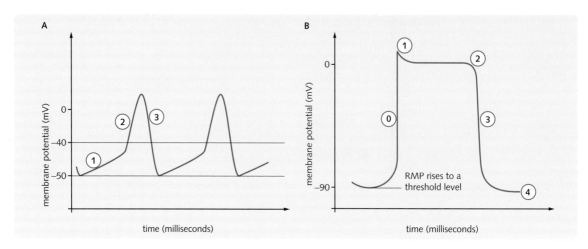

Fig. 3.4 (A) Characteristics of the action potential seen in sinoatrial node cells. (1) Drifting RMP caused by slow Na^+ influx, or 'pacemaker potential'; (2) influx of Ca^{2+}; (3) repolarization because of K^+ efflux. (B) Phases of the cardiac action potential in ventricular contractile myocytes. (0) Depolarization because of rapid Na^+ influx; (1) initial rapid depolarization due to inactivation of Na^+ channels and a passive influx of Cl^-; (2) prolonged plateau phase with opening of slow Ca^{2+}/Na^+ exchangers. This prolongs depolarization because of the Ca^{2+} influx and results in contraction of the myocyte; (3) late repolarization caused by closure of Ca^{2+}/Na^+ channels and K^+ efflux owing to opening of K^+ channels; (4) restoration of RMP. RMP, resting membrane potential.

There are some differences in the contractile apparatus:

- Cardiac T-tubules are much wider than those of skeletal muscle
- There is less organized association of sarcoplasmic reticulum to the T-tubules
- Sarcoplasmic reticulum forms dyads rather than triads around the T-tubules. Instead of being located around the junction of the A band and the I band (the AI junction), as they are in skeletal muscle, they are found around the Z line.

Bioenergetics of cardiac contraction

Cardiac muscle is mainly dependent on oxidative phosphorylation for contraction, sourcing its energy from aerobic metabolism, as totally anaerobic conditions would not provide sufficient energy to sustain ventricular contraction.

Energy substrates vary according to dietary intake, but lipid and carbohydrate tend to be utilized.

Cardiac muscle has a rich blood supply derived from the coronary arteries (Fig. 3.5) that branch out to surround the entire heart. They stem from just above the aortic valve and fill with blood during diastole.

Cardiac muscle differs from skeletal muscle in that:

- The cardiac AP is 100 times longer
- There is a long refractory period and therefore tetanus does not occur. However, when the frequency of APs is increased there is an increase in intracellular Ca^{2+} levels. This results in an increase in the force of successive contractions and is known as the *treppe* or staircase effect
- It has the potential to be self-excitatory
- The sarcoplasmic reticulum and T-tubules are organized in dyads (at the Z lines), not in triads
- The sarcoplasmic reticulum is not as well developed and therefore stores less Ca^{2+}. Additionally, extracellular Ca^{2+} enters the cell directly through the T-tubules via slow Ca^{2+} channels. Hence, the force of contraction in cardiac muscle is largely dependent on the extracellular Ca^{2+} concentration.

Factors affecting contractility

Factors can affect either the rate or the force of contraction. Factors that increase the force of contraction are said to have positive inotropic action, and those that decrease it have a negative inotropic action (Fig. 3.6). They exert their effect by affecting the intracellular calcium concentration.

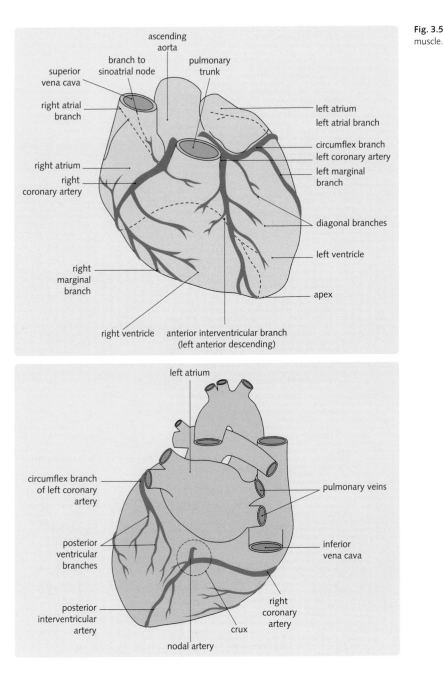

Fig. 3.5 The blood supply to cardiac muscle.

Positive inotropes increase the intracellular Ca^{2+} concentration by:

- Increasing Ca^{2+} influx by opening the Ca^{2+} channels, e.g. noradrenaline
- Decreasing Ca^{2+} removal, e.g. digitalis glycosides such as digoxin inhibit the Na^+/K^+ ATPase pump. This results in an increase in intracellular Na^+, causing less calcium to be secreted by the Ca^{2+}/Na^+ exchanger. This causes an increase in intracellular calcium concentration. The intracellular calcium is stored in the sarcoplasmic reticulum, thus an increased amount of calcium is released with each AP.

Examples of positive inotropes include:

- Hormones released upon activation of the sympathetic nervous system, e.g. epinephrine, norepinephrine
- Thyroid hormones
- Glucagon

Fig. 3.6 Inotropic drugs and their sites of action in the cardiac cell. PDE, phosphodiesterase; ECF, extracellular fluid; ICF, intracellular fluid.

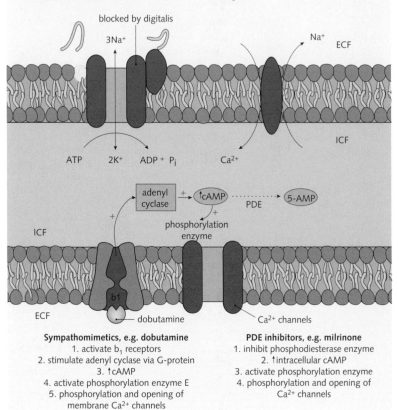

Cardiac glycosides, e.g. digoxin
- inhibit Na^+/K^+-ATPase pump
- increase intracellular Na^+
- increase intracellular Ca^{2+} due to Ca^{2+}/Na^+ exchanger

Sympathomimetics, e.g. dobutamine
1. activate b_1 receptors
2. stimulate adenyl cyclase via G-protein
3. ↑cAMP
4. activate phosphorylation enzyme E
5. phosphorylation and opening of membrane Ca^{2+} channels

PDE inhibitors, e.g. milrinone
1. inhibit phosphodiesterase enzyme
2. ↑intracellular cAMP
3. activate phosphorylation enzyme
4. phosphorylation and opening of Ca^{2+} channels

Palpitations are, by definition, an awareness of the sensation of the heart beating. It is vital to clarify what patients mean when they describe having palpitations, as the term is used by many to describe different sensations. Ask the patient to tap out the rate and rhythm as he or she is aware of it.

- Drugs, e.g. cardiac glycosides such as digoxin, phosphodiesterase inhibitors such as milrinone, and β_1 agonists such as dobutamine.

Negative inotropes may block Ca^{2+} movement or depress cardiac muscle metabolism in some way. Examples of negative inotropes include:

- Disease, e.g. hypoxia, ischaemia
- Drugs such as β-blockers, calcium channel antagonists (many of the drugs used to treat hypertension have a negative inotropic action), barbiturates and most anaesthetic agents

- Hormones released upon activation of the parasympathetic nervous system, e.g. ACh.

Chronotropes

Chronotropes are agents that affect the rate of contraction.

Autonomic nervous system and the heart

Activation of the parasympathetic (vagal) nerves

Activation of the parasympathetic (vagal) nerves has the effect of decreasing heart rate, decreasing contractility and slowing transmission of the cardiac impulse. Activation of the parasympathetic (vagal) nerves causes hyperpolarization of the myocytic membrane via muscarinic ACh receptors. Primarily, this causes a slowing of the heart rate through its effects at the SA and AV nodes. It can also cause some decrease in force of contraction. Anticholinergic drugs antagonize this effect.

Activation of the sympathetic system

Sympathetic system activation causes the release of norepinephrine from postganglionic fibres, and release of norepinephrine and epinephrine from the adrenal medullae. Activation of the sympathetic system has the effect of increasing heart rate and force of contractility:

- It influences the SA node, causing an increased rate of decay of the RMP, thereby causing more frequent action potentials to be produced, increasing the heart rate
- Epinephrine opens calcium channels, producing an enhanced plateau in the AP of a contractile myocyte, ultimately resulting in increased force of contraction
- Norepinephrine binds the β_1 subtype of adrenoceptors on myocytes, causing cAMP-mediated increase in intracellular calcium concentration and an increase in the force of contraction.

> β_2-Adrenoceptor antagonists reduce the formation of cAMP and calcium currents, reducing the rate and force of myocardial contraction. These drugs are used clinically to treat hypertension, angina, arrhythmias, heart failure and thyrotoxicosis. Side effects arise from blocking β-adrenoceptors which are also present in the peripheral vasculature, the bronchi, pancreas and liver.

Starling's law

As with skeletal muscle, the force of contraction increases with muscle fibre length.

Starling's law follows the principle of 'more in = more out'. It states that the force of contraction is proportional to the initial length of the cardiac muscle fibre. As the end-diastolic volume (measured and recorded as the end-diastolic pressure) increases, the greater the length of the ventricular muscle fibres and the greater the energy of contraction (stroke work). Thus, within physiological limits, the heart is able to pump out all the blood entering it (stroke volume). This is represented by the Starling curve (Fig. 3.7).

The curve can be displaced upwards (positive inotropic effect, e.g. exercise) or downwards (negative inotropic effect, e.g. heart failure).

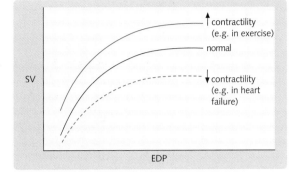

Fig. 3.7 Starling curve. EDP, end-diastolic pressure; SV, stroke volume.

Starling's law does not hold in situations where excessive stretching of cardiac muscle fibres causes a decrease in actin–myosin interaction.

SMOOTH MUSCLE

The majority of smooth muscle found in the body is of the single-unit type (Fig. 3.8).

Organization of smooth muscle

Microstructure of smooth muscle

Smooth muscle cells are around 15 μm wide and vary from 30 to 200 μm in length. Each cell is spindle shaped, with a single, centrally placed nucleus. They are organized into small groups or bunches within the muscle (Fig. 3.8). These are surrounded by connective tissue containing the nerves and blood vessels.

Within a bunch the cells are arranged parallel to one another and surrounded by an external lamina. Similar to cardiac cells, they adhere to one another at multiple sites and communicate with each other via gap (nexus) junctions at sites where the external lamina is deficient. This facilitates the movement of membrane excitation from cell to cell, allowing them to contract together as a single functional unit.

Arrangement of smooth muscle in different tissues

The arrangement of smooth muscle differs in different structures.

In blood vessels it is arranged circumferentially, where it helps to control the distribution of blood and to regulate blood pressure. In the airways it alters

Fig. 3.8 Microstructure of a single unit of smooth muscle in longitudinal section.

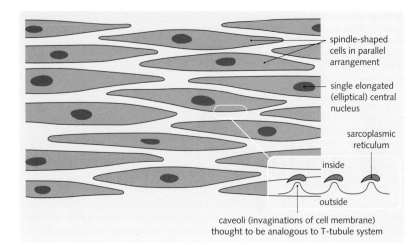

spindle-shaped cells in parallel arrangement

single elongated (elliptical) central nucleus

sarcoplasmic reticulum

inside

outside

caveoli (invaginations of cell membrane) thought to be analogous to T-tubule system

the diameter of the respiratory airways and alters resistance to airflow (Fig. 3.9).

In the intestines and lower two-thirds of the oesophagus (the upper third comprises skeletal muscle), smooth muscle is arranged in two layers (Fig. 3.10):

- In the inner layer, cells are arranged circumferentially and alter the diameter of the lumen.
- In the outer layer cells are arranged longitudinally and influence the length of the muscle forming the walls of the intestines.

In this way both the diameter and length of the tract can be altered, causing movement of contents by peristalsis.

In the stomach, smooth muscle cells are arranged in three layers:

- Inner oblique
- Middle circular
- Outer longitudinal.

Here they play an essential role in peristalsis, mixing food and digestive enzymes to break down the food and move materials along the gastrointestinal tract.

In the bladder, smooth muscle cells are arranged in three layers:

- Inner longitudinal
- Middle circular
- Outer longitudinal.

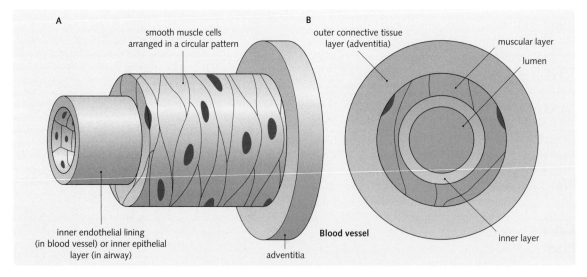

A

smooth muscle cells arranged in a circular pattern

B

outer connective tissue layer (adventitia)

muscular layer

lumen

inner endothelial lining (in blood vessel) or inner epithelial layer (in airway)

adventitia

Blood vessel

inner layer

Fig. 3.9 Circumferential arrangement of smooth muscle cells in the respiratory airways. (A) Longitudinal section; (B) transverse section.

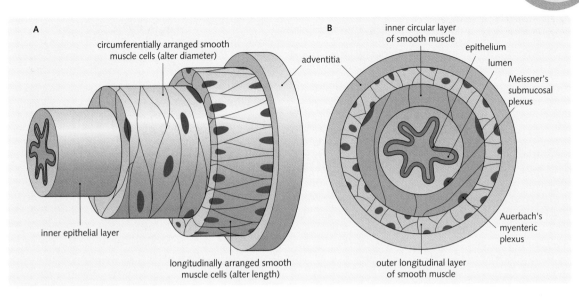

Fig. 3.10 Arrangement of smooth muscle cells in the intestine. (A) Longitudinal section; (B) transverse section.

Contraction of the muscle expels urine from the body via the micturition process.

Sphincters controlling the rate and volume of substances passing from one system to another are formed by circumferential rings of smooth muscle around a structure, contraction controlling the rate and volume of a substance beyond it. Examples include the lower oesophageal sphincter between the lower oesophagus and the stomach, and the vesicoureteric sphincters at the lower end of the ureters and the base of the bladder.

There are two anal sphincters controlling the passage of faeces: internal and external. The internal anal sphincter is composed of smooth muscle and gates the distal colon and the rectum, and is under autonomic control. The external anal sphincter is composed of skeletal muscle and is located around the opening of the anal canal and is under voluntary control, allowing an individual control over when to defecate.

Control of smooth muscle contraction

Initiation of contraction of smooth muscle may result from several mechanisms.

Autonomic nervous system stimulation

In smooth muscle, branching nerve fibres contain neurotransmitter within swellings called varicosities. Released neurotransmitter diffuses to receptors on smooth muscle fibre, so there is usually no direct contact between nerve fibres and muscle cells (Fig. 3.11).

According to the type of receptor activated, the effect will be either excitatory or inhibitory.

The neurotransmitter released by a parasympathetic nerve may be ACh or, if released by a sympathetic nerve, noradrenaline. The two types of neurotransmitter have opposite effects in any one tissue.

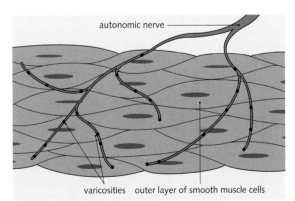

Fig. 3.11 Arrangement of autonomic nerve fibres in smooth muscle.

If a section of smooth muscle has many layers, usually only the outer one is innervated. The resulting AP is conducted to other layers via gap junctions. In the intestinal tract, peristalsis is coordinated by Auerbach's (myenteric) and Meissner's (submucosal) plexuses, which lie on either side of the inner circular layer of smooth muscle, closest to the epithelium.

Action of circulating hormones

The most common hormones influencing smooth muscle contraction are ACh, adrenaline, noradrenaline, angiotensin and vasopressin; others include serotonin and histamine. These act on receptors on the muscle fibre membrane, opening/closing ion channels and thereby initiating or inhibiting APs and changes within the cell due to activation of second-messenger pathways, e.g. the release of Ca^{2+} from the sarcoplasmic reticulum.

A hormone may have an excitatory effect in one tissue type yet an inhibitory effect in another, depending on the receptor activated.

Local tissue factors

Local tissue factors involved in smooth muscle tone are carbon dioxide, H^+ and Ca^{2+} (Fig. 3.12). However, the mechanism by which these produce contraction is unclear.

Cellular physiology of smooth muscle

Contractile apparatus

Smooth muscle has two types of contractile protein: actin and myosin. In addition, a network of intermediate filaments composed of the protein desmin, which produces dense bodies analogous to Z discs in skeletal muscle, is firmly attached to the sarcolemma. These intermediate filaments provide a site of attachment and anchorage to thin filaments that allows the cell to uniformly shorten upon contraction. Dense bodies also transmit the force of contraction to surrounding smooth muscle cells,

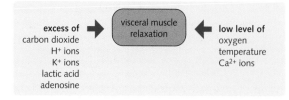

Fig. 3.12 Effect of local tissue factors on the tone of smooth muscle.

allowing smooth muscle cells to contract as a single unit.

Smooth muscle AP

In smooth muscle, the RMP is usually about –50 to –60 mV (i.e. less negative than skeletal muscle), and Ca^{2+}, not Na^+, is usually responsible for the AP. The AP can be a spike (like skeletal muscle) or plateau-like.

Excitation–contraction coupling

During excitation–contraction coupling of smooth muscle there is a rise in intracellular Ca^{2+}. This can be mediated by:

- Response to an AP: calcium enters through voltage-gated calcium channels
- Independent of AP: through ligand-gated Ca^{2+} channels or Ca^{2+} channels mediated by the second messenger inositol triphosphate (IP3), which is itself produced by a G-protein coupled receptor in response to agonist binding
- Caveolae: these are invaginations in the sarcolemma and are believed to be analogous to T-tubules in skeletal muscle. The exact mechanism by which they control the entry of Ca^{2+} into the cell is unknown.

Four Ca^{2+} bind to calmodulin protein present in the cytoplasm. This results in the formation of a myosin kinase–calmodulin–Ca^{2+} complex.

The contractile apparatus is activated when the myosin light chain is phosphorylated by the enzyme myosin light chain kinase, resulting in its detachment from one part of the actin molecule and allowing it to form cross-bridges with another part as part of contraction. Myosin light chain kinase is itself activated when it is bound in a complex with calcium and calmodulin.

The muscle relaxes when the myosin light chain is dephosphorylated by a second enzyme, myosin phosphatase. The actions of the two enzymes work in tandem to produce contraction.

A decrease in myoplasmic Ca^{2+} concentration inactivates myosin kinase, preventing contraction from occurring.

Intracellular Ca^{2+} concentration is restored by:

- Active pumping back into the sarcoplasmic reticulum
- Active pumping of Ca^{2+} out of the cell
- Na^+/Ca^{2+} exchange across the sarcolemma.

Smooth muscle contraction differs from skeletal muscle in that troponin is not a component of the thin filament. Instead, Ca^{2+} binds to the cytoplasmic protein calmodulin.

Disadvantages of smooth muscle contraction are that:

- Phosphorylation is a relatively slow process, therefore cross-bridge interactions and speed of contraction are low
- ATP is required for both phosphorylation and powering of cross-bridges. Therefore, smooth muscle contraction is less efficient.

Advantages of slow cross-bridge turnover are that:

- The lower ATP consumption is adequately provided by oxidative phosphorylation, so smooth muscles are not fatigued.
- There is prolonged contraction.

Drugs affecting smooth muscle

Organic nitrates
Examples of organic nitrates include glyceryl trinitrate and isosorbide dinitrate.

Mechanism of action   Organic nitrates act in the same way as the vasodilator nitric oxide (NO), produced by endothelial cells (eNO). Organic nitrates relax smooth muscle indirectly by acting on the endothelial cells lining blood vessels to produce the molecule guanylate cyclase, which crosses the endothelial cell membrane and passes into the underlying smooth muscle, where it mediates its relaxation. They cause potent vasodilation, desirable in an angina attack as it decreases venous return and the subsequent work of the left ventricle.

Indications   Organic nitrates are drugs used in both the prophylaxis and symptomatic treatment of angina, and in left ventricular failure (LVF).

Adverse effects   They can cause flushing, headache and postural hypotension by affecting smooth muscle elsewhere in the body.

> The body can develop tolerance to many drugs, including nitrates, with the result that their therapeutic effect is reduced. This can affect many patients on long-acting or transdermal nitrates. When a patient develops tolerance the prescription is changed, with the aim of producing a reduced blood–nitrate concentration for 4–8 hours per day, so that the level of tolerance can subside.

Myoepithelial cells
Myoepithelial cells are contractile cells found in mammary glands, sweat glands, salivary glands and the iris. They comprise a layer of flat cells arranged around acini and ducts. The arrangement of contractile proteins is similar to that in smooth muscle.

Upon stimulation, myoepithelial cells contract and cause the expulsion of glandular secretions.

DISORDERS OF CARDIAC MUSCLE

There is a wide spectrum of cardiac disorders affecting different aspects of the functioning cardiovascular system. This section considers some of those disorders that specifically affect cardiac muscle.

Myocardial disease that is not secondary to ischaemic, valvular or hypertensive heart disease can be classified by its causative factors:

- Inflammatory
- Genetic
- Idiopathic.

This encompasses the cardiomyopathies and myocarditis.

Cardiomyopathy
Cardiomyopathy is defined as disease of the myocardium associated with cardiac dysfunction. There are four functional types: dilated (or congestive), hypertrophic (obstructive), restrictive and arrhythmogenic right ventricular cardiomyopathy. All of the cardiomyopathies are rare.

Hypertrophic obstructive cardiomyopathy
Epidemiology   Hypertrophic obstructive cardio-myopathy (HOCM) occurs more commonly in young adults.

Aetiology   An established cause of HOCM is genetic, with autosomal dominant inheritance. Chromosomal abnormalities can be identified in up to 50% of cases, with genetic mutations in more than seven cardiac muscle proteins having been identified.

Pathology   The main feature is massive hyper-trophy of the left ventricle, particularly around the interventricular septum close to the aortic valve outlet.

Clinical features Patients usually present with chest pain, dyspnoea, syncope or presyncope (usually occurring on exertion), the incidental finding of cardiac arrhythmias, or sudden death with the diagnosis being made post mortem (occurring in up to 6% of cases in adolescents).

Diagnosis Physical examination can find a double apical pulsation and fourth heart sound due to forceful contraction. Also, an ejection systolic murmur and jerky carotid pulse due to obstruction of the left ventricular outflow tract.

ECG demonstrates abnormal Q waves in 25–50% of patients, left ventricular hypertrophy (LVH), and changes in ST and T waves. Echocardiography is diagnostic, revealing asymmetrical LVH mostly involving the septum.

Atrial fibrillation (AF) can occur in association with decreasing ventricular filling, with deterioration in symptoms.

Complications Risk factors identified for sudden death include massive LVH (>30 mm) as well as genotype, a family history of sudden death, abnormal blood pressure during exercise and recurrent syncope. Two or more risk factors put the individual at significant risk.

Management Treatment is concerned primarily with preventing sudden death. Implantable defibrillators are used in those at high risk of sudden death, or treatment with amiodarone in those identified as at lesser risk. Chest pain and dyspnoea are treated with β-blockers and/or verapamil.

Prognosis The course of the disease is very variable. Most patients remain stable for years.

Dilated cardiomyopathy

Epidemiology There is an incidence of 2–8 cases per 100 000 per year in Europe and North America. The median age of those diagnosed is in the 50s but the disease can affect people of any age.

Aetiology It can occur as a complication of many systemic or other cardiac diseases (Fig. 3.13), but in most cases no cause is found (idiopathic).

Pathology The heart is enlarged (cardiomegaly), but the ventricles are dilated and hypertrophied, and mural thrombi can develop. The muscle fibres can fibrose and hypertrophy in an irregular fashion. Pathology is similar to that of chronic alcoholic heart disease. There is no significant atherosclerosis.

Clinical features Individuals tend to present with congestive heart failure. They may also be affected by

Fig. 3.13 Causes of dilated cardiomyopathy (DCM)

genetic	e.g. autosomal dominant DCM, X-linked cardiomyopathy
inflammatory	post-infective, autoimmune, connective tissue diseases (systemic lupus erythematosus, systemic sclerosis)
metabolic	e.g. glycogen storage disease
nutritional	thiamin, selenium deficiency
endocrine	acromegaly, thyrotoxicosis, myxoedema, diabetes mellitus
infiltrative	hereditary haemochromatosis
neuromuscular	e.g. muscular dystrophy, Friedreich's ataxia, mitochondrial myopathies
toxic	alcohol, cocaine, doxorubicin, cyclophosphamide, cobalt
haematological	sickle-cell anaemia, thrombotic thrombocytopenic purpura

syncope due to ventricular arrhythmia or conduction disease.

Diagnosis Chest X-ray can reveal cardiomegaly. ECG findings include diffuse non-segment ST segment and T-wave changes, with sinus tachycardia and conduction abnormalities. Echocardiography can show left and/or right ventricle dilatation with poor overall contractile function. Patients should have an angiogram to exclude coronary artery disease.

Complications Sudden death can occur, and is occasionally the means by which the condition presents.

Management Treatment is aimed at relieving symptoms and the heart failure and preventing disease progression. Diuretics can be given to relieve symptoms of congestive heart failure, alongside suppression of the renin–aldosterone system and sympathetic activation with ACE inhibitors and β-blockers. In severe cases, implantable defibrillators, antiarrhythmic therapy and, where medical treatment fails, cardiac transplantation are used.

Prognosis The prognosis is poor, with only 50–60% of patients surviving 2 years after diagnosis.

Myocarditis

Myocarditis is an acute inflammation of the myocardium.

Fig. 3.14 Causes of myocarditis

idiopathic	
infective	*viral*: Coxsackievirus, adenovirus, cytomegalovirus, echovirus, influenza, polio, hepatitis, HIV
	parasitic: *Trypanosoma cruzi*,*Toxoplasma gondii* (acause of myocarditis in the newborn or immunocompromised)
	bacterial: Streptococcus (most commonly rheumatic carditis), diphtheria (toxin-mediated heart block common)
	spirochaetal: Lyme disease (heart block common), leptospirosis
	fungal
	rickettsial
toxic	**drugs** causing hypersensitivity reactions, e.g. methyldopa, penicillin, sulphonamides, antituberculous
	radiation may cause myocarditis but pericarditis more common

Aetiology   There is a wide range of causative factors (Fig. 3.14), including viral, bacterial, parasitic and fungal infective organisms, as well as toxins and drugs. Myocarditis can also occur in autoimmune form.

Pathology   In the acute stage, myocytes are destroyed by a combination of cell-mediated cytotoxicity and cytokine release in response to the assault of the causative agent, leading to myocardial damage and dysfunction. This leads to autoimmune destruction of myocytes.

Clinical features   Presentation varies with the stage of the disease. Patients may complain of chest pain, fatigue, dyspnoea and palpitations, although they may be asymptomatic and present with incidental ECG abnormalities. Indeed, it is believed that myocarditis is responsible for 20% of sudden unexpected deaths in those under 40 years of age. It can also present acutely with fever and cardiac failure, possibly with a recent history of a respiratory infection. Features on examination include soft heart sounds, a prominent third heart sound, and tachycardia creating the 'gallop' rhythm.

Diagnosis   ECG can reveal ST segment elevation or depression and T-wave inversion, atrial arrhythmias and transient atrioventricular block. Blood cardiac markers such as creatine kinase (CK) and troponin I can be raised, implicating myocardial damage. Chest X-ray may show cardiac enlargement in virulent or severe disease. Serology for viruses and autoantibodies can be performed to look for causative factors. Endomyocardial biopsy can reveal acute inflammation but is of limited specificity and sensitivity.

Management   Management is supportive, with bed rest and treatment of any arrhythmias, heart failure and any underlying infection.

Prognosis   The prognosis depends on the cause of the disease. Those suffering mild disease usually make a full recovery. A third of patients can go on to develop dilated cardiomyopathy, and some may progress into intractable heart failure.

DISORDERS OF SMOOTH MUSCLE

Disorders affecting smooth muscle are less common than those affecting the other types of muscle. However, they do include some important conditions.

Leiomyoma (fibroids)

Epidemiology   These are the most common benign growth to occur in the female reproductive tract. They are more prevalent in the third and fourth decades and approaching the menopause.

Aetiology   The cause of fibroids is unknown. Some associated factors include:

- Low parity
- Afro-Caribbean race.

Pathology   They are usually multiple, round, well-circumscribed masses of interlaced bundles of smooth muscle fibres, their diameter varying anywhere from 5 mm upwards. They are prone to progressive enlargement, displaying cystic development or focal necrosis, but showing little or no mitotic activity. They can be demonstrated as having steroid hormone receptors, which respond to oestrogen and therefore make them hormone dependent.

Clinical features Women commonly present with abnormally heavy uterine bleeding and/or pain. Sometimes a mass is palpable on bimanual vaginal or even abdominal examination. They can become large enough to cause symptoms of urinary dysfunction due to intra-abdominal pressure effects.

Diagnosis They can be visualized on vaginal or pelvic ultrasound examination. Tissue can be biopsied for histological analysis by hysteroscopic instrumentation with or without ultrasound guidance. Small, asymptomatic fibroids are often an incidental finding at hysterectomy.

Complications There is an established correlation between the mitotic activity of leiomyomas and their clinical behaviour, with higher counts suggesting unpredictable behaviour and possible malignant progression and metastasis. A leiomyoma with mitotic counts of 10 or more per 10 high power fields (hpf) (normal being 0–3) should be regarded as a malignant leiomyosarcoma and should be removed.

Occasionally fibroids can develop around the fundal region of the uterus and occlude the fallopian tubes as they enlarge, which can create fertility problems in women of reproductive age.

Management First-line management is medical, using medication to reduce pain and blood loss. Where conservative medical therapy fails to control symptoms, or their removal is desired (e.g. where they are causing difficulties in attempting to conceive), the fibroids can be removed by myomectomy. However, where symptoms are causing poor quality of life, the woman may wish to have a hysterectomy, particularly where they cause chronic heavy bleeding and/or pain.

Prognosis As fibroid growth is partly oestrogen dependent, they usually regress without recurrence after the menopause.

Gastro-oesophageal reflux disease (GORD)

The lower oesophageal sphincter consists of smooth muscle along the last 4 cm of the oesophagus. It prevents food from regurgitating back up into the oesophagus. Although reflux of gastric contents into the lower oesophagus does occur in healthy individuals, GORD develops where prolonged reflux causes symptoms of reflux to persist.

Epidemiology An estimated 10% of people suffer from heartburn on a daily basis, of which an estimated 20–40% actually experience abnormal oesophageal exposure to gastric juice. It is likely to be underreported, as many can control symptoms with over-the-counter medication.

Aetiology Gastro-oesophageal reflux is exacerbated by certain factors. Pregnancy and obesity are important ones, as there is an increase in intra-abdominal pressure associated with a relaxation of the lower oesophageal sphincter. Alcohol and smoking can exacerbate symptoms, and large meals predispose to reflux due to mechanical factors of digestion. Other associated factors include hiatus hernia, systemic sclerosis and medications that affect smooth muscle, such as anticholinergic drugs, calcium channel blockers and nitrates.

Pathology Numerous factors have been implicated in GORD. Mechanical factors involve the sphincter itself. Intermittent relaxation has been implicated, as well as reduced resting pressure of the sphincter when intra-abdominal pressure rises, such as in pregnancy. There may be abnormal intestinal peristalsis, resulting in reduced clearance of stomach contents from the oesophagus and stomach, thereby increasing the likelihood of reflux occurring. In addition, the oesophageal mucosa is relatively more sensitive to gastric acid.

Clinical features Pain and heartburn are important presenting complaints, which are worse on bending or lying down and taking alcohol or hot drinks. They are relieved by antacid medication. The patient may report an acidic taste in the mouth or regurgitation of food after a meal, and a nocturnal cough may occur due to regurgitation. The patient may rarely present with vomiting blood (haematemesis) or develop a chronic iron-deficiency anaemia when they have developed oesophagitis.

Diagnosis GORD is a clinical diagnosis, and patients younger than 45 are initially treated on diagnosis without further investigations. Older patients and those whose disease is refractory to treatment are usually investigated with a combination of an OGD (oesophagogastric–duodenal endoscopy) alongside 24-hour pH and manometry studies

Complications Long-term disease can result in transformation (metaplasia) of the normal oesophageal squamous epithelium to gastric columnar epithelium, termed Barrett's oesophagus. This is a premalignant change, requiring endoscopic surveillance and surgical ablation if it progresses. Peptic strictures can also form in chronic, untreated disease, most commonly in patients over 60, producing symptoms of intermittent dysphagia. Strictures are treated by balloon dilatation as well as treatment of the underlying condition.

Management Proton pump inhibitors reduce the amount of acid that the stomach produces, and relieves symptoms in many sufferers. Lifestyle factors that exacerbate the disease, including diet and alcohol consumption, should be addressed. Surgery is an option for those whose reflux does not respond to treatment or lifestyle modifications.

Objectives

By the end of this chapter you should be able to:

- List the functions of the skeleton
- Describe the classifications, growth and microstructure of cartilage
- Describe the classifications, growth and microstructure of bone
- List the factors that affect bone growth
- Describe remodelling of immature bone
- Explain how calcium levels are maintained by parathyroid hormone (PTH) and calatonin
- List hormonal influences on bone
- List the causes of hereditary abnormalities of bone
- Describe the features of pyogenic osteomyelitis
- List the different types of fracture and how they heal
- Explain the causes and pathology of osteoporosis
- Give a simple classification of hyperparathyroidism and its effects
- Describe the effects of renal disease on bone
- Describe the features of Paget's disease of bone
- List common tumours of the skeleton
- Distinguish between benign and malignant tumours
- Understand the cause and pathophysiology of rickets and osteomalacia.

OVERVIEW OF THE SKELETON

The skeletal system is composed of various types of connective tissue, including bone and cartilage.

Bone and cartilage consist of cells embedded in an extracellular matrix. This matrix consists of an amorphous ground substance permeated by a system of collagen and elastic fibres. These fibres differ from general connective tissue because their matrices are solid, although they do share the same origin from embryonic cellular connective tissue, the mesenchyme.

X-rays are a type of electromagnetic radiation that are used to image body structures. When a photographic plate is placed behind the area being imaged, the emitted X-rays are blocked by dense tissues such as bone, producing a shadow outlining the structure, but pass through soft tissues such as muscle and cartilage, these areas appearing black when the plate is developed.

Functions of the skeleton

The skeleton performs the following functions:

- Support for the body, as it is a rigid framework
- Protection for organs, e.g. the cranium over the brain and the thoracic cage over the heart and lungs
- A mechanical basis for locomotion
- Mineral storage—the majority of calcium, phosphorus and magnesium salts are found in bone
- Provides the site for bone marrow, where the development of blood cells, or haemopoiesis, occurs.

Red bone marrow produces red blood cells, some lymphocytes, granulocytic white blood cells and platelets. In adults, yellow bone marrow is mature bone marrow that has filled with adipocytes.

ORGANIZATION OF BONE AND CARTILAGE

Distribution of bone and cartilage

The human skeleton is bilaterally symmetrical. It is composed of two separate skeletons: axial and appendicular (Fig. 4.1).

The axial skeleton consists of the bones of the head (skull), neck (hyoid bone and cervical vertebrae) and trunk (ribs, sternum, thoracic and lumbar vertebrae, and sacrum).

The appendicular skeleton consists of the bones of the upper and lower limbs and includes those that form the pectoral and pelvic girdles.

With age, the proportion of bone and cartilage in the skeleton changes. In the fetus, most long bones are initially represented by cartilage that resembles the shape of adult bone. In the adult, the only remnants of hyaline cartilage are the articular cartilages of joints and the cartilage rings of the trachea.

Cartilage

Cartilage microstructure

Cartilage is a very special support tissue composed mainly of large, unbranched polysaccharide molecules called glycosaminoglycans, intricately arranged in association with collagen fibres. The collagen is mainly type II and gives cartilage its mechanical stability, whereas the glycosaminoglycans hydrate the matrix, helping it to resist compressive mechanical forces. The glycosaminoglycans are produced by cells called chondroblasts and maintained by chondrocytes, with these cells becoming embedded in the extensive cartilaginous matrix along with fibrous elements and a ground substance.

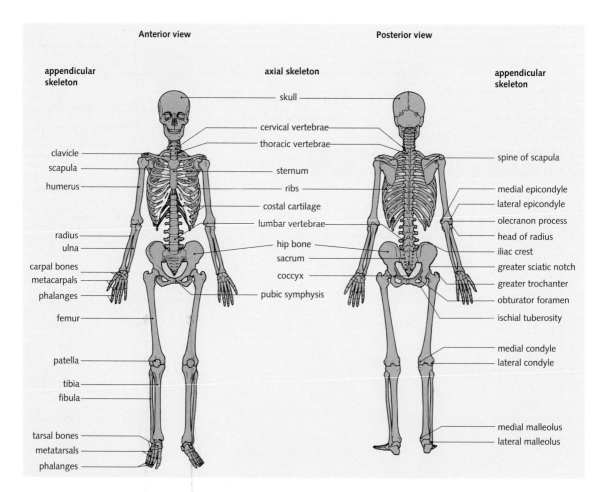

Anterior view · Posterior view

appendicular skeleton · axial skeleton · appendicular skeleton

skull
cervical vertebrae
thoracic vertebrae
clavicle
scapula
sternum
humerus
ribs
costal cartilage
lumbar vertebrae
radius
ulna
hip bone
sacrum
carpal bones
coccyx
metacarpals
phalanges
pubic symphysis
femur
patella
tibia
fibula
tarsal bones
metatarsals
phalanges

spine of scapula
medial epicondyle
lateral epicondyle
olecranon process
head of radius
iliac crest
greater sciatic notch
greater trochanter
obturator foramen
ischial tuberosity
medial condyle
lateral condyle
medial malleolus
lateral malleolus

Fig. 4.1 Anterior and posterior views of the adult axial and appendicular skeletons.

A radical surgical approach in the management of full-thickness cartilage damage of the knee is autologous cartilage transplantation. A small amount of normal cartilage is biopsied from the joint margin, cultured under laboratory conditions for 6 weeks and then transplanted back into the area of the defect. Although it gives good results, because of the strict suitability criteria, the vigorous rehabilitation that follows and cost issues, it is not appropriate for everyone.

Cartilage formation and cell types

Cartilage derives from mesenchyme, embryonic cellular connective tissue. During development, the primitive mesenchymal cells retract, become round in shape and undergo rapid mitotic division, forming clusters of vacuolated cells. The undifferentiated mesenchyme surrounding these islands develops into fibroblasts and forms confining sheets of cells called the perichondrium.

Chondroblasts

Chondroblasts are the precursors of cartilage and are derived from the differentiation of mesenchyme. They secrete cartilage matrix. They have a high glycogen and lipid content, with a basophilic cytoplasm and lots of rough endoplasmic reticulum, which is necessary to maintain active synthesis of the extracellular matrix.

Proliferation of metabolically active chondroblasts within the matrix results in the deposition and growth of cartilage. As they lay down cartilaginous matrix, chondroblasts become less metabolically active, turning into chondrocytes.

Chondrocytes

Chondrocytes are mature cartilage cells occupying small cavities, or lacunae, within the matrix. Chondrocytes maintain the integrity of the matrix. They can be distinguished from chondroblasts on histological examination as their cells are smaller, they have a pale cytoplasm and a reduced Golgi complex (Fig. 4.2).

Perichondrial cells differentiate into chondroblasts and eventually become chondrocytes, growing inwards from the periphery, with the secreted cartilage matrix, rich in collagen, lying between the cells. The lacunae surrounding the chondroblasts and chondrocytes are rich in glycosaminoglycans.

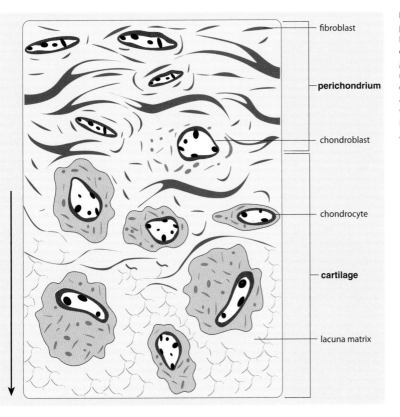

fibroblast

perichondrium

chondroblast

chondrocyte

cartilage

lacuna matrix

Fig. 4.2 Diagram of an area of perichondrium overlying hyaline cartilage. Perichondrial cells differentiate into chondroblasts, then chondrocytes, growing in from the periphery. Cartilage matrix lies between the cells; it is rich in collagen, apart from the lacunae, which are rich in glycosaminoglycans. (Adapted with permission from Junqueira LC. Basic histology, 8th edn. Stamford, CN: Appleton & Lange, 1995.)

Matrix

Cartilage matrix is firm and solid, but pliable and hence resilient. Its main constituent is glycosaminoglycan molecules. These have an important role in hydrating cartilage and making it resilient to compressive forces. The major glycosaminoglycans are hyaluronic acid, chondroitin sulphate and keratin sulphate, which are joined to a core protein called aggrecan to form a large proteoglycan. Cross-linking glycoproteins bind these proteoglycans to the collagen fibrils in the tissue.

Perichondrium

All hyaline cartilage, apart from articular cartilage, is covered by a layer of perichondrium. This is a dense connective tissue that is rich in type I collagen fibres, and it merges with the outer layer of extracellular cartilage matrix. It contains peripheral layers of spindle-shaped fibroblasts and an inner layer of chondroblasts.

Growth

Cartilage can increase in size by either interstitial or appositional growth.

Interstitial growth

Interstitial growth takes place in the middle of cartilage. As the chondroblasts proliferate they secrete extracellular matrix around them, resulting in the matrix growing and expanding outwards from around the cells. This is the main way in which cartilage grows.

Appositional growth

Appositional growth occurs when chondroblasts lying on the periphery of cartilage within the perichondrium differentiate and produce cartilage.

Blood supply

As mature cartilage is an avascular tissue, the exchange of metabolites between chondrocytes and surrounding tissue occurs by diffusion through the matrix.

In sites where cartilage is particularly thick, e.g. costal cartilage, small blood vessels are carried into the centre of the tissue by cartilage canals.

Poor blood supply to cartilage:

- Limits the extent of its thickness, as the innermost cells need to be maintained
- Makes repair after injury difficult. Although minor injury to cartilage can stimulate reparative appositional growth, damage usually results in injured areas being replaced by fibrous tissue.

Cauliflower ear is a complication of injury to the cartilage in the ear, commonly occurring from a blow to the side of the head. A blood clot forms under the perichondrium, separating the underlying cartilage from it and depriving it of nutrients so that it dies. The outer ear becomes permanently swollen and deformed. It is common among rugby players, boxers and wrestlers.

Cartilage types

Cartilage type depends on the composition of its matrix components. Three types of cartilage occur: hyaline, elastic and fibrocartilage.

Hyaline cartilage

Hyaline is the most common type of cartilage. Type II collagen fibres are orientated along lines of stress.

Throughout childhood and adolescence, hyaline cartilage is present in the epiphyseal plates of long bones. It has a great resistance to wear and covers the surface of nearly all synovial joints, areas that are subjected to a great deal of mechanical stress.

Elastic cartilage

Elastic cartilage is structurally arranged in a similar way to hyaline cartilage. It contains large numbers of elastic fibres and elastic lamellae embedded in matrix, giving it the properties of resilience and recoil. It is found in the auricle of the ear, the external auditory meatus, the auditory tube and the epiglottis.

Fibrocartilage

Fibrocartilage consists mostly of type I collagen fibres embedded in a fibrocollagenous support matrix. It is found in discs within joints, e.g. the temporomandibular, sternoclavicular and knee joints, and also on the articular surfaces of the clavicle and the mandible.

Costochondritis, or Tietze's syndrome, is an inflammation of the costal cartilage that connects each rib to the sternum, producing pain that is reproducible on palpation of the affected area. Occasionally, swelling can be apparent. The cause is not clear, although it can result from physical strain or minor injury. It is considered benign and resolves spontaneously within 6–8 weeks.

Bone

Bone is another form of specialized tissue that functions to provide mechanical support, allow movement, provide protection, and store mineral salts as part of the body's mechanisms that maintain metabolic homoeostasis. It is composed of:

- Support cells (osteoprogenitor cells, osteoblasts, osteoclasts and osteocytes)
- A non-mineral matrix of osteoid
- Inorganic minerals stored within the matrix.

It undergoes constant remodelling throughout life.

> Just like skin, bone can be surgically harvested from a donor site and grafted to fill a defect elsewhere. This is commonly used for dental implants.

Anatomy of bone

Long bone

Long bone comprises a shaft called the diaphysis, each end of which is expanded into an epiphysis (Fig. 4.3). The diaphysis contains a large central medullary cavity surrounded by a thick-walled tube of compact bone. A small amount of cancellous bone lines the inner surface of the compact bone, forming a network of trabeculae.

In adults, the medullary cavity is filled with yellow (inactive) marrow, which is mostly adipose tissue; red (active) marrow is confined to the proximal epiphyses of larger adult long bones.

The epiphyses consist mainly of cancellous bone and have a thin outer shell of compact bone. The articulating surfaces are covered with a layer of hyaline cartilage.

In growing bone, the site of elongation is known as the epiphyseal cartilage (growth plate). When bone stops growing, the epiphyseal growth plate becomes ossified and forms the epiphyseal line.

The metaphysis, the flared epiphyseal end of the diaphysis, is very vascular.

Long bone is covered by periosteum and lined by endosteum.

Short, flat and irregular bone

Short, flat and irregular bone is composed of compact bone surrounding cancellous bone.

Microstructure of bone

Bone is supported by specialized cells embedded in the extracellular matrix, namely:

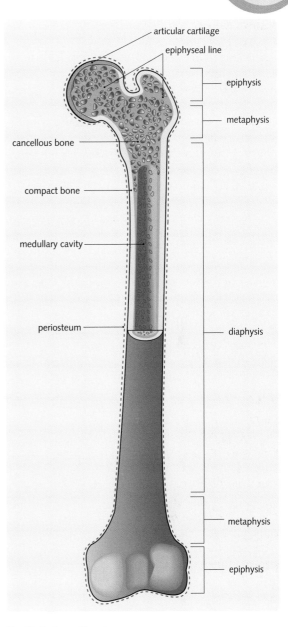

Fig. 4.3 Features of long bone.

- Osteoprogenitor cells
- Osteoblasts
- Osteocytes
- Osteoclasts.

Bone cells

Osteoprogenitor cells   These are stem cells derived from mesenchyme, committed to differentiate into the specialized bone support cells called osteoblasts. They are large, numerous, and actively convert into osteoblasts in actively growing bone, e.g. in the fetus or during the process of fracture repair. They are flat and dormant in mature bone, applied closely to the surface of the bone.

Osteoblasts Osteoblasts lie on the inner periosteum and the endosteum. They secrete an organic bone matrix and help to process the deposit of mineral salts into it. After they have completed their burst of activity they convert into osteocytes. Active, protein-secreting osteoblasts have a large Golgi complex, plenty of rough endoplasmic reticulum and a basophilic cytoplasm. Resting (inactive) osteoblasts are smaller, flattened and have a paler cytoplasm.

Osteocytes Osteocytes are applied to the surface of inactive bone. However, some become embedded in the bone matrix they have produced and come to lie in small cavities called lacunae. Each has many processes, which run along canaliculi, both to receive nutrients and connect with other cells via gap junctions. The function of osteocytes is unknown, although each maintains the narrow area of osteoid that surrounds it. They retain less rough endoplasmic reticulum and a smaller Golgi complex than osteoblasts, which suggests that they maintain the organic matrix. When the cells die, the lacunae remain empty and the matrix is resorbed.

Osteoclasts Osteoclasts are large, multinucleated cells with many branched processes. They are derived from blood monocytes. Osteoclasts resorb bone and are found in troughs, called Howship's lacunae, attached to the surfaces where bone is being eroded. Cells in the process of active resorption have a pale, acidophilic cytoplasm and many vacuoles and lysosomes for enzymatic digestion. They also have a ruffled border of cytoplasmic protrusions facing the bone matrix, interlacing into the osteoid matrix and providing a suitable environment of low pH for the lysosomal enzymes.

Bone matrix

Bone matrix has an organic component (osteoid), responsible for flexible strength, and an inorganic component of minerals, responsible for rigidity and mechanical strength.

Osteoid is a functional support tissue composed of type I collagen embedded in a glycosaminoglycan gel with specific glycoproteins such as osteonectin, osteopontin and osteocalcin, which strongly bind calcium.

The inorganic matrix is composed of deposited mineral salts, which make up around two-thirds of the weight of dried matrix. The most abundant minerals in the inorganic matrix are calcium and phosphate. These form hydroxyapatite crystals $(Ca_{10}(PO_4)_6(OH)_2)$, the surface ions of which are hydrated to facilitate the exchange of water between the mineral crystals and body fluids. Bicarbonate, citrate, potassium and sodium are also found, but in smaller quantities.

Periosteum

Periosteum covers the outer surface of bone. Its outer layer contains blood vessels, nerves and lymphatics, and its inner layer a few osteoblasts and osteoclasts.

Sharpey's fibres penetrate into the outer layer of bone to attach the periosteum to ligaments and tendons, holding them in place.

The enthesis is the site of insertion of ligaments and tendons, and of the articular capsule. Inflammation of an enthesis is called enthesitis. Rheumatoid arthritis commonly begins at the enthesis by producing enthesitis.

Endosteum

Endosteum is a single layer of tissue containing osteoblasts and osteoclasts. It lies between the cortical bone plate and the outer surfaces of the bone trabeculae, as well as lining the inside of the haversian canals.

Blood supply and lymph drainage of bone

Several arteries provide bone with a rich blood supply, entering it by penetrating the periosteum (Fig. 4.4). These blood vessels include periosteal arteries, which enter the bone shaft at many points, running in tunnels called Volkmann's canals that connect neighbouring Haversian canals, to supply the compact bone.

At the midshaft of the bone, nutrient arteries branch from those in the Volkmann's canals, passing through the compact bone to supply the cancellous bone and the marrow beneath. Metaphyseal and epiphyseal arterial branches supply the ends of the bone.

The arteries are accompanied by nerves and veins. The veins are large and numerous both in long bone and in areas of red bone marrow. They exit through vascular foramina near the articular ends of bones.

Lymph vessels are most abundant in the periosteum. They drain into the regional lymph nodes.

Nerve supply of bone

Many nerve fibres travel with the blood vessels to bone. They are mostly vasomotor, i.e. causing constriction or dilatation of blood vessels.

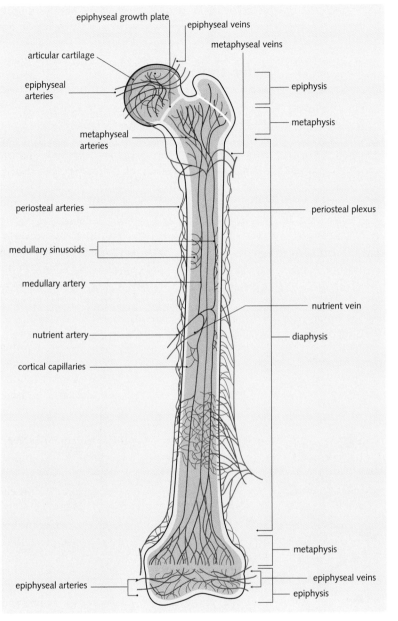

Fig. 4.4 Blood supply of bone. The periosteal, epiphyseal and nutrient arteries supply the bone.

Labels on figure:
epiphyseal growth plate
epiphyseal veins
metaphyseal veins
articular cartilage
epiphyseal arteries
epiphysis
metaphysis
metaphyseal arteries
periosteal arteries
periosteal plexus
medullary sinusoids
medullary artery
nutrient vein
nutrient artery
diaphysis
cortical capillaries
metaphysis
epiphyseal arteries
epiphyseal veins
epiphysis

Periosteal nerves are sensory and contain pain fibres. They are sensitive to tearing or tension.

Classification of bone

There are two patterns of bone, depending on the pattern of collagen deposited:

- Immature or woven bone
- Mature or lamellar bone.

Immature (woven) bone

An irregular array of coarse collagen fibres and a low mineral content make immature (woven) bone mechanically weak. Immature bone is produced in situations when osteoid is produced rapidly, such as when a fracture is being repaired, and during embryonic development of the skeleton, and is gradually remodelled and replaced by lamellar bone.

Mature (lamellar) bone

In mature (lamellar) bone, collagen fibres appear in a regular parallel arrangement and have a highly organized infrastructure, which makes the bone mechanically strong (Fig. 4.5).

Lamellar bone may be formed either as compact or cancellous bone.

Compact bone This forms a rigid outer shell with hard outer and inner circumferential layers, between which lie parallel neurovascular canals called Haversian canals, which run the length of the bone, supported by interstitial lamellar bone. Each canal is made of concentric layers of osteocytes fixed in the matrix in cavities called lacunae. The units of lamellae and canals together are known as haversian systems or osteons. The vertical haversian canals communicate directly with each other, with the endosteum, and with the periosteum via transverse Volkmann's canals.

Cancellous bone This consists of lamellae that together form lattices called trabeculae. They are orientated along lines of stress, scaffolding the bone cavity to provide structural strength. Cancellous bone has greater metabolic activity, and so is more affected in conditions such as osteoporosis.

Bone shape

The functions of bone are defined largely according to its structure and shape, i.e. long, short, flat, irregular or sesamoid. Most bones share a similar architecture, with an outer layer of compact bone and an inner trabecular zone, with variations according to its function and design.

Long bone

Long bone is longer than it is wide. Most of the bones in the appendicular skeleton are long bones. The ends and the central core of long bones are composed of cancellous (spongy) bone surrounded by concentric layers of compact bone. Their shafts contain a bony network along stress-bearing lines and surround cavities filled with bone marrow. The articular surfaces are covered by hyaline (articular) cartilage.

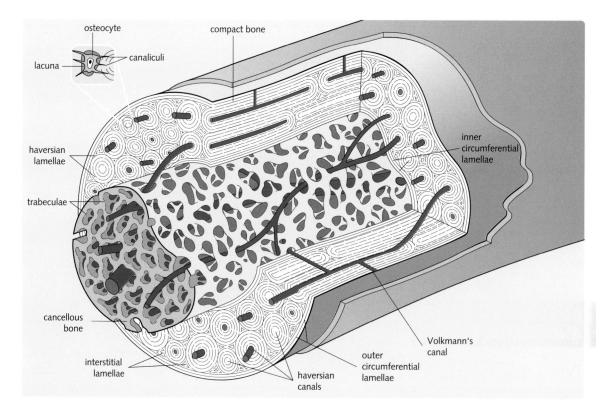

Fig. 4.5 Arrangement of mature bone.

Short bone

Short bone is similar in length and width and roughly cuboidal or round in shape. Such bones are found in the wrist and midfoot. Short bone is composed of cancellous bone surrounded by a thin layer of compact bone, and is covered by periosteum. Hyaline cartilage covers the articulating surfaces.

Flat bone

Flat bone is usually thin, flat and curved. It is found in the vault of the skull, ribs, sternum and scapula. It consists of thin inner and outer layers of compact bone separated by a layer of cancellous bone called the diploë.

Irregular bone

Irregular bone does not fit into any of the previous groups. Vertebrae and the sphenoid bones are examples of this type. Irregular bone is composed of cancellous bone with a covering of thin compact bone.

Sesamoid bone

Sesamoids are small bones found in some tendons, where they rub over bony surfaces. Tendons such as quadriceps femoris and flexor pollicis brevis contain the patella and the sesamoid bones, respectively. Most of a sesamoid bone is buried in the tendon; the free surface is covered with cartilage. Sesamoid bone reduces friction on the tendon, and may also alter its direction of pull.

> The scaphoid bone in the hand receives the majority of its blood supply interosseously from the distal through to the proximal pole. Fractures of the scaphoid predispose to avascular necrosis. This produces pain and swelling of the radial portion of the wrist after trauma, with reduced range of movement, pain on movement and reduced grip strength. Casting is sufficient in most cases, but surgical reduction and fixation are sometimes required.

BONE FORMATION, GROWTH AND REMODELLING

Types of ossification

All bones are derived from mesenchyme, but develop through one of two mechanisms. Bone can develop directly from primitive mesenchymal cells, sheets of which act as bone-forming membranes (intramembranous ossification): examples of these are the skull bones and the clavicle. Alternatively, it can develop indirectly by converting a cartilage model into bone (endochondral ossification). This occurs in most human bones.

The two processes result in an identical bone microstructure—both compact and cancellous bone can develop from either mechanism.

After ossification, immature bone grows and is continuously remodelled by osteoclasts and osteoblasts until it is mature. This process continues throughout life in a homoeostatic fashion.

The development of bone is controlled by hormones: growth hormone, thyroid hormones and sex hormones.

Intramembranous ossification

Intramembranous ossification occurs between 'membranes' of condensed mesenchyme tissue. Ossification takes place from the centre outwards (Fig. 4.6).

Clusters of mesenchymal spindle cells differentiate into osteoprogenitor cells and osteoblasts at primary ossification centres. Osteoblasts secrete clusters of new bone matrix, becoming encapsulated in lacunae within it and transforming into osteocytes. Surrounding mesenchymal tissue develops blood vessels and haemopoietic bone marrow which penetrate the islands of developing tissue. The new bone matrix is further remodelled by osteoclasts and osteoblasts to produce flat sheets of bone.

Intramembranous ossification results in the production of flat bones, such as those in the skull, and the development of some of the cortical bone.

As bone formation progresses, there is fusion of adjacent centres of ossification to form immature bone with a woven appearance.

Endochondral ossification

Endochondral ossification is the process of forming new bone from cartilage models that are formed prenatally in the developing fetus.

Chondroblasts develop in the immature mesenchyme (Fig. 4.7A), producing hyaline cartilage that is roughly modelled into the shape of the required bone (Fig. 4.7B).

Osteoprogenitor cells, osteoblasts and chondroblasts surround the midshaft of the diaphysis of this model, creating a periosteum and a mineralized collar of bone by the process of intramembranous ossification.

Fig. 4.6 Intramembranous ossification. Some mesenchymal cells differentiate into osteoblasts within the primary ossification centre. The islands of bone formed within the mesenchyme that will eventually become bone marrow are known as spicules. (Adapted with permission from Junqueira LC. Basic histology, 8th edn. Stamford, CN: Appleton & Lange, 1995.)

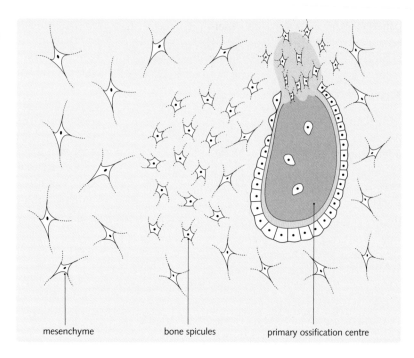

mesenchyme   bone spicules   primary ossification centre

Calcium begins to be deposited in the cartilage matrix (Fig. 4.7C).

Blood vessels grow from the periosteum and the bone collar, penetrating the bone to transport osteoprogenitor cells into the middle of the diaphysis. These cells differentiate to create a primary ossification centre (Fig. 4.7D).

The osteoblasts form lamellar trabecular bone on the calcified cartilage model, in a growth process that spreads from the centre outwards. The outer bone collar becomes cortical bone (Fig. 4.7E). All of this occurs before birth in the developing fetus.

After birth, blood vessels penetrate the club-shaped epiphyses at the ends of each bone, transporting

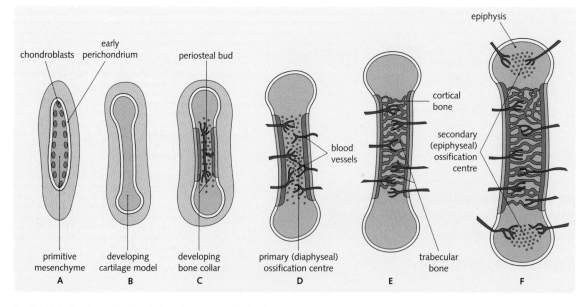

Fig. 4.7 Endochondral ossification. Parts A–F are explained in the text.

osteoprogenitor cells into them to establish secondary ossification centres (Fig. 4.7F). This occurs at different times/ages in different bones.

Bone growth
Endochondral growth
Activity at the secondary ossification centre establishes a cartilaginous zone at the junction between the epiphysis and the diaphysis, with the secondary ossification centre on the outer (epiphyseal) side and the developing inner (diaphyseal) trabecular bone on the other. This is called an epiphyseal growth plate (Fig. 4.8A). The actively proliferating cartilage results in the apposition of cartilage to the ends of the diaphyses, which is converted to trabecular bone in a series of steps:

- From the resting zone on the epiphyseal side of the growth plate, cartilage proliferates, producing columns of chondrocytes embedded in matrix
- The chondrocytes enlarge and hypertrophy, and produce alkaline phosphatase to induce calcification of the matrix
- Onto this, osteoblasts begin adding osteoid, and ossification begins
- The deposited trabecular bone is remodelled and incorporated into the diaphysis.

At the growth plate, the diaphysis lengthens. The plate also expands outwards, facilitating an increase in width as well as length. Growth continues throughout childhood, until growth activity stops and the plate fuses, forming an epiphyseal line that is detectable on plain radiographs. Fusion of the epiphyses occurs at around 25 years of age.

In addition to forming a growth plate, the secondary ossification centre produces a surround of cartilage that becomes the outer articular cartilage.

Appositional growth
Appositional growth involves bone formation on the outer surface of bone, contributed to by the periosteum. In long bone this results in an increase in width, whereas in short, flat and irregular bone there is an increase in general size.

Factors affecting growth
Factors that have an influence on bone growth include:

- Genetic influences, which determine bone shape and size
- Environmental factors, such as adequate diet and absorption of nutrients such as vitamins D and C, which affect the formation of the organic and inorganic components of bone matrix. Health and happiness are also very important factors during childhood growth

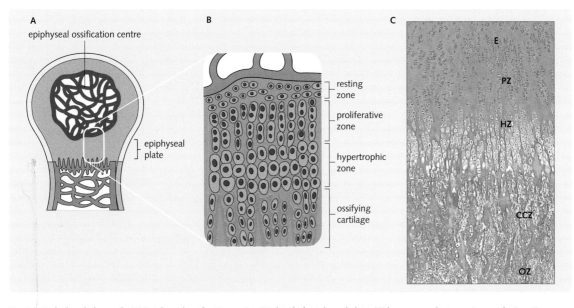

Fig. 4.8 Endochondral growth. (A) Epiphyseal ossification centre; (B) detail of epiphyseal plate; (C) low-power electron micrograph. E, resting zone of the epiphyseal plate cartilage; PZ, proliferative zone; HZ, hypertrophic zone; CCZ, calcified cartilage zone; OZ, beginning of the ossification zone. (Courtesy of Dr A Stevens and Professor J Lowe.)

- Hormones: growth hormone, thyroid hormones, sex hormones and glucocorticoids usually stimulate bone growth, and also cause fusion of the epiphyseal plates to stop bone growth.

Bone remodelling

Bone remodelling consists of a balance between:

- Deposition and mineralization by osteoblasts
- Resorption by osteoclasts (Fig. 4.9).

The level of remodelling is determined by:

- Mechanical stresses applied to bone, creating an increase in demand for mechanical strength, for example increased levels of physical activity
- The requirements of fracture repair.

In addition, osteoclasts can be influenced independently by hormones involved in maintaining metabolic homoeostasis.

BONE AND METABOLIC HOMOEOSTASIS

Maintenance of calcium levels

Calcium homeostasis depends on:

- Systemic calcium balance through absorption (intake) and excretion (output) at the kidney or gastrointestinal tract

- Distribution of calcium between extracellular fluid (ECF) and bone, with calcium mobilized from bones when blood calcium levels are low, and stored when levels are raised.

In health, the skeleton contains 99% of the body's calcium. It maintains the levels of calcium in the blood within narrow limits to ensure a constant, stable level so that effective muscle contraction and membrane potential activity can occur.

Normally, calcium levels in blood and tissues are stable and there is a continuous interchange of calcium between the blood and bone (Fig. 4.10).

When levels of calcium in the blood decrease, calcium is mobilized from bones. Conversely, excess levels of calcium in the blood can be removed and stored in bone.

One mechanism by which blood calcium levels are regulated is the active transfer of calcium ions, first from hydroxyapatite crystals to interstitial fluid, and then into blood. This takes place in cancellous bone. It occurs rapidly, helped by the large surface area of the hydroxyapatite crystals.

Two major hormones involved in calcium homoeostasis are parathyroid hormone and vitamin D, with calcitonin playing a more limited role (Fig. 4.11). (Refer to *Crash Course: Endocrine and reproductive systems* for more details of hormones.)

Fig. 4.9 Osteoclastic resorption in bone remodelling. (Adapted with permission from Junqueira LC. Basic histology, 8th edn. Stamford, CN: Appleton & Lange, 1995.)

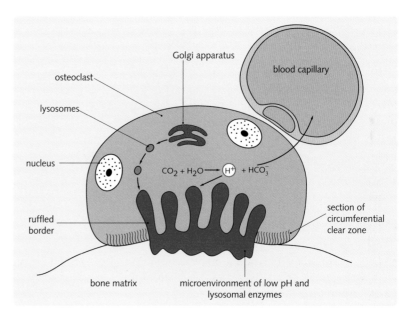

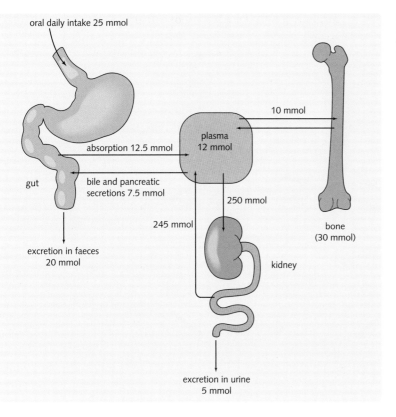

Fig. 4.10 Daily calcium exchange in the body tissues. A continuous exchange of calcium between blood and bone takes place to keep calcium levels stable.

oral daily intake 25 mmol

10 mmol

plasma 12 mmol

absorption 12.5 mmol

bile and pancreatic secretions 7.5 mmol

gut

250 mmol

245 mmol

bone (30 mmol)

excretion in faeces 20 mmol

kidney

excretion in urine 5 mmol

Parathyroid hormone

Parathyroid hormone (PTH) is the main regulator of calcium levels in blood. It is responsible for restoring low blood calcium levels to normal (Fig. 4.11A).

- Low blood calcium levels stimulate PTH release
- Elevated blood calcium levels inhibit PTH release.

PTH is a peptide made of 84 amino acids. It is secreted from the parathyroid glands in response to low blood calcium levels, which the glands detect via plasma membrane calcium receptors.

Mechanism of action

PTH:

- Stimulates osteoclast activity, resulting in bone resorption with calcium and PO_4^{2-} released into the blood
- Directly increases renal reabsorption so that less calcium is lost in the urine
- Directly stimulates the formation of vitamin D in the kidneys. Vitamin D increases the absorption of calcium from the small intestine.

In hyperparathyroidism there is an excessive production of PTH, which results in demineralization of bone and elevated blood calcium levels. The excess calcium is eventually deposited at other sites, such as arterial walls and the kidneys.

Vitamin D

Small amounts of vitamin D occur in foods such as fish liver oil and egg yolks. Most, however, is produced in the epidermis from 7-dehydrocholesterol via a photolytic reaction mediated by the ultraviolet light that is present in sunlight (Fig. 4.12). This is metabolized into the active substrate 1,25-dihydroxyvitamin D_3 by two steps of hydroxylation, the first occurring in the liver and the second in the kidney. This most active form of vitamin D is called calcitriol. Vitamin D is responsible for maintaining calcium balance, acting to restore low calcium levels.

Mechanism of action

- Vitamin D primarily increases the absorption of calcium from the diet through the GI tract
- To a lesser extent it reduces renal calcium excretion.

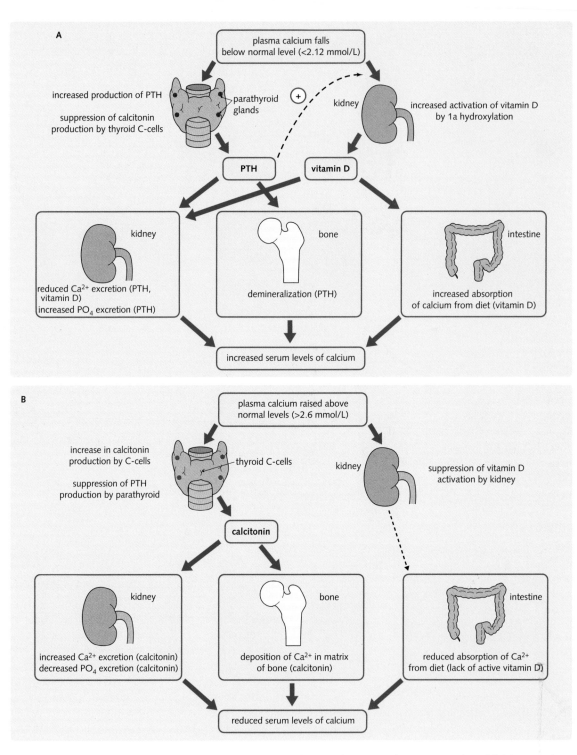

Fig. 4.11 Control of serum calcium levels by parathyroid hormone (PTH), calcitonin and vitamin D, where (A) serum calcium falls below normal levels; (B) serum calcium rises above normal levels. (Adapted with permission from Depopoulous A. Colour atlas of physiology. Stuttgart: Thieme, 1991.)

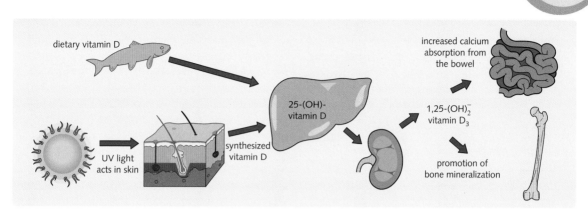

Fig. 4.12 Formation and actions of vitamin D.

The enzyme that catalyses renal hydroxylation of vitamin D is also stimulated by PTH. In this way, PTH secretion in response to low plasma calcium enhances the production of $1,25\text{-}(OH)_2$ vitamin D_3, with both hormones jointly contributing to the restoration of plasma calcium levels.

Vitamin D levels can be reduced by lack of exposure to sunlight and poor dietary intake, and this can lead to demineralization and poor calcification of bone. In adults this condition is called osteomalacia, whereas in children whose epiphyseal lines have yet to fuse it is known as rickets. Both conditions involve a loss of bone density, large epiphyses and bowing of the legs.

Calcitonin

Calcitonin is a peptide hormone comprising 32 amino acids and secreted from the parafollicular cells of the thyroid gland in response to high plasma calcium levels. It is responsible for reducing high blood calcium levels to normal (Fig 11.4B).

Mechanism of action

- Calcitonin inhibits osteoclast activity and so opposes the action of PTH.
- It decreases calcium and phosphate reabsorption in the kidney.

Other factors

Nutrition

During growth, bone is sensitive to nutritional factors. For bone and matrix formation to occur, the diet needs to contain adequate amounts of proteins, calcium, and vitamins D and C.

Vitamin C

Vitamin C is found in many fresh fruit and vegetables. It is essential for the synthesis of collagen by osteoblasts in the bone matrix. It is a reducing agent, required for the hydroxylation of collagen residues, to allow calcification to occur.

A deficiency of vitamin C results in scurvy. The defective connective tissue leads to sore, spongy gums, loose teeth, fragile blood vessels, swollen joints and anaemia. There is also interference with bone growth and slowed tissue repair.

Hormonal influences on bone growth

Growth hormone

Growth hormone is a peptide hormone released from the anterior pituitary gland and regulated by growth hormone-releasing hormone and the inhibiting hormone somatostatin.

Mechanism of action

Growth hormone increases bone growth:

- Directly: by stimulating prechondrocytes at the growth plate to develop into chondrocytes
- Indirectly: as these chondrocytes then secrete insulin-like growth factor (IGF)-1, which stimulates the chondrocytes to divide and produce cartilage.

Growth hormone also stimulates appositional bone growth and general tissue growth.

During the growing years, too much growth hormone results in an abnormal increase in the length of the long bones, causing gigantism. Adults with elevated growth hormone levels develop acromegaly. In acromegaly, the epiphyseal plates have closed, so the bones cannot grow longer and therefore become wider. This causes disfiguring bone thickening, along with overgrowth of other organs.

A lack of growth hormone gives rise to pituitary dwarfism.

Sex hormones

Sex hormones influence the time at which the ossification centres develop, and stimulate closure of the epiphyses.

Sex hormones initially stimulate bone growth by stimulating the secretion of growth hormone, normally during puberty, when their production is increased. This accounts for the growth spurts seen at this time. However, they also stimulate closure of the epiphyseal plates, so that growth stops. Oestrogens cause faster ossification of the epiphyseal plates than does testosterone, which is why girls stop growing earlier than boys and are normally shorter than boys.

Precocious sexual development caused by hormone-secreting tumours or iatrogenic administration of sex hormones tends to retard growth by causing early epiphyseal closure, whereas deficiencies of sex hormones caused by abnormal gonadal development tend to delay epiphyseal closure, prolonging the growth phase and resulting in tall stature.

> In precocious puberty, although the growth spurt initially produces tall stature, it ultimately leads to reduced height in relation to peers. As pubertal growth begins earlier, it also ceases earlier, producing fusion of the epiphyseal growth plates at an earlier age and reduced height. Treatment is aimed at suppressing pituitary production with gonadotrophin-releasing hormone agonists.

A low oestrogen level gives rise to osteoporosis, which is commonly found in postmenopausal women. In osteoporosis, although bone morphology is normal there is a net decrease in bone mass, caused by less bone formation and more resorption.

Thyroid hormones

Thyroid hormones regulate gene expression, metabolism, and the general development of all tissues.

Triiodothyronine (T_3) and tetraiodothyronine (T_4; thyroxine) are peptide hormones released by the follicular cells of the thyroid gland. They are regulated by thyroid-stimulating hormone (TSH), which is released from the anterior pituitary gland. They are required for the synthesis of growth hormone and for its subsequent growth-promoting effects during growth and development. In the fetus they play a principal role in the development of the central nervous system.

If thyroid hormone deficiency is undetected in the neonate it can lead to mental retardation (cretinism). A hypothyroid state in infants and children can cause growth delay, as bone growth is slowed, resulting in dwarfism. Thyroid hormone levels are one of several tests performed on babies around 7 days after birth in the Guthrie 'heel-prick' test.

Haemopoiesis in bone

Haemopoiesis is the formation of mature blood cells from precursor cells. In humans, haemopoiesis occurs in the medullary cavities of bone.

Red bone marrow is actively haematopoietic, whereas yellow bone marrow (former red marrow) has become filled with adipocytes and is therefore inactive. When stress is applied to the haematopoietic system, yellow bone marrow can revert to red marrow.

Location of haemopoiesis

In humans, haemopoiesis takes place in various sites according to the stage of development.

In the embryo, primitive blood cells arise in the yolk sac within 4 weeks of conception.

At 6 weeks' gestation, the embryonic liver becomes the major site of haemopoiesis. The spleen and lymph nodes also show some activity.

Bone marrow starts to produce blood cells when bones form medullary cavities after 20 weeks' gestation; by birth, when all marrow is red, it is the only site to do so.

In children, the diaphyses of long bone—but not the epiphyses—show replacement of red marrow by yellow marrow.

In adults, haemopoiesis occurs only in certain bones, e.g. the vertebrae, sternum, ribs, clavicles, hip bones and upper femora, with some activity in the upper portions of the limbs (Fig. 4.13). However, all bone marrow retains some haematopoietic potential, and haematopoietic activity can reappear in critical situations, such as anaemia, resulting in extramedullary haemopoiesis.

The bone marrow receives its blood supply from vessels that supply cancellous bone. Nutrient arteries

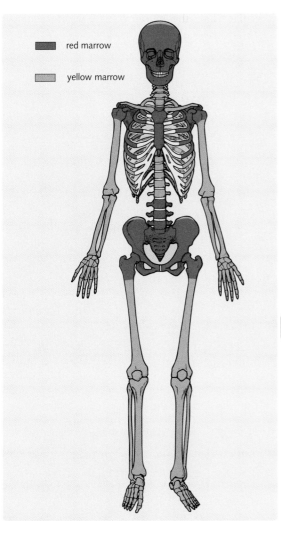

red marrow

yellow marrow

Fig. 4.13 Sites of haemopoiesis in an adult. (Adapted with permission from Seeley RR, Stephens TD, Tate P. Anatomy and physiology, 3rd edn. Chicago: Mosby Year Book, 1995.)

enter the midshaft of bone through the periosteum and pass through compact bone to reach the medullary space.

Response of bone to stress

Within limits, bone is a labile tissue that is capable of remodelling its internal structure according to different stresses (Fig. 4.14). The two main mechanical stresses on bone are those from:

- The pull of skeletal muscles
- The pull of gravity.

In response to mechanical stress, the increased deposition of mineral salts and production of collagen fibres make the bone stronger. In sites that are frequently stressed, bone is thicker, develops heavier prominences, and the trabeculae are rearranged (Fig. 4.15). Stress also increases the production of calcitonin, which inhibits bone resorption.

The bones of athletes, which are repeatedly subjected to high stresses, are notably thicker than those of non-athletes. Weightbearing activities, such as walking, help build and retain bone mass.

The removal of mechanical stress results in weakening of the bone. Bone is unable to remodel normally, as resorption outstrips bone formation, resulting in demineralization and collagen reduction.

People who are bedridden or wear a cast lose strength in their unstressed bones. Astronauts subjected to the weightlessness of space also lose bone mass. In these situations bone loss can be as much as 1% per week.

DISORDERS OF BONE

Genetic abnormalities

Osteogenesis imperfecta

Osteogenesis imperfecta, or brittle bone disease, is a group of disorders caused by genetic abnormalities that lead to abnormally fragile bones. There are several genetic subtypes, each with varying degrees of severity (Fig. 4.16). Most, however, are due to point mutations in the genes that encode type I collagen. The incidence of osteogenesis imperfecta is 1 in 20 000.

Pathology In osteogenesis imperfecta there is an abnormal synthesis of type I collagen, which makes up 90% of bone matrix. Some forms of the disorder are fatal in the perinatal period, whereas others are not but do predispose to repeated fractures on minor trauma.

Morphology Osteopenia (decreased bone) occurs in osteogenesis imperfecta, with thinning of the cortex and trabeculae.

Other features As type I collagen is a component of many of the tissues of the body, osteogenesis imperfecta has a wide range of systemic manifestations, including a blue uveal pigment that can be seen through thin sclerae, deafness and dental abnormalities. The prognosis is variable and depends on the severity of the disease.

Osteopetrosis

Osteopetrosis, also known as Albers–Schönberg or marble bone disease, is a very rare clinical syndrome

Fig. 4.14 Factors affecting bone remodelling in response to stress. $1,25(OH)_2D_3$,1,25-dihydroxyvitamin D_3; PGE_2, prostaglandin E_2; PTH, parathyroid hormone. (Adapted with permission from Laycock J, Wise P. Essential endocrinology. Oxford: Oxford University Press, 1996.)

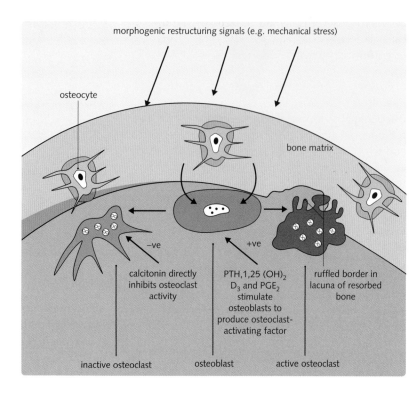

morphogenic restructuring signals (e.g. mechanical stress)

osteocyte

bone matrix

−ve   +ve

calcitonin directly inhibits osteoclast activity

PTH,1,25 (OH)$_2$ D$_3$ and PGE$_2$ stimulate osteoblasts to produce osteoclast-activating factor

ruffled border in lacuna of resorbed bone

inactive osteoclast   osteoblast   active osteoclast

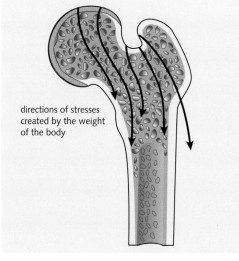

directions of stresses created by the weight of the body

Fig. 4.15 Orientation of trabeculae along lines of stress. (Adapted with permission from Seeley RR, Stephens TD, Tate P. Anatomy and physiology, 3rd edn. Chicago: Mosby Year Book, 1995.)

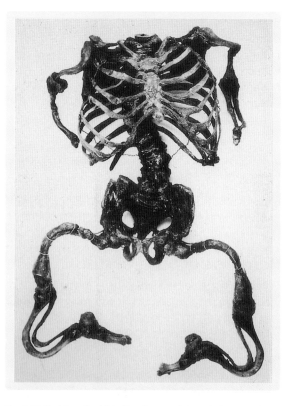

Fig. 4.16 Skeleton of a child with osteogenesis imperfecta congenita. Note the deformed limbs, scoliosis, and chest and pelvic deformities. (Courtesy of Dr PG Bullough and Dr VJ. Vigorita.)

of varying severity characterized by failure of osteoclasts to resorb bone (Fig. 4.17). If the condition is autosomal recessive it presents from birth as anaemia and leukocytopenia. Adult types predispose to fractures and infection.

Pathology Osteopetrosis is caused by failure of osteoclast function, with consequent impaired bone remodelling and resorption. There is overgrowth and sclerosis of bone with marked thickening of the cortex, producing skeletal fragility and a tendency to fracture. Medullary cavities can narrow and are filled with defective osseous tissue, inhibiting haemopoiesis.

Clinical features Infantile osteopetrosis tends to present with nasal stuffiness owing to the failure of the mastoid and paranasal sinuses to develop. Other features include skeletal fragility, anaemia and immune deficiencies arising from haematopoietic insufficiency, delayed tooth eruption, growth impairment and nerve entrapment syndromes.

Presentation, clinical features and prognosis depend on the mode of inheritance. In the severe autosomal recessive form there is failure to thrive, recurrent infection, anaemia, thrombocytopenia, hypocalcaemia and mental retardation, for which the prognosis is poor. In the less severe autosomal dominant form there may only be changes in radiography detectable, presenting during childhood with fractures.

Management A bone marrow transplant can cure the disorder.

Bone marrow transplants involve transplantation of haematopoietic stem cells. They can be autologous, using stem cells isolated from the patient, or allogeneic, where stem cells are harvested from a donor and transplanted into the patient. Allogeneic stem cell donors must have a human leukocyte antigen that matches that of the recipient, otherwise graft-versus-host disease will develop and the graft will be rejected.

Achondroplasia

Achondroplasia is also known as dwarfism. It is a disorder inherited in an autosomal dominant manner that displays complete penetrance, although around 50% of cases are caused by new mutations. The incidence of achondroplasia is 1 in 25 000.

Homozygotes die soon after birth, whereas heterozygotes have a normal lifespan and normal mental, sexual and reproductive development.

Pathology In achondroplasia there is derangement of endochondral ossification.

Clinical features Achondroplastic heterozygotes have short stature due to marked shortening of the limbs, although there is a normal-sized trunk. The skull is enlarged and there is a big forehead with frontal bossing and depression of the nasal bridge. Occasionally there is hydrocephalus and short, broad hands. The epiphyses are abnormally wide (appositional growth is unaffected).

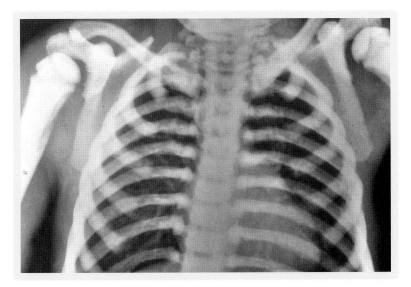

Fig. 4.17 Radiograph of the upper body of a child with osteopetrosis, showing a marked increase in the density of all bones. (Courtesy of Dr PG Bullough and Dr VJ Vigorita.)

Sufferers can develop a marked lumbar kyphosis, recurrent otitis media and neurodevelopmental delay.

Malformations Occasionally, malformations of the skeletal bones occur. These result from either:

- Failure of formation
- Extra bones (in fingers and toes)
- Fusion of bones (skull sutures).

Generally these malformations are of no consequence, although cosmetic correction is possible if the patient wishes.

INFECTIONS AND TRAUMA

Osteomyelitis

Osteomyelitis is a common problem. It is an infection of the metaphyses of long bones. It can be caused by any bacterial agent, especially in people who are immunosuppressed (Fig. 4.18). The incidence of the disease is higher in areas with poor hygiene and living standards. In two-thirds of cases it occurs in the:

- Distal femur
- Proximal tibia.

Pyogenic osteomyelitis

Causes Most infections are caused by *Staphylococcus aureus*. Other causative agents include *Streptococcus spp.* and *Haemophilus influenzae*.

In immunocompromised people and intravenous (IV) drug users, pyogenic osteomyelitis can be caused by *Staphylococcus aureus*, *Escherichia coli*, *Klebsiella* spp., *Pseudomonas* spp., *Salmonellae* spp., *Haemophilus influenzae* and *Streptococcus* spp.

In neonates, common causative agents are encountered during passage through the birth canal, i.e. group B streptococcus and *Escherichia coli*.

The differential diagnosis should include *Mycobacterium tuberculosis*.

Spread This is usually haematogenous (i.e. due to pathogens being transported in the blood). It can also occur directly from infected wounds, open fractures or surgery.

> Often in osteomyelitis no primary site of infection is found. However, it most commonly affects bone with a rich, diverse blood supply, in particular the long bone metaphyses of the distal femur, the upper tibia and the humerus, as well as the vertebral bodies.

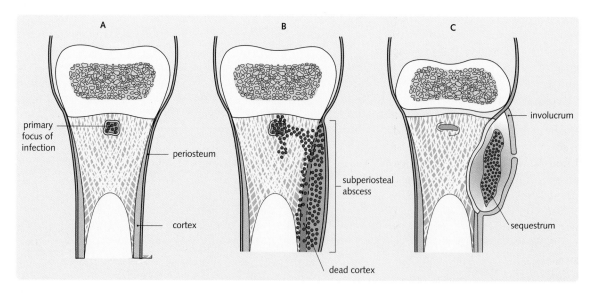

Fig. 4.18 Sequence of osteomyelitis. The primary focus of infection (A) has spread through the bone, causing the death of cortical bone and the formation of a subperiosteal abscess (B). Death of a segment of bone (sequestrum) occurs (C), and the area is surrounded by new subperiosteal bone (involucrum).

(Continued)

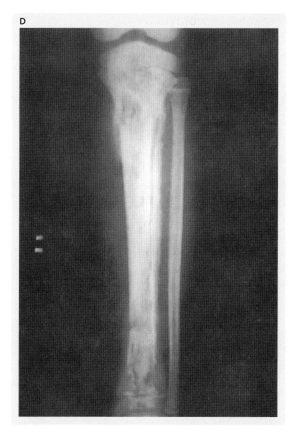

Fig. 4.18 cont'd (D). Plain x-ray showing osteomyelitis. This chronic case shows a periosteal reaction along the lateral shaft of the tibia and multiple hypodense areas within the metaphyseal region (Courtesy of Dr T. Lissauer).

Histology   In adults, cancellous (spongy) bone is usually affected. The focus of infection starts initially around small vessels in the metaphysis, where the good blood supply encourages bacterial growth and enables spread to other areas. Cortex erosion can occur, creating holes (cloacae) through which pus can channel, lifting the periosteum and causing the original bone to necrose and die (sequestrum). A sheath of new subperiosteal bone formed by the lifted periosteum creates an involucrum. A lytic area surrounded by a zone of reactive new bone can eventually be seen on radiographs.

Infection of bone leads to a progression through ischaemic necrosis, fibrosis and bony repair. There may be formation of sinus tracts (these are sometimes sterile).

Clinical features   These include acute bone pain and fever. The skin is swollen, red, tender and warm directly over the site of infection, with swelling of the nearest joint.

Other features depend on the site of infection, e.g. there is back pain when there is vertebral involvement. Infection can occasionally occur at multiple sites.

Signs are more marked in children, who present with a painful, immobile limb and an acute, febrile illness.

Complications   Short-term complications can occur locally or systemically. Local complications include fractures and abscesses, called Brodie's abscesses, forming in the sinus tracts. These become surrounded by sclerotic bone, giving a halo effect on MRI scans.

Pus may discharge into adjacent joint spaces. Alternatively, the joint capsule may insert distally to the growth plate, e.g. the hip. In these instances, septic arthritis can develop.

Systemic complications include septicaemia and endocarditis.

Long-term complications can include an alteration in growth rate and deformity.

Investigations   When osteomyelitis is suspected, blood cultures should be taken, as these are positive in 60% of cases. White cell count, erythrocyte sedimentation rate (ESR) and the acute-phase protein C-reactive protein (CRP) are raised. Pus cultures should be sought—e.g. bone aspiration, discharging sinus—in order to determine the organism and its antibiotic sensitivity.

X-rays are normal for the initial 7–10 days but after this features become visible; these include haziness and loss of bone density around the affected area. Later, new subperiosteal bone formation, sequestrum and involucrum can be identified. Ultrasound can be considered at presentation as it can show periosteal elevation.

MRI is sensitive to the pathological changes that occur in the disease.

Management   Antibiotic treatment is critical to the management of osteomyelitis. If the diagnosis is suspected, IV broad-spectrum antibiotics against the most likely causative organisms must be started immediately and cultures sought. Antibiotics that achieve high concentrations in bone should be used, such as fusidic acid. Once the causative organism and its antibiotic sensitivity are identified from appropriate tissue or pus samples, the antibiotics can be adjusted accordingly. Intravenous antibiotics should be given until there is clinical recovery and normal acute-phase proteins (usually around 2 weeks). Treatment can then be changed to an oral course, usually for a further 4 weeks. Surgical drainage may be required if there is no immediate response to IV treatment, the patient is immunocompromised, or it is an atypical case.

Management of a Brodie's abscess requires drainage of the abscess and a 6-week course of antibiotics.

Surgery should only be undertaken if there is dead bone present, which acts as a nidus of infection and may lead to recurrence.

Tuberculosis of bone

Tuberculosis of bone (tuberculous osteomyelitis) is a complication of tuberculosis infection. It is relatively uncommon in people who are immunocompetent. About 2% of all cases of tuberculosis have bone involvement, and the incidence is increasing.

Spread Tuberculous osteomyelitis is spread from primary sources of infection, either haematogenously or from nearby lymph nodes. It is more destructive and resistant to control than pyogenic osteomyelitis caused by other organisms.

It commonly occurs in long bones. When it occurs in the thoracic and lumbar vertebrae it is called Pott's disease.

Clinical features Tuberculous osteomyelitis is usually a chronic condition with involvement of a single bone (except in patients with AIDS). Chronic infection causes remitting episodes of pain, fever and sinus formation. Signs of bone infection may be present, such as swelling, local pain, 'cold abscess' formation and joint effusion. Signs of joint infection include pain, swelling, pain on movement and muscle wasting. Systemic signs of the disease include weight loss, malaise, fever and lethargy.

Complications Tuberculous osteomyelitis can cause fractures and nerve compression. Involvement of the joint space can lead to septic arthritis.

Investigations Plain radiographs show thick irregular bone with periostitic changes, cysts and bone rarefaction. Later in the infection loss of joint space, erosions and bony alkylosis is visible.

Pus can be aspirated and will be positive on culture and Ziehl–Nielsen stain.

Management Prompt, rigorous treatment aims to prevent chronic osteomyelitis developing. The management of tuberculous osteomyelitis is both medical and surgical. Surgical excision of tuberculous cavities is required, together with a prolonged course of antibiotics. Combination chemotherapy with rifampicin, isoniazid and pyrazinamide is administered for an initial 6 months

under the guidance of infectious disease specialists, after which time the regimen is tapered to the patient's response.

If the spine is involved, prolonged bed rest, administration of a plaster cast to prevent deformity, and surgical stabilization may be required. Where joints have been destroyed by the infection arthrodesis may be required.

Fractures

Fractures can be described in a number of ways.

Types There are several types of bone fracture:

- Simple (clean break)
- Comminuted (more than one bone fragment)
- Compound (breaks through overlying skin)
- Stress (small linear fragments)
- Pathological (bones weakened by disease, e.g. osteoporosis, bony metastases, Paget's disease of bone)
- Impacted (crush) fracture (affects cancellous bone, caused by compression forces)
- Avulsion (a piece of bone is detached by a tendon/ligament due to traction force).

They can be described according to the way in which the bone is fractured, which can be identified on radiographs. They can be:

- Transverse
- Oblique
- Spiral.

The bone can also be identified as being:

- Dislocated
- Subluxed (partial loss of contact of the joint surfaces).

Causes Fractures are usually caused by trauma, which can be substantial or repeated minor forces. Trivial forces produce pathological fracture in diseased bone.

Clinical features These include pain, tenderness, swelling, deformity and loss of function.

Healing Healing of fractures requires immobilization of approximated bone ends and good alignment. Where joints are involved, open reduction and internal fixation are required to allow immediate movement, otherwise secondary osteoarthritis will invariably occur. Comminuted fractures require external fixation with screws inserted into the bone to realign and stabilize the fractured pieces to optimize healing, e.g. with an Ilizarov frame.

Delayed or imperfect healing   Delayed or imperfect healing of fractures can be caused by malalignment, movement during healing, poor blood supply and soft tissue interposition in the fracture gap. These can occur in the elderly, those in poor general health, and in people who are immunosuppressed.

Histology of healing   Healing of a fracture follows a sequence (Fig. 4.19). The histological changes that take place during healing include:

- Development of a haematoma, which forms a soft procallus (Fig. 4.19A)

- Conversion of the procallus to a fibrocartilaginous callus (Fig. 4.19B)
- Replacement of fibrocartilaginous callus to an osseous callus consisting of trabecular lamellar bone (Figs 4.19C and D)
- Remodelling along weightbearing lines by osteoclasts (Fig. 4.19E).

Complications   In the short-term, localized complications include internal or external bleeding, and injury to nerves, skin or blood vessels. After the event, localized skin necrosis, gangrene and infection can

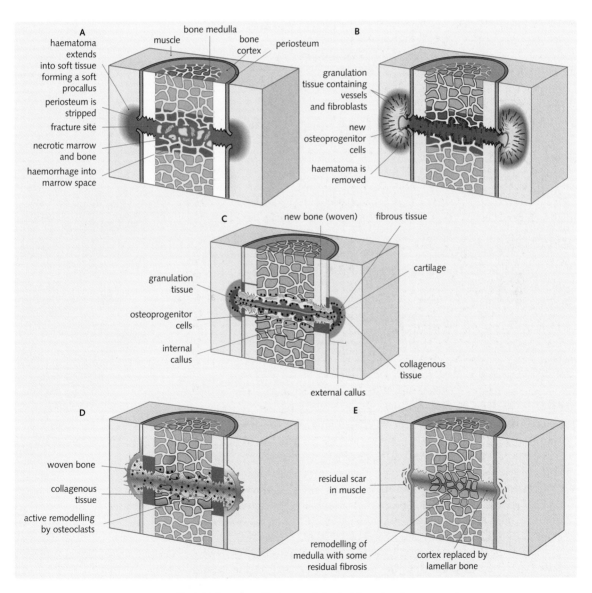

Fig. 4.19 Sequence of fracture repair. See text for explanation.

occur, and treatment should aim to minimize the chance of this. Systemic complications include generalized venous thrombosis and pulmonary embolus. Serious complications requiring vigorous management include crush or compartment syndromes and fat embolus.

In the long term, if the patient may suffer from wound infection (particularly internal fixation was required), failure to fixate, joint stiffness, contractures and malunion. There may be patchy osteoporosis and psychological problems in mobilizing.

Management Immediate management involves stabilizing the patient. Look for signs of shock and correct/stop any bleeding. Appropriate pain relief should be administered.

Individual management of fractures depends on the age and expectations of the patient, the pathology present, and the patient's personal requirements in terms of occupation, etc. The basic principles of fracture management are:

- Immobilization and reduction of bone fragments in their previous anatomical position—external or internal fixation may be necessary to achieve this, depending on the type of injury and fracture
- Maintenance of reduction until the fractured bone reunites; by a plaster cast, a brace and/or traction
- Encouraging the healing of the fracture and surrounding tissues, minimizing complications by optimizing conditions, e.g. wound sterility and hygiene, especially with open wounds. Educate on the effects of smoking on wound healing, Antibiotics should be administered and a tetanus booster to prevent infection
- Rehabilitation, including early mobilization of adjacent joints to prevent stiffness and wasting.

Avascular necrosis

Pathology Avascular necrosis involves the death of bone and marrow without infection, and is caused by a poor blood supply. It is most commonly seen in the hip (head of femur), scapula, scaphoid bone and the knee, occurring when fractures deprive adjacent areas of their blood supply (Fig. 4.20). Medullary infarctions affect cancellous bone and bone marrow, with cortical sparing. Subchondral infarctions lead to wedge-shaped areas of damage.

Causes Avascular necrosis can be idiopathic or occur secondary to local or systemic predisposing conditions.

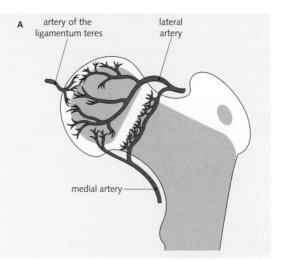

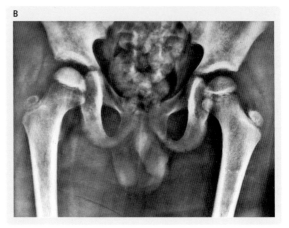

Fig. 4.20 Avascular necrosis of the femoral head (Perthes' disease). (A) Normal blood supply; (B) radiograph of the (patient's) left femoral head showing widened joint space, cessation of growth of the bony epiphyses and increased growth of cartilage. (Courtesy of Dr PG Bullough and Dr VJ Vigorita.)

Important local causes include trauma (e.g. fractured neck of femur), as well as rheumatoid arthritis, psoriatic arthropathy or septic arthritis, and in neuropathic joints.

Systemic causes include sickle-cell disease, systemic lupus erythematosus (SLE), thromboembolism, large-scale burns, diabetes, polycythaemia and corticosteroid therapy.

Idiopathic osteonecrosis of the femoral head in children occurring before skeletal maturity is called Perthes' disease.

Histology Dead bone is identified by empty lacunae surrounded by necrotic adipocytes. The adipocytes may rupture to release fatty acids, which bind calcium and form deposits. There is osteoclastic resorption of trabeculae and the articular cartilage is distorted.

Clinical features   There is pain and immobility.

Management   Medical management is unable to arrest the progression of avascular necrosis. Appropriate analgesia should be given to control pain, and patients should be advised to avoid using the affected bone, e.g. where the neck of femur is affected avoid weightbearing and use crutches. In early disease, surgical decompression and bone grafting may be required. In late stages, where bone collapse, deformity or secondary osteoarthritis has occurred, arthroplasty may be performed.

METABOLIC DISEASES OF BONE

Osteoporosis

Osteoporosis is a disease that results in abnormally decreased bone mass affecting all components of bone. It is relatively common, with a prevalence of 5%, becoming more common with increasing age, especially in postmenopausal women. It has a female to male ratio of 4:1. Osteoporosis causes major social and economic problems.

Classification   Osteoporosis can be localized to one bone or generalized, affecting many bones. It can occur secondary to conditions that interfere with bone metabolism, such as endocrine abnormalities, gut malabsorption and neoplasia.

Aetiology   Risk factors for osteoporosis are those that cause a decrease in peak bone mass or those that cause increased bone loss. Possible causes of osteoporosis include decreased exercise, oestrogen deficiency, lack of calcium and vitamin D, hyperadrenocorticism, hypogonadism, thyrotoxicosis, hypopituitarism, pregnancy, immobilization, diabetes, and long-term heparin administration.

Histology   In osteoporosis there is thinning of the bone cortex, the trabeculae are attenuated, and there are wide haversian canals (Fig. 4.21). There is increased osteoclastic resorption, with slowed bone formation. The main sites affected are the vertebrae, femoral necks, wrists and pelvis. In the spine there may be disc herniation and nerve root compression.

Clinical features   Symptoms commonly arise due to fractures, which occur most commonly at three sites: thoracolumbar vertebrae, neck of femur and distal radius (Colles' fracture).

Fractures cause bone pain and can cause loss of height and deformities such as dowager's hump, lumbar hyperlordosis and kyphoscoliosis, where there is vertebral collapse.

A dual emission X-ray absorptiometry (DEXA) scan is the gold standard of diagnosis—these measure the bone density of the lumbar spine and proximal femur. A 30% loss of bone mass is required before radiographs show osteoporosis. Radiography will detect fractures and osteopenia. Serum biochemistry does not reveal

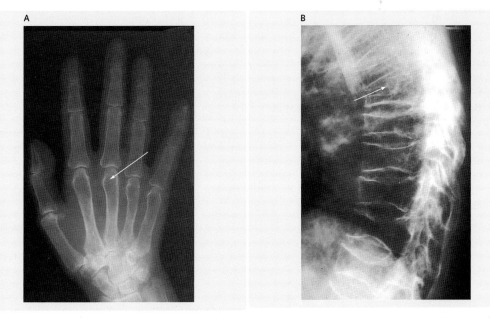

Fig. 4.21 Features of osteoporosis. (A) Loss of cortical thickening and reduction of trabeculae in the hand; (B) wedge-shaped flattening of vertebral bodies leading to loss of height;

(Continued)

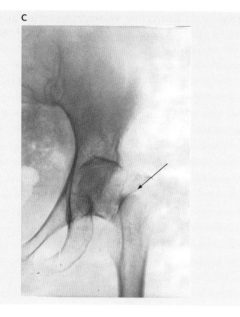

Fig. 4.21 cont'd (C) fracture of the neck of the femur in an elderly person. (Courtesy of Dr PG Bullough and Dr VJ Vigorita.)

any significant abnormality: calcium, phosphate and alkaline phosphatase levels are normal.

Complications

- Increased mortality (especially in the first year following hip fractures)
- Chronic pain and deformity
- Limited mobility and loss of independence.

Management Primarily, the patient should be counselled on lifestyle factors that can increase the rate of disease progression, such as smoking, alcohol and immobility, and the importance of avoiding them, as well as the benefits of staying physically active. They should be given dietary advice, in addition to calcium and vitamin D supplements where these are required. The rapid bone loss in postmenopausal women may be countered to some extent by hormone replacement therapy (HRT). However, the UK's Committee on Safety of Medicines no longer advises prescribing HRT as prophylaxis for osteoporosis in women over 50 years of age. Bisphosphonates inhibit osteoclast action and increase bone density. They may be given orally or intravenously.

Rickets and osteomalacia

These diseases are caused by either vitamin D deficiency or phosphate depletion, the latter being less common. Rickets occurs in growing children, and osteomalacia occurs in adults whose growth plates have closed.

Aetiology Vitamin D deficiency can be caused by low dietary intake, insufficient exposure to sunlight, malabsorption (e.g. coeliac disease, small bowel resection), or deranged liver or kidney metabolism.

Phosphate depletion can be caused by renal disease that disrupts vitamin D activation, liver failure, X-linked phosphataemia, neoplasia, or poisoning from heavy metals. Anticonvulsant therapy can cause an increase in vitamin D inactivation by inducing those liver enzymes that break down the vitamin D precursor.

Pathology Rickets and osteomalacia arise from a failure of bone mineralization, which leads to softer and wider channels of matrix. Excess unmineralized matrix and underdeveloped epiphyseal cartilage calcification leads to endochondral bone that is deranged and overgrown.

Clinical features Rickets presents with bowing of the legs and a 'knocked-kneed' appearance, overgrowth of costochondral junctions (forming a 'rachitic rosary'), widened epiphyses and either a flattened ('bossed') square skull or craniotabes (the skull snaps back into shape after being pressed in). Children presenting with rickets are systemically ill (Fig. 4.22).

Osteomalacia presents with muscle and bone pain, spontaneous incomplete fractures ('Looser's zones') in long bones and the pelvis (especially the neck of femur), and a proximal myopathy that causes a waddling gait and Gower's sign.

Investigations Bone biopsy is definitive for the diagnosis of rickets or osteomalacia, revealing an increased proportion of non-mineralized bone.

Serum biochemistry reveals low phosphate, low/low-normal calcium and raised alkaline phosphatase. Serum 25-hydroxyvitamin D is usually low.

In osteomalacia, radiography reveals defective mineralization and a loss of cortical bone. There may be apparent partial fractures without displacement (Looser's zones).

In rickets, radiography reveals cupped, ragged metaphyseal surfaces.

Management Treatment involves monitored prescription of oral vitamin D therapy to regulate bone formation, the dose and formulation being dependent on the cause of the condition.

Vitamin D therapy can cause dangerous hypercalcaemia, so plasma calcium should be closely

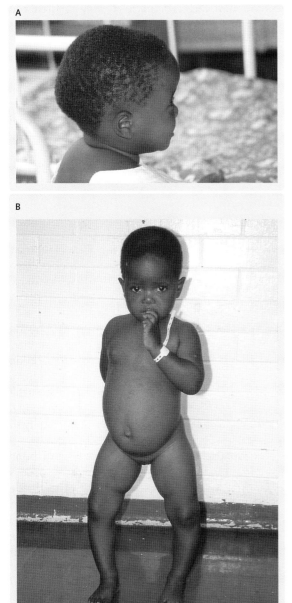

monitored. Corrective osteotomies may also be required if the deformities are severe and established.

Signs of hypercalcaemia commonly feature in clinical examinations. They include muscle weakness, lethargy, confusion, polyuria and dehydration. Common causes include bone malignancy, e.g. metastases and hyperparathyroidism. Less common causes include thyrotoxicosis and sarcoidosis. Severe hypercalcaemia can be extremely dangerous as it causes gross dehydration from polyuria. Management requires rehydration and intravenous bisphosphonates to reduce the loss of bone calcium.

Hyperparathyroidism

Classification   Hyperparathyroidism can be classified as:

- Primary—caused by a lesion of the parathyroid gland, usually an adenoma, rarely a carcinoma, which increases PTH and thus raises calcium levels. It is the most common cause of hypercalcaemia. It affects 0.1% of the population
- Secondary—a physiological response to hypocalcaemia, e.g. renal failure, vitamin D deficiency
- Tertiary—the result of the development of autonomous hyperplasia in the parathyroid glands, which occurs in chronic secondary hyperparathyroidism, most commonly in renal disease. There is a raised plasma calcium and PTH. Treatment requires parathyroidectomy.

Pathology   Increased PTH levels cause an increase in osteoclast activity that leads to increased bone resorption. The net effect is raised plasma calcium and low plasma phosphate.

Histology   In hyperparathyroidism, demineralization leads to increased osteoclast activity and resorption. There is characteristic peritrabecular fibrosis, called osteitis fibrosa, and more marked fibrosis and cyst formation within the marrow (osteitis fibrosa cystica or von Recklinghausen's disease of the bone). 'Brown tumours' of osteoclasts, fibrosis and haemorrhage

Fig. 4.22 Rickets and osteomalacia. (A) Skull 'bossing' in rickets; (B) lateral and forward bowing of legs in rickets; (C) radiograph showing pseudofractures (Looser's zones) in the forearm in osteomalacia. (A and B courtesy of Dr S Taylor and Dr A Raffles; C courtesy of Dr PG Bullough and Dr VJ Vigorita.)

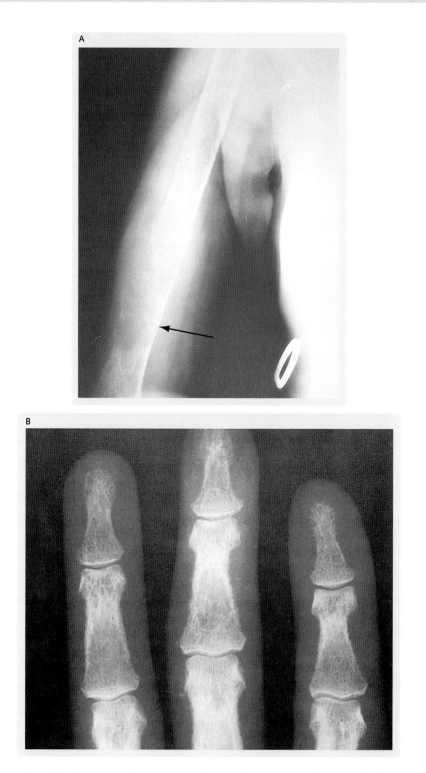

Fig. 4.23 Hyperparathyroidism. (A) Radiograph showing a large destructive lesion (brown tumour) in the lower half of the humerus. (Courtesy of Dr PG Bullough.) (B) Radiograph showing subperiosteal erosion of the cortical surfaces of the phalanges. (Courtesy of Dr PM Bouloux.)

are also seen (Fig. 4.23). These resemble giant-cell granulomas.

Clinical features   These are associated with raised calcium levels—thirst, anorexia, nocturia, dehydration and confusion; and the effects of elevated PTH on the skeleton—decreased mobility and joint stiffness.

Signs include raised blood pressure.

Investigations   Serum biochemistry reveals elevated calcium and alkaline phosphatase, and low phosphate levels (unless in renal failure). PTH is usually elevated.

Radiography will show subperiosteal reabsorption, especially in the hand, where the phalanges show 'moth-eaten' erosions (Fig. 4.23B), and in the skull, where it produces a pepper-pot effect. This bone damage can be reversed by treating the cause of the elevated PTH.

Management   With primary and tertiary hyper-parathyroidism, if symptoms are mild or the patient is asymptomatic, with a mild elevation of calcium (between 2.65 and 3 mmol/L), surgery is not required. Where surgery is required, removal of the affected gland (parathyroidectomy) can be performed. In secondary hyperparathyroidism, a subtotal parathyroidectomy is performed, which involves removal of three and a half of the four glands. Surgical risks include inducing hypocalcaemia if too much gland tissue is removed, so plasma calcium levels should be monitored for 2 weeks or more. There is also a surgical risk of damage to the recurrent laryngeal nerve owing to its proximity to the thyroid and parathyroid glands.

Renal osteodystrophy

Renal osteodystrophy is a bone disease that results from poor mineralization due to chronic renal failure.

Pathology   Renal osteodystrophy is caused by:

- Inadequate renal tissue for making vitamin D, leading to osteomalacia
- High serum phosphate (in severe chronic renal failure; CRF), which results in hypocalcaemia and precipitates hyperparathyroidism, with subsequent bone resorption to release calcium stores
- Haemodialysis—those patients undergoing prolonged haemodialysis suffer from inhibition of calcification of the bone matrix, producing osteomalacia
- Steroid treatments, which may also induce osteoporosis or avascular necrosis.

Clinical features   The clinical picture is similar to that of osteomalacia and rickets, with low PTH and

hence low bone turnover. In severe CRF [glomerular filtration rate (GFR) < 25% of normal] the body can no longer compensate to increase phosphate excretion so phosphate levels rise, causing a decreased calcium level and a subsequent rise in PTH, enhancing bone resorption in order to release calcium. The elevated PTH causes fibrosis of the bone marrow (known as osteitis fibrosis cystica).

Failing kidneys cannot activate vitamin D and so calcium cannot be reabsorbed from the GI tract, further exacerbating the hypocalcaemia.

Osteosclerosis occurs and chronically there are metastatic calcifications in the skin, eyes, joints and arterial walls.

Management   This aims to normalize calcium and phosphate levels. The patient is advised to reduce dietary phosphate (e.g. milk, cheese, eggs) and is prescribed phosphate binders to be taken before meals, e.g. Calcichew, which stimulates faecal phosphate excretion. Where calcium levels are low, vitamin D analogues are prescribed, e.g. alfacalcidol and calcium supplements.

TUMOURS OF THE SKELETON

Metastatic tumours

Metastatic tumours of the skeleton are much more common than primary bone tumours, particularly in adults.

Metastases arising from the breast, lung, kidney and thyroid are lytic, whereas those from the prostate are sclerotic.

Cartilage-forming tumours

Chondroma and endochondroma

Cartilage-forming tumours are benign tumours composed of mature hyaline cartilage. Those within bone are called endochondromas and those on the surface are subperiosteal chondromas (Fig. 4.24).

Epidemiology   Males are more likely to develop cartilage-forming tumours than females—usually between 20 and 50 years of age.

Classification   There are two types of cartilage-forming tumour: solitary and multiple.

Multiple tumours involve non-familial types (endochromatosis or Ollier's disease) and familial types (Mafucci's syndrome). Familial types are associated with haemangiomas.

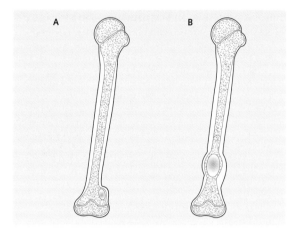

Fig. 4.24 Benign bone tumours. (A) Endochondroma and (B) chondroma.

Clinical features Features of cartilage-forming tumours include bone pain and fractures. The tumours consist of cartilage nests and arise at the epiphyses. There is a risk of chondrosarcoma in multiple lesions, especially if the condition is familial.

Management Many of these lesions do not require treatment. When needed, treatment consists of curettage of the cartilage tissue and the grafting of bone onto the subsequent defect.

Common sites of bony metastases include the thoracic and lumbar spine, the proximal femur and the proximal humerus. Patients often present with pathological fractures—breaks in the bone caused by minimal stress. Patients may also present with hypercalcaemia. All patients with back pain, especially that which is unremitting and frequently severe at night, must have a full systemic examination, including assessment of the most likely primary tumour sites, in particular the lung and the breast.

Osteosarcoma

Osteosarcomas are the most common type of primary bone tumour (Fig. 4.25A). They are composed of osteocytes and osteoid. Osteosarcomas are thought to be related to the retinoblastoma and p53 genes. They grow quickly. With combination therapy they have a 60% 5-year survival rate. Some histological

variants, such as juxtacortical and periosteal types, have a better prognosis.

Epidemiology Males are more likely to develop osteosarcomas than are females—usually up to 20 years of age, although the elderly with pre-existing bone tumours are also at risk.

Clinical features Osteosarcomas are found in the medullary cavity of metaphyses of long bones (especially near the knee) and, in the elderly, in flat bones. They produce bone pain, tenderness and swelling. Osteosarcomas are usually a complication of Paget's disease of bone. Radiographs show elevated periosteum (Codman's triangle) caused by new bone growth under the periosteum. There may be haematogenous spread to the lungs.

Management Over the past 25 years, new multidrug chemotherapy has been introduced and has led to a reduction in the mortality rate of patients with osteosarcomas. The adoption of aggressive surgical treatment has also led to an increase in survival; cure rates vary, but may reach up to 80%.

Miscellaneous tumours

Ewing's sarcoma

Ewing's sarcomas are aggressive malignant tumours of primitive neural differentiation (see Fig. 4.25B).

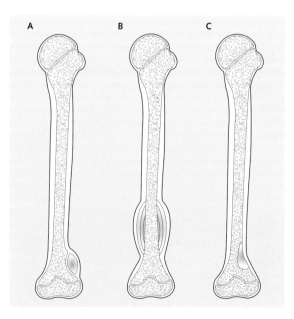

Fig. 4.25 Malignant bone tumours. (A) Osteosarcoma; (B) Ewing's sarcoma; (C) metastatic bone tumour.

These grey tumours contain small, round cells growing in sheets around blood vessels, and show focal necrosis and haemorrhage. However, they respond to drugs and have an overall 5-year survival of 60%. The tumour metastasizes to lungs and lymph nodes.

Epidemiology   Females are more likely to develop Ewing's sarcoma than are males—usually under 25 years of age. Ewing's sarcoma is very rare in Afro-Caribbean children.

Clinical features   Ewing's sarcoma presents as a soft-tissue mass—periosteal 'onion-skinning' is seen on radiographs. This is often followed by a 'moth-eaten' or mottled appearance of the bone, accompanied by the extension of the lesion into soft tissue.

Management   Management for Ewing's sarcoma is medical and surgical. Preoperatively, chemotherapy with vincristine, adriamycin and cyclophosphamide (VAC), and radiation is used. Following tumour resection, chemotherapy is used to reduce the chance of recurrence.

Giant-cell tumour

Giant-cell tumours, or osteoclastomas, are low-grade malignant tumours of giant multinucleate cells and stroma; 10% form metastases.

Epidemiology   Females are more likely than males to develop giant-cell tumours, usually between 20 and 40 years of age.

Clinical features   Radiographs of giant-cell tumours show large lytic 'soap-bubble' lesions with absent calcified spots. These can often be mistaken for the 'brown tumours' that occur in hyperparathyroidism. Giant-cell tumours are found at the metaphyses and epiphyses of long bones, especially the knees.

Management   Management depends on the history and the histological grading of the lesion. Recommended methods of removal include curettage

Treatment of bone pain caused by tumours is palliative. Bones at risk of fracture because of malignant pathology are often treated prophylactically by internal fixation, as the risk of fracture is substantial if more than one-third of the bone's width is destroyed by tumour lesions.

and bone grafting, and cryosurgery involving the use of liquid nitrogen to destroy residual tumour cells.

OTHER DISEASES OF BONE

Paget's disease of bone

Paget's disease of bone is a disease of disordered bone formation characterized by increased turnover and resorption. It commonly occurs in people over 40 years of age and its incidence increases with age. It affects males more than females. Paget's disease of bone is more common in temperate climates in Anglo-Saxon populations.

Classification   Paget's disease of bone affects either one bone (15%) or several (85%). Bones affected are the tibia, femur, ileum, vertebrae, humerus and skull (Fig. 4.26).

Causes   The cause of Paget's disease of bone is unknown, but may be due to infection of osteoclasts by paramyxovirus, measles virus or respiratory syncytial virus.

Pathology   Paget's disease of bone occurs in three phases:

- Initial osteolytic phase, when there is a huge increase in osteoclast activity
- Mixed osteoclast/osteoblast phase, when there is disordered activity as osteoblasts try to fill the erosions left by osteoclasts, producing a mosaic pattern of woven bone
- Osteosclerotic phase, when new sclerotic bone is produced.

Histology   In Paget's disease the new bone deposited is thick and haphazard, not constructed in an organized manner, making it more prone to fracture. There is intertrabecular fibrosis and a mosaic pattern of new bone, as the osteoid is very bulky and porous.

Clinical features   The disease may be asymptomatic or it may cause pain, with enlargement of the bones affected by the disease process, and pathological fractures. Deafness can develop as a result of nerve compression by bone overgrowth in the skull.

Investigations   Serum calcium and phosphate levels are normal. Serum alkaline phosphatase and calcium levels are raised; hydroxyproline is present in the urine.

Complications   Complications of Paget's disease of bone include secondary osteoarthritis and high-output heart failure caused by new blood vessels

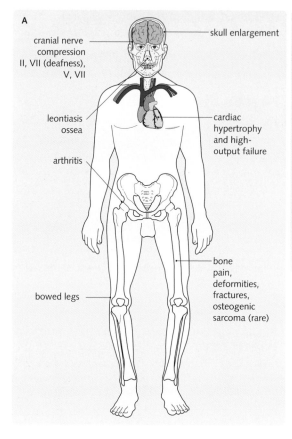

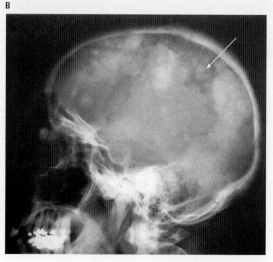

Fig. 4.26 Paget's disease of bone. (A) General features; (B) radiograph of skull in late stage showing patchy sclerosis and loss of diploic architecture. (Courtesy of Dr PG Bullough.)

forming shunts. Bone sarcoma can occur in around 10% of those suffering with Paget's for more than 10 years.

Management Treatment is required where the disease is symptomatic. Treatment aims to prevent fractures and nerve compression developing. Drugs to decrease bone turnover are used, such as IV pamidronate in 6-weekly cycles. Oral bisphosphonates can be given. Surgical correction of severe deformities is also sometimes performed. As bone heals poorly in this condition, intramedullary fixation devices are usually applied at the end of the operation.

Hypertrophic pulmonary osteoarthropathy

Hypertrophic pulmonary osteoarthropathy is an uncommon, idiopathic condition causing changes to bones and joints.

Pathology In hypertrophic pulmonary osteoarthropathy there is:

- New periosteal bone formation in the distal long bones, wrists, ankles and proximal phalanges
- Arthritis of adjacent joints
- Clubbing of digits.

Clinical features Hypertrophic pulmonary osteoarthropathy is associated with lung cancer or pleural mesothelioma, and there is usually an increased blood flow to the limbs.

Management Resection of the tumours usually leads to regression of the condition.

Joints and related structures

Objectives

By the end of this chapter you should be able to:

- Give a simple classification of all joints
- Describe the different types of joints, with examples
- Describe the structure and function of synovial joints
- Describe the blood and nerve supply and lymph drainage of joints
- Classify the arthropathies
- Differentiate between osteoarthritis and rheumatoid arthritis
- Understand the pathologies of important rheumatological conditions and how these produce features of the disease
- Have a good understanding of conditions that commonly affect the joints.

CLASSIFICATION OF JOINTS

Joints are classified into fibrous, cartilaginous or synovial, according to the type of tissue between the bones (Figs. 5.1–5.3).

Fibrous

Fibrous joints have fibrous tissue uniting the bones. This type of joint allows very little movement.

Cartilaginous

There are two types of cartilaginous joint, primary and secondary.

Primary cartilaginous

Primary cartilaginous joints unite two bones with a plate of hyaline cartilage. No movement is possible with this type of joint.

Secondary cartilaginous

Secondary cartilaginous joints unite two bones with a plate of fibrocartilage; there is also a thin layer of hyaline cartilage on the articular surfaces. A small amount of movement is possible with this type of joint.

Synovial

Synovial joints have a thin layer of hyaline cartilage on the articulating surfaces of the bones, which are separated by a joint cavity and covered by a joint capsule. The cells of the synovial membrane lining the capsule secrete a lubricating nutritive medium called synovial fluid. An extensive range of movement is possible with this type of joint.

There are several types of synovial joint, based on the shape of the articulating surfaces and the range of movements possible.

STRUCTURE AND FUNCTION OF JOINTS

The structure and function of joints are closely related. The range of movements available at a joint is related to its stability. This, in turn, depends on the shape, size and arrangement of the bones, and the flexibility of the ligaments and the tone of muscles around the joint.

Generally, the more stable a joint, the less movement it permits. If a joint is solid (no cavity), then it has limited mobility. If a cavity exists between the two ends of bone, movement can occur.

Fibrous and cartilaginous joints are both known as synarthroses, i.e. solid joints. Synovial joints are diarthroses, i.e. cavitated joints.

Fig. 5.1 Fibrous joint.

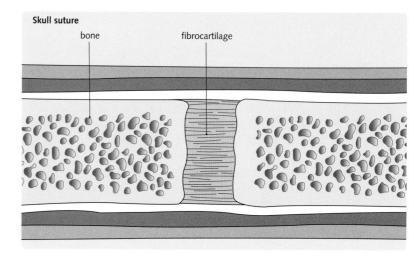

Fig. 5.2 Secondary cartilaginous joint.

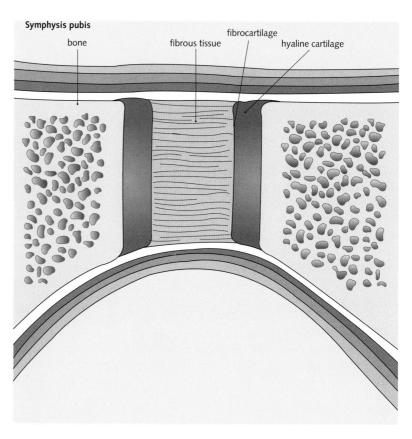

During pregnancy, hormones soften the ligaments of the body, allowing them to stretch so that the pelvis can accommodate the growing fetus and eventually facilitate the birth of the baby. Pregnant women should therefore be advised to avoid strenuous activities or overstretching, and to modify their physical activities.

Fibrous joints

Fibrous joints consist of two bones united by fibrous tissue. These types of joint have no cavity, and little or no movement is exhibited.

Fibrous joints are further classified into sutures, syndesmoses and gomphoses.

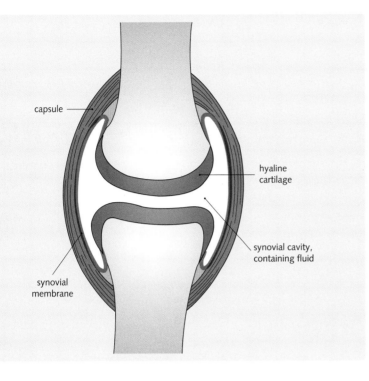

Fig. 5.3 Synovial joint.

capsule

hyaline cartilage

synovial cavity, containing fluid

synovial membrane

Sutures

Sutures are interdigitating bones held together by dense fibrous connective tissue. This type of joint occurs in the skull. The inner and outer layers of periosteum of the adjacent bones are continuous over the joint; these two layers and the fibrous tissue form the sutural ligament.

In newborn infants, the bone sutures are called fontanelles. The bones within the sutures undergo intramembranous ossification, forming a synostosis. In normal adults, this happens between the frontal bones. However, in old age there can be fusion between the coronal, sagittal and lambdoid sutures, and also in the sternum. This is of no clinical consequence.

Syndesmoses

Syndesmoses are where bones are separated by a larger distance than in sutures, and are joined by a sheet of fibrous tissue—either a ligament or a membrane. This type of joint occurs in the radioulnar interosseous membrane.

A small amount of movement may be achieved with syndesmoses. The degree of movement depends on the distance between the bones and the flexibility of the fibrous ligaments.

Gomphoses

Gomphoses are specialized joints that occur between teeth and their sockets, and the alveolar processes of the maxillae and mandible. Gomphoses are anchored by the fibrous tissue of the periodontal ligament.

Movement of a gomphosis is usually pathological, e.g. disease loosening a tooth.

Two important fontanelles to palpate for on a newborn baby are the anterior and posterior fontanelles. The posterior fontanelle is formed by the junction of the lambdoid and sagittal sutures and closes (or fuses) within 2 months of birth. The anterior fontanelle is formed by the junction of the coronal and sagittal sutures and fuses by 8 months.

Primary cartilaginous joints

Primary cartilaginous joints are also known as synchondroses. The bones are united by hyaline cartilage. They are found in the epiphyseal growth plate and costosternal joints. Synchondroses appear in the normal development of long bones, so most are temporary unions.

This type of joint is slightly moveable.

Secondary cartilaginous joints

Secondary cartilaginous joints are also known as symphyses. The bone-articulating surfaces are covered with hyaline cartilage and joined by fibrocartilage. They are found in the manubriosternal joint, symphysis pubis, intervertebral discs and the mandibular symphysis in the newborn.

This type of joint is slightly moveable and is strong.

Separation of the symphysis pubis can occur during pregnancy and is called diastasis symphysis pubis. It occurs as a result of increasing intra-abdominal pressure and the physiological softening of the pelvic ligaments. It can cause palpable pain over the symphysis pubis, worse on movement, and sometimes a clicking sound can be heard. It can be detected on ultrasound and usually improves with anti-inflammatory medication.

Synovial joints

Synovial joints are the most common joint in the skeleton and also the most functionally important (Fig. 5.4).

Fully formed synovial joints can be characterized by six features, namely:

- The articular surfaces of the bones involved are covered by a thin layer of hyaline cartilage
- Lubrication is by a viscous synovial fluid
- There is a joint cavity
- The cavity is lined by synovial membrane
- The joint is surrounded by a capsule
- The capsule is reinforced externally or internally (or both) by fibrous ligaments.

Synovial joints are classified according to the shape of the articular surfaces of the bones involved and the movements that are possible.

The movements at synovial joints can be described as:

- Monoaxial, i.e. occur in one direction or plane
- Biaxial, i.e. occur in two directions or planes
- Multiaxial, i.e. occur in many directions or planes.

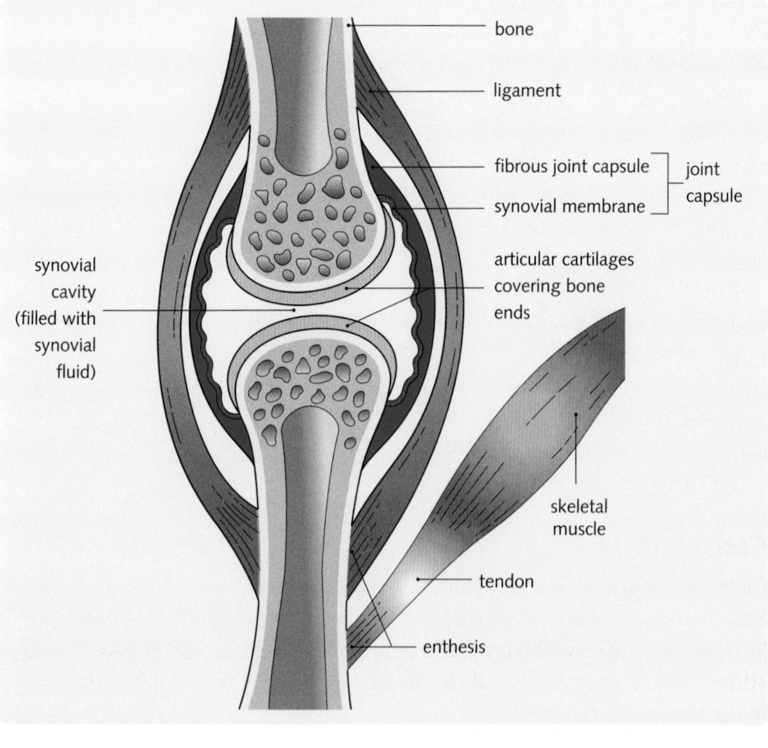

Fig. 5.4 Features of a synovial joint. The articular cartilages and fluid-filled synovial cavity prevent bone from rubbing against bone.

Plane joints

Plane joints are shaped like two flat surfaces (Fig. 5.5A). They allow a sliding movement, i.e. they are monoaxial.

Examples of plane joints are the sternoclavicular and acromioclavicular joints.

Hinge joints

Hinge joints have concave and convex surfaces (Fig. 5.5B). They allow flexion and extension movements, i.e. they are monoaxial.

Hinge joints are located in the elbow, knee and ankle.

Pivot joints

Pivot joints consist of a cylindrical projection inside a ring (Fig. 5.5C). They allow rotation movements, i.e. they are monoaxial.

Pivot joints are located in the atlantoaxial and superior radioulnar joints.

Saddle joints

Saddle joints have concave and convex surfaces that are saddle shaped (see Fig. 5.5D). They allow flexion, extension, abduction and rotation movements, i.e. they are biaxial.

The carpometacarpal joint of the thumb is a saddle joint.

Ball and socket joints

Ball and socket joints are shaped like a ball sitting in a dip or a socket (see Fig. 5.5E). They allow flexion, extension, abduction, and medial and lateral rotation movements, i.e. they are multiaxial.

Examples of the ball and socket joint is that located at the glenohumeral joint of the shoulder, and the hip joint.

Ellipsoid joints

Ellipsoid joints have ellipsoid concave and convex surfaces (Fig. 5.5F). They allow flexion, extension, abduction and adduction movements, but no rotation, i.e. they are biaxial.

Ellipsoid joints are located at the wrist.

Condyloid joints

Condyloid joints are shaped like two sets of concave and convex surfaces at right-angles to each other (Fig. 5.5G). They allow flexion, extension, abduction, adduction, and a small amount of rotation, i.e. biaxial movements.

Condyloid joints are located in the metacarpophalangeal (MCP) and metatarsophalangeal joints.

> The anterior fontanelle is usually soft, but can bulge or sink in certain conditions. It can bulge because of an increase in intracranial pressure, such as in hydrocephalus or meningitis, or when the baby is crying or vomiting. Sinking of the anterior fontanelle is a sign of dehydration.

BLOOD SUPPLY AND LYMPH DRAINAGE OF JOINTS

Periarticular arterial plexuses supply blood to the joints and branch into articular arteries. They pierce the joint capsule to reach the synovium, and communicate with one another to create rich anastomoses around and inside the joint.

Articular veins accompany the arteries, so they too are present in the joint capsule and synovial membrane.

Lymphatic vessels are present in the synovial membrane and drain along the blood vessels to the regional deep lymph nodes.

NERVE SUPPLY OF JOINTS

Joints are richly supplied with articular nerves whose endings are located in both the fibrous capsule and the synovial membrane. Articular nerves arise from the nerves supplying the overlying skin and the muscles that move a joint. This is known as Hilton's Law.

Both myelinated and non-myelinated nerve fibres are present in articular nerves. They have different endings that correspond to their roles in sensory input. The main types of input are proprioception and pain.

Myelinated nerves have Ruffini endings, lamellated corpuscles (rather like pacinian corpuscles), and some like Golgi neurotendinous organs. These provide information about the movement and position of the joint relative to the body. Non-myelinated and finely myelinated nerves have free endings, which are thought to mediate pain.

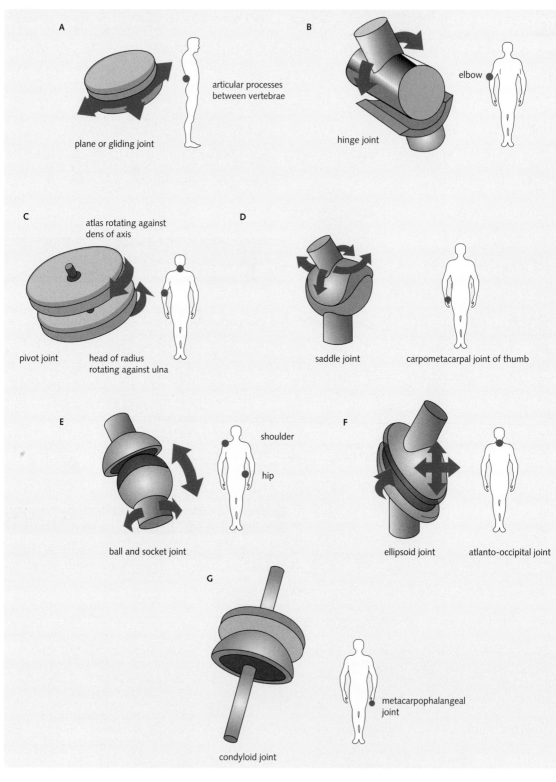

Fig. 5.5 Types of synovial joint. (A) Plane; (B) hinge; (C) pivot; (D) saddle; (E) ball and socket; (F) ellipsoid; (G) condyloid.

ARTHROPATHIES

Degenerative arthropathy

Osteoarthritis

Osteoarthritis is characterized by loss of the articular cartilage and the formation of new bone in an attempt at repair.

Epidemiology Osteoarthritis is the most common type of arthritis. It affects more than 20% of the population of the UK, and most people over the age of 65 will have some osteoarthritic changes on radiography. The true prevalence of symptomatic osteoarthritis is only 20%. It is twice as common in women as in men.

Osteoarthritis is particularly common in the elderly and usually presents around 50 years of age, although secondary osteoarthritis can develop earlier. Although it occurs worldwide, it is less common in black populations. The condition tends to run in families.

Aetiology Osteoarthritis can be either primary or secondary (idiopathic).

Osteoarthritis arising from no obvious cause is known as primary osteoarthritis. Predisposing factors include age (it is most common in the elderly), genetic factors, biomechanical factors, and systemic factors such as obesity. Some genes that encode for type II cartilage have been proposed as candidate genes for familial osteoarthritis.

Secondary osteoarthritis is less common than primary osteoarthritis and tends to affect younger people. Causes include congenital abnormalities, trauma, occupational hazards (e.g. the knee joint in footballers), avascular necrosis (e.g. sickle-cell disease) and other associated arthropathies or bone diseases.

There are several additional factors that predispose to osteoarthritis. These include family history, obesity, occupation (heavy physical work), age and hypermobility.

Pathology Osteoarthritis affects synovial joints, most commonly the distal interphalangeal (DIP) and thumb carpometacarpal joints in the hand, the metatarsophalangeal joints in the foot, the apophyseal joints of the spine, and weightbearing joints such as the hip and knee.

In the early stages of osteoarthritis there is a loss of balance between cartilage production and degradation, so there is destruction and loss of articular cartilage (Fig. 5.6). This involves:

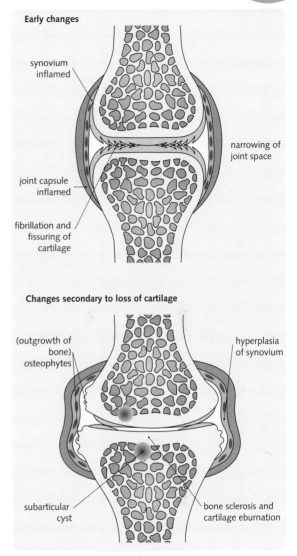

Early changes

synovium inflamed

joint capsule inflamed

fibrillation and fissuring of cartilage

narrowing of joint space

Changes secondary to loss of cartilage

(outgrowth of bone) osteophytes

hyperplasia of synovium

subarticular cyst

bone sclerosis and cartilage eburnation

Fig. 5.6 Pathological changes in osteoarthritis. Early changes and changes secondary to loss of cartilage.

- Focal breakdown of cartilage, caused by chondrocytes
- The loss of cartilage is variable, ranging from an irregular cartilage surface to full-thickness loss
- The inflammation of synovium and joint capsule due to the presence of debris from the cartilage.

In later stages, there are secondary changes in bone occurring as a result of cartilage destruction:

- Articulation of bone on bone due to loss of cartilage results in thickening and polishing (eburnation) of subarticular bone

- Cysts develop in the exposed, sclerotic subarticular bone
- Attempts to repair bone produce cartilaginous overgrowths at the joint margins, which eventually calcify to form osteophytes
- Synovial hyperplasia due to inflammation
- Development of deformity owing to loss of joint space
- Immobility of a joint.

Clinical features   Characteristic symptoms are joint pain, stiffness and joint swelling. It affects many joints.

Symptoms include:

- Intermittent or chronic pain at affected joints, which is worse upon exertion, e.g. at the end of the day
- Early-morning stiffness and pain, which only lasts for a few minutes (in contrast to inflammatory arthritis, in which stiffness lasts much longer)
- Joint tenderness and instability
- Loss of function, deformity and disability, e.g. hip, knee.

Joints are usually affected bilaterally although a unilateral pattern can occur. When only one joint is involved there may be a history of previous pathology at that specific joint, i.e. injury.

Signs include:

- Swelling and effusion of the affected joints due to osteophyte formation
- Joint deformities with crepitus upon movement and limited range of movement
- Muscular wasting due to limited use of a joint
- Bony swelling.

Complications   Osteoarthritis has the potential to cause disability as a consequence of pain and decreased mobility.

Management   Management aims to alleviate symptoms and minimize disability arising from clinical disease, rather than managing bone disease detected by radiological examination. The patient is educated about the disease and its progressive nature. Treatment is patient centred, encouraging lifestyle changes such as weight loss, and providing physiotherapy support with exercises to build strength and stability in the muscles that support the joints.

Medication to control pain can be given where required. Analgesics such as paracetamol are given before non-steroidal anti-inflammatory drugs (NSAIDs). Intra-articular corticosteroid injections can be used intermittently, as they appear to give short-term symptomatic improvement and reduce inflammation.

Surgery may be needed on certain joints that become severely diseased, for instance the hip and knee joints.

> Joint replacement carries many risks. As with most major surgery, a major risk is deep vein thrombosis (DVT), which occurs in over two-thirds of orthopaedic operations, although fatal pulmonary embolism occurs in only 0.1–0.2%. Prophylactic low-molecular-weight heparin is given to patients, with the first dose within 12 hours prior to surgery and then for 7–10 days afterwards. Contraindications include those with or at risk of uncontrolled bleeding, e.g. peptic ulcers.

Prognosis   Osteoarthritis is frequently a progressive disease— the affected joints slowly get worse and other joints also become involved.

Consider the joints affected by osteoarthritis.

Osteoarthritis of the wrist and hand

The joints of the hand are commonly affected by osteoarthritis, usually one at a time over the years. DIP joints are more involved than proximal interphalangeal (PIP) joints. The carpometacarpal joint of the thumb can be affected.

Clinical features   The onset of osteoarthritis in the wrist and hand is painful, causing tender, swollen, inflamed joints and impairment of function. The inflammation settles over months and years, leaving painless swellings (osteophytes) at the DIP joints (Heberden's nodes) and at the PIP joints (Bouchard's nodes). Bony swelling of the carpometacarpal (CMC) joint can develop, with fixed adduction and limited abduction of the thumb, creating a squared hand. In the long term, PIP joint involvement restricts gripping. CMC joint involvement can cause pain.

The wrists are usually affected at a later stage after trauma (lower radius or scaphoid fracture).

Osteoarthritic involvement is diagnosed on X-ray, showing marginal osteophytes and loss of joint space.

Osteoarthritis of the hip

Aetiology Osteoarthritis of the hip is a very common cause of disability, especially in the elderly. It may develop from general wear and tear, or as a consequence of acetabular injuries, Perthes' disease, coxa vara or slipped femoral epiphysis.

Pathology In osteoarthritis of the hip, the articular cartilage is worn away where stress is applied. The underlying bone becomes sclerotic and there is cyst formation; there is also synovial hypertrophy, capsular fibrosis and osteophytes in the joint margins. Pain occurs in the groin and may also radiate to the knee; this is made worse by walking and relieved by rest. All hip movements are limited.

Clinical features At the hip, internal rotation is the first movement to be affected; passive movements also become painful at the end of the range of movement. There is also frequently a fixed flexion deformity (detected by Thomas' test).

Joints are usually affected bilaterally and symmetrically, although a unilateral pattern may be seen.

Management Management of osteoarthritis of the hip depends on its severity. It is either conservative, i.e. analgesics and hydrocortisone injections, or surgical, by osteotomy, joint replacement or arthrodesis.

> The most commonly performed joint replacement is that of the hip, with knee replacements becoming as common. Other joints that can be surgically replaced include finger joints using joint spacers, the elbow and shoulder joints.

Osteoarthritis of the knee

The knee is more affected by osteoarthritis than other joints, especially in overweight and elderly patients, affecting 40% of those over 75. It occurs more commonly in women than men. It generally affects both joints, and has a strong association with osteoarthritis of the hand. Other risk factors include previous trauma to the joint, meniscal injury, cruciate ligament tears and obesity.

Clinical features There is joint pain on use, and swelling, leading to knee locking. It most commonly affects the medial compartment of the knee, leading to a genu varus (bow-legged) deformity. It can also affect the retropatellar region.

Diagnosis A plain X-ray demonstrates features including narrowing of the joint space and the presence of osteophytes, subchondral cysts and osteosclerosis. MRI can show early cartilage changes.

Blood tests are negative for rheumatoid factor and antinuclear antibodies (ANAs). The acute inflammatory proteins erythrocyte sedimentation rate (ESR) and C-reactive protein (CRP) are normal.

Culture is negative. Arthroscopy will demonstrate early fissuring and erosion of surface cartilage.

Management Management of osteoarthritis of the knee depends on the severity of the disease. It may be managed conservatively with analgesics and physiotherapy, or surgically by debridement, osteotomy or joint replacement.

Osteoarthritis in the spine

Osteoarthritis in the back tends to affect the cervical and lumbar vertebrae (Fig. 5.7). It usually occurs in people who lift heavy objects or those with previous injuries, such as disc prolapse or degeneration. There is narrowing of the intervertebral discs and osteophyte formation in the lateral joint margins; these predispose to spinal stenosis and spondylolisthesis.

Inflammatory arthropathies

Rheumatoid arthritis

Rheumatoid arthritis is a systemic inflammatory disease characterized by a chronic symmetrical polyarthritis. It also affects many non-articular parts of the body. It has a variable course, with periods of exacerbation and remission. Some patients have a self-limiting mild form of the condition, but the majority progress to a chronic destructive joint disease.

Epidemiology Rheumatoid arthritis is a significant cause of morbidity and disability. It affects at least 1% of Caucasians; the male:female ratio is 1:3. The disease can present at any age, although the peak age of onset is between 30 and 50 years.

Aetiology The cause of rheumatoid arthritis is unknown, although the disease process is believed to be due to an immunological response to an unknown stimulus. There are a number of possible hypotheses.

Evidence supporting autoimmune mechanisms in rheumatoid arthritis includes:

- The presence of an autoantibody called rheumatoid factor, produced by plasma cells and present in synovium

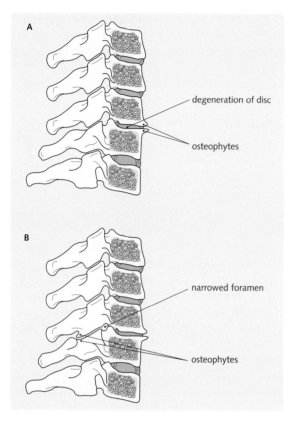

Fig. 5.7 Osteoarthritis of the spine. (A) Degeneration and narrowing of intervertebral disc, forming osteophytes anteriorly; (B) articular cartilage is worn away and marginal osteophytes surround the intervertebral foramen.

- Circulating immune complexes—these are believed to be responsible for the extra-articular features
- Defective T-cell-mediated immunity results in continuous T-cell activation
- The frequent co-occurance of other autoimmune diseases.

Genetic factors affecting susceptibility to rheumatoid arthritis and an association between human leukocyte antigen (HLA) DR4 and DR1. It should be noted that HLAs are not diagnostic: their presence does not guarantee that the disease will develop, but they do give prognostic information in those diagnosed with rheumatoid arthritis, and are generally associated with a poorer prognosis. Fifty to 75% of patients have HLA-DR4.

The initiating factor in rheumatoid arthritis has not been determined, although possible candidates include viral infections such as the Epstein–Barr virus (EBV) and parvoviruses.

Pathology The most common sites affected by rheumatoid arthritis are the small joints of the hands (i.e. the PIP joints, as opposed to the DIP joints in osteoarthritis). The wrist, elbow, shoulder, cervical spine, hip and knee may also become involved.

The disease process can be split into three stages (Fig. 5.8):

- Inflammation and thickening of the synovium, with inflammation and infiltration of lymphocytes and macrophages
- Destruction of cartilage as the infiltrate spreads onto the cartilage surface, creating a pannus (a layer of chronically inflamed fibrous tissue) that extends across the cartilage, thinning it out and eventually destroying it
- Destruction of bone due to the pannus interfering with nutrient supply to the bone. This creates juxta-articular osteoporosis during active inflammation. In chronic disease it results in joint deformities (e.g. ulnar deviation, swan-neck and Boutonnière deformities in the hand).

Secondary changes include muscle wasting of the surrounding muscles due to disuse of the joint.

Clinical features Seventy per cent present with progressive, symmetrical, peripheral polyarthritis that progresses over a few months.

Symptoms include:

- Joint pain, with prolonged early morning stiffness and 'gelling' of the joint after activity
- Weight loss during active disease
- Fatigue and general malaise
- Extra-articular symptoms (Fig. 5.9).

Signs include:

- Warm and tender joints, with insidious onset, first affecting the small joints of the hands and feet. Rheumatoid arthritis usually affects the metacarpophalangeal (MCP) and PIP joints, but not the DIP joints. It frequently progresses to affect other joints
- Swelling
- Decreased, limited range of movement.

Deformities of the hands characteristic of the disease include:

- Subluxation of the DIP joints, creating a flexed PIP joint and a hyperextended DIP joint with

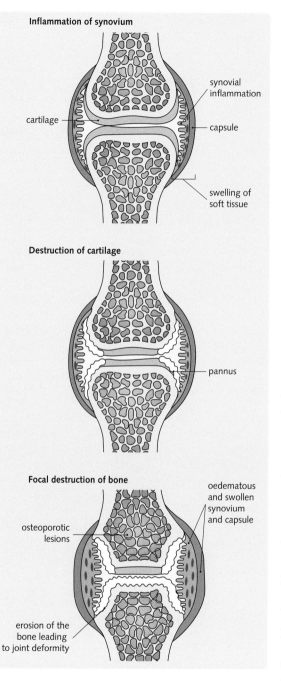

Inflammation of synovium

cartilage

synovial inflammation

capsule

swelling of soft tissue

Destruction of cartilage

pannus

Focal destruction of bone

osteoporotic lesions

oedematous and swollen synovium and capsule

erosion of the bone leading to joint deformity

Fig. 5.8 Pathological changes in rheumatoid arthritis. Inflammation of synovium, destruction of cartilage and focal destruction of bone.

extension of the MCP joint (Boutonnière deformity) (Fig. 5.10)
- Subluxation of the PIP joints, creating a hyperextended PIP joint and a flexed DIP joint (swan-neck deformity) (Fig. 5.10)
- The thumb acquires a Z-deformity

- The MCP joints and wrists undergo subluxation so that the fingers show ulnar deviation. The ulnar styloid and radial head become prominent
- Firm rheumatoid nodules can develop on the extensor surfaces and the flexor tendons.

Complications   The wrists and hands usually suffer a major loss of function and deformities in rheumatoid arthritis. Progressively, there is synovitis of the proximal joints and tendon sheaths, then erosions, and finally joint derangement and tendon rupture, leading to structural and functional loss.

Rheumatoid arthritis of the elbow

The elbow joint is involved in over half of all patients with rheumatoid arthritis. There is pain and limitation of movement in both the elbow and the superior radiohumeral joints.

Management is conservative; removal of the synovium or joint replacement may be considered in severe cases.

Rheumatoid arthritis of the hip

The hip is frequently affected in rheumatoid arthritis. There is progressive femoral head erosion that leads to leg shortening, limited range of movement, gluteal and thigh muscle wasting, and gradual pain. Rheumatoid arthritis is treated conservatively with NSAIDs and immunosuppressants, or by hip replacement.

Rheumatoid arthritis of the spine

When rheumatoid arthritis occurs in the spine, it often affects the cervical vertebrae. There is diffuse pain and impaired movement.

In the later stages joint deformities and muscle wasting may develop.

Periarticular features   Periarticular features that may be seen include:

- Bursitis
- Development of subcutaneous rheumatoid nodules
- Tenosynovitis.

Extra-articular features   Rheumatoid arthritis causes a wide range of extra-articular features, most commonly:

- Fever and fatigue
- Anaemia

Fig. 5.9 Extra-articular features of rheumatoid disease

Site	Manifestation
nerves	carpal tunnel syndrome, peripheral neuropathy ('glove and stocking' sensory loss)
skin	subcutaneous nodules (particularly on extensor aspect of forearm near elbow), vasculitic lesions
blood vessels	vasculitis
eyes	episcleritis, scleritis, secondary Sjögren's syndrome (i.e. triad of dry mouth, dry eyes, and arthritis)
chest	intrapulmonary nodules, pleural effusions, fibrosing alveolitis, Caplan's syndrome
heart	myocarditis, pericarditis, pericardial effusion
kidney	amyloidosis, impaired renal function may be a side effect of drug treatment
soft tissues around joints	bursitis, tenosynovitis

- Pericarditis
- Lymphadenopathy
- Carpal tunnel syndrome
- Secondary Sjögren's syndrome
- Atlantoaxial subluxation (apparent on X-ray).

Diagnosis The diagnosis of rheumatoid arthritis is made clinically using criteria set by the American College of Rheumatology.

About 80% of patients have rheumatoid factor present and 30% have ANAs, although it should

Fig. 5.10 Finger deformities in rheumatoid arthritis: normal finger, swan-neck and boutonnière deformities.

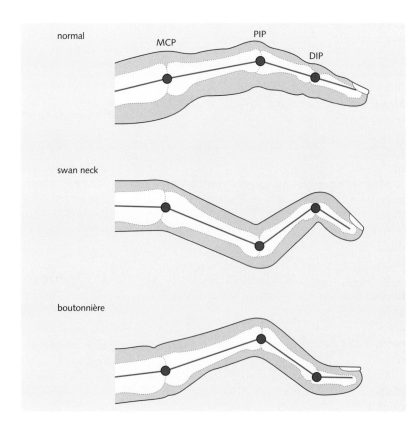

be noted that ANAs are not specific to rheumatoid arthritis. The ESR and C-reactive protein levels are frequently raised. There is an associated anaemia and thrombocytosis.

A plain X-ray will demonstrate changes, depending on the stage of the disease and the joint under investigation. Narrowing of joint spaces and subchondral cysts can be seen. In addition, there may be osteoporosis in bone adjacent to the affected joint, focal erosions of bone, and cysts.

Synovial fluid is sterile, with a raised neutrophil count.

C-reactive protein (CRP) is an acute-phase reactant, a protein that is produced by the liver. The liver is stimulated to increase the production of acute-phase reactants such as CRP in response to cytokines released from cells such as macrophages at the site of injury or inflammation. This makes CRP a more sensitive test than erythrocyte sedimentation rate (ESR) as an indicator of inflammatory processes in a wide range of diseases.

Complications Rheumatoid arthritis can lead to secondary osteoarthritis and may be complicated by septic arthritis. In addition, it can become severely disabling, markedly reducing the patient's quality of life.

Management Management of the condition requires a multidisciplinary approach. Treatment is aimed at controlling the symptoms and at modifying disease activity rather than eradicating the cause.

Medical management aims to control symptoms, in particular the use of NSAIDs and COX2 inhibitors to reduce inflammation.

In early disease, disease-modifying antirheumatic drugs (DMARDs), e.g. sulfasalazine, can be used to reduce joint damage.

In severe cases, corticosteroids and gold can be injected into the joint to suppress disease progression and alleviate symptoms. All of these drugs are associated with serious side effects and the patient needs to be educated about these, and monitored closely.

Surgical management aims to restore function in severe disease (e.g. joint replacement) or help to control disease (e.g. arthroplasty).

Physiotherapy is essential to improve muscle power, maintain mobility and minimize deformities and disability.

Prognosis Long-term prognosis is variable, ranging from minimal symptoms to severe disability.

Juvenile idiopathic arthritis

Arthritis affects around 1 in 1000 children, the most common form being juvenile idiopathic arthritis (JIA). This condition of unknown aetiology presents before the age of 16 years, with a prognosis worse than that of adult disease. It causes chronic synovial inflammation, which can be progressive and destroy the affected joint(s). It is classified according to the pattern of onset seen within the first 6 months: pauciarticular (up to four joints affected), polyarticular (over five joints affected), or systemic (causing spiking fevers, a systemic rash and arthralgia). Onset is abrupt, with morning stiffness and arthralgia. Investigations characteristically reveal a raised ESR, and anaemia may be present in chronic disease. ANAs are present in up to 25% of affected children. Management of the condition requires input from a multidisciplinary team with the aim of establishing an optimal quality of life, including physiotherapy and encouraging the child to remain active. NSAIDs are the first line of treatment for all subtypes of disease, with more aggressive disease requiring immunosuppressant agents and pulsed steroid therapy.

Sjögren's syndrome

Sjögren's syndrome is a chronic autoimmune inflammatory disease in which the body's epithelial exocrine glands are destroyed. It can occur alone (primary Sjögren's syndrome) or secondary to other systemic diseases, the most common of these being rheumatoid arthritis, but also systemic lupus erythematosus, scleroderma and primary biliary cirrhosis.

Clinical features The lymphatic infiltration of exocrine glands leads to keratoconjunctivitis sicca (dry eyes) and xerostomia (dry mouth).

Investigations ANAs are found in 60–70% of patients. In primary disease over two-thirds are found to have anti-Ro and anti-La ANAs.

Management The condition is treated symptomatically with artificial tears and pilocarpine hydrochloride tablets, which increase secretion from the salivary glands.

Seronegative arthritides

The seronegative arthritides are a group of related disorders, termed seronegative as no rheumatoid factors are produced. They are similar because they:

- Are often associated with certain human leukocyte antigens (HLAs), in particular HLA-B27
- Are negative for rheumatoid factor and other autoantibodies
- Have a familial tendency
- Are more common in white people.

Conditions include:

- Ankylosing spondylitis
- Psoriatic arthritis
- Reactive arthritis
- Enteropathic arthritis.

Patients may present with several different disorders, occurring either simultaneously or at different times. The patterns of joint involvement are different from those seen in rheumatoid arthritis, and are generally more limited.

Ankylosing spondylitis

Ankylosing spondylitis is a chronic autoimmune inflammatory disorder that affects the back, most commonly in young adults (Fig. 5.11).

Epidemiology   The male:female ratio in ankylosing spondylitis is estimated to be of the order of 9:1. Women tend to show milder symptoms. Most patients present in their late teens or early adulthood.

Aetiology   There is a familial tendency in ankylosing spondylitis, with the HLA B27 association occurring in 90% of affected individuals.

Pathology   The spinal joints are affected. Inflammation starts in the lumbar vertebral and sacroiliac joints, and extends proximally. The pathology begins at sites of ligamentous insertion (entheses), resulting in enthesiopathy—the hallmark of spondyloarthro-pathies.

There are initial erosive lesions on the articular cartilage and the underlying vertebral body, which lead to the growth of bony spurs across the annulus fibrosis, called syndesmophytes. The upper and lower syndesmophytes across each intervertebral disc fuse together and ossify, thereby fusing the spine. On X-ray there is 'squaring' of the vertebral bodies, giving rise to a 'bamboo spine' appearance.

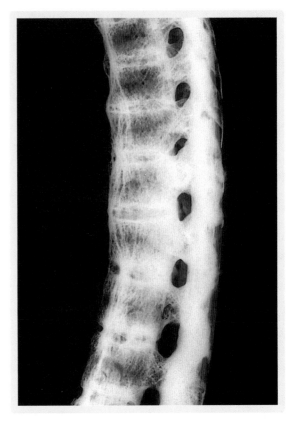

Fig. 5.11 Radiograph of a sagittal section through the vertebral column showing ankylosing spondylitis. There is complete fusion of the spine and apophyseal joints, and across the intervertebral disc. (Courtesy of Dr PG Bullough.)

Clinical features   Symptoms include:

- Diffuse pain in the back, pelvis and joints of the lower limbs
- Pain and stiffness in the lower back that is worse in the mornings
- Progressive loss of movement of the spine.

Signs that may be present include:

- Kyphosis with hyperflexion of the neck
- Loss of normal lumbar lordosis
- Limited spinal flexion
- Progressive fixed flexion deformity of the hips
- Decreased chest expansion.

Other features include Achilles tendonitis and plantar fasciitis.

Ankylosing spondylitis can have systemic manifestations. Notably, iritis occurs in 25% and, less commonly, aortic regurgitation and apical lung fibrosis.

Diagnosis Ankylosing spondylitis is diagnosed clinically.

A spinal X-ray may be normal, or demonstrate erosion and sclerosis of sacroiliac joints, which can develop into ankylosis (immobility of the joint). There may also be vertebral squaring and calcification of the spinous ligaments—the so-called tramline or bamboo spine appearance. ESR and CRP levels are often raised.

Management Ankylosing spondylitis is usually treated with slow-release NSAIDs, taken at night to relieve night pain and early morning stiffness. Immunosuppressive drugs such as sulfasalazine can help in peripheral arthritis. Patients undergo physiotherapy and are taught daily exercises to perform to maintain movement and posture. Anti-TNF is very effective therapy for Ankylosing spondylitis.

Prognosis Although ankylosing spondylitis is progressive, most patients are able to lead a normal life. In cases of severe kyphosis, breathing can become difficult. Severe spinal involvement can increase the risk of fractures and cord compression.

Arthritis associated with gastrointestinal disease

Enteropathic arthritis

This is relatively uncommon, presenting as a large-joint monoarthritis or an asymmetrical oligoarthritis affecting the knees, ankles and elbows. It is associated with inflammatory bowel disease (IBD) and affects 10–15% of patients with ulcerative colitis or Crohn's disease. The severity of the arthritis reflects the activity of the IBD, with most episodes resolving within a few months. Successful treatment of the IBD usually leads to remission of enteropathic arthritis.

Arthritis associated with other systemic disease

Reactive arthritis

Reactive arthritis presents acutely in response to infection at a distant site, unlike septic arthritis, where organisms can be isolated from the joint itself. The main causative organisms are:

- *Chlamydia*, causing genital infection
- *Salmonella, Campylobacter* or *Shigella* spp., causing gastrointestinal infection.

Reactive arthritis is more common in males.

About 80% of patients show an association with HLA B27, suggesting an autoimmune process.

Rarely, reactive arthritis occurs in Reiter's syndrome, when it follows a diarrhoeal or sexually transmitted infection where it is present in a triad with non-specific urethritis/cervicitis and conjunctivitis.

The arthritis usually affects the knees or ankles causing an asymmetrical oligoarthritis, although axial disease may occur.

It is diagnosed clinically. In acute disease there may be a raised ESR. Synovial fluid aspirate is sterile, with a raised neutrophil count.

Although symptoms may clear spontaneously within a few months, 50% of sufferers will suffer recurrences. A minority may develop severe spondylitis. In patients who are HIV positive, a very severe form of reactive arthritis may result.

Management involves treating the underlying infection with antibiotics, and inflammation with NSAIDs.

Psoriatic arthritis

Psoriatic arthritis occurs in 5–10% of psoriasis sufferers, especially those with nail involvement. It may also occur in individuals with a family history of psoriasis (see Chapter 7 for more information about psoriasis). Psoriatic arthritis can occur before or after clinical cutaneous manifestations of the disease.

Clinical features There are several patterns of disease. The small joints of the hand can be involved asymmetrically. Axial involvement may also occur. Symmetrical polyarthritis can occur, and is often indistinguishable from rheumatoid arthritis.

There is also an association with ankylosing spondylitis and HLA B27.

Investigations Routine blood tests are often normal. Radiography may show bone erosion and periarticular osteoporosis in the DIP joints.

Management Treatment is with NSAIDs and analgesics. Immunosuppressive drugs may also be used in severe cases, as they control both the arthritis and the skin disease.

Prognosis Severe disease can result in arthritis mutilans, an uncommon complication in which the small bones in the hands and feet are destroyed.

Still's disease

Still's disease accounts for 10% of cases of JIA, the arthritis occurring in a person under 16 years of age.

Clinical features include a salmon-coloured maculopapular rash with a spiking fever. Generalized lymphadenopathy, splenomegaly, arthralgia and pericarditis can occur.

The number of joints affected is variable, depending on the type of Still's disease.

Blood tests reveal a raised ESR or CRP, a raised neutrophil count and thrombocytosis, with negative autoantibodies.

Most patients recover spontaneously before early adulthood.

Sarcoid arthritis

This can present as a transient polyarthritis or an acute monoarthritis, which occurs in early-onset sarcoidosis, and it can be a presenting feature of the condition. It is often accompanied by erythema nodosum and hilar lymphadenopathy. The sites affected are usually large joints such as the ankles and knees, although the patterns of joint involvement can change later in the disease. Treatment is with NSAIDs, or steroids where NSAIDs fail to control symptoms. Sarcoidosis that presents with arthritis has a good prognosis and is usually self-remitting.

Neuropathic joint disease (Charcot's joint)

In neuropathic joint disease, or Charcot's joint, conditions that produce loss of sensation in the lower limbs results in traumatic joint damage.

This condition is most commonly associated with diabetes mellitus, where joints in the feet are affected. There can be gross deformity and swelling.

Systemic lupus erythematosus

Systemic lupus erythematosus (SLE) is a chronic, multisystem inflammatory disease and the most common of the systemic connective tissue disorders. It can develop at any age, affecting women eight times more often than men.

The aetiology is unclear, although it has a major genetic component. There is a dysregulated immune response to cellular antigens that become expressed on the surface of apoptosing cells. The resulting immune response produces immune complexes within the blood vessels, producing vascular inflammation that may affected any organ.

Clinical features Rheumatological presentation is with joint symptoms that resemble those of rheumatoid arthritis. Patients develop migrating asymmetrical arthralgia, one of the commonest presenting complaints of SLE. There can also be myalgia and arthritis, initially affecting the small joints of the hands and wrists and later affecting the knees. Synovitis, joint effusions and joint destruction are rare. Patients may also develop Raynaud's phenomenon. Refer to Chapter 7 for cutaneous involvement of the disease.

Diagnosis The diagnosis is based on history, clinical features and investigations. Blood tests can detect ANAs, which can be present against double-stranded DNA and complement, as well as ANA subtypes against Sm, SSA (Ro) and SSB (La). In active disease, inflammatory markers such as ESR are raised, whereas complement C3 and C4 levels are low. A full blood count can show leukopenia, anaemia or thrombocytopenia. Liver function tests are raised in active disease and creatine kinase is raised in myositis.

Joint radiography does not reveal many changes beyond periarticular osteopenia and soft tissue swelling. Blood tests and imaging (including radiography, MRI and CT) can be used to assess involvement of other systems.

Complications Ten per cent of patients develop Jaccoud arthropathy, non-erosive hand deformities similar to those occurring in rheumatoid arthritis as a complication of chronic arthritis.

Management Medical management aims to slow the progression of the disease with disease-modifying antirheumatic drugs (DMARDs), inclu- ding corticosteroids and immunosuppressants. Aspirin and NSAIDs can reduce the inflammation and pain.

Scleroderma

Scleroderma is a systemic, multisystem disease characterized by tight, thickened and indurated skin developing over the fingers, limbs, trunks and face. It can be classified according to the distribution of skin involvement and systemic involvement into localized and systemic scleroderma (also known as systemic sclerosis). It occurs worldwide, affecting females five times more than men. The peak age of onset is between 30 and 50 years of age. See also Chapter 7 for details of cutaneous involvement of scleroderma. Joint involvement can occur in systemic scleroderma.

Aetiology The cause is unclear, although it is believed to be associated with endothelial cell injury and fibroblast activation in the presence of a disordered immunological response. Some environmental factors have been identified, including silica and exposure to industrial solvents.

Pathophysiology There is an excessive production of types I and III collagen, which are then deposited in the microvasculature supplying the skin as well as all of the body's systems, producing an inflammatory response and progressive fibrosis. The small arteries, arterioles and capillaries frequently become occluded at an early stage.

Clinical features Symptoms arise as a consequence of the inflammatory response, fibrosis and vascular dysfunction. Three-quarters of patients have Raynaud's phenomenon at first presentation, and almost all will develop it during the course of the disease. Patients complain of generalized arthralgia, joint stiffness that is worse in the mornings, and muscle weakness. On examination there may be a reduced range of movement of affected joints, muscle wasting and flexion contractures. Patients may present with features of carpal tunnel syndrome arising as a consequence of peripheral nerve entrapment.

Vascular dysfunction and fibrosis can affect all other systems, producing a diverse range of symptoms, including shortness of breath, chest pain, persistent cough, gastro-oesophageal reflux disease, erectile dysfunction and dyspareunia.

Diagnosis Diagnosis is made primarily on history and examination. Blood tests can detect autoantibodies: 40% of those with diffuse systemic sclerosis develop antibodies against anti-topoisomerase-1 or anti-Scl-70. Up to 90% of those with limited sclerosis develop anticentromere antibodies. There may also be raised creatine kinase in myositis.

Imaging, including radiography, MRI or CT scans, can be used to assess the level of systemic fibrosis and disease progression.

Complications Systemic complications include congestive cardiac failure, pulmonary fibrosis and pulmonary hypertension, chronic renal failure and systemic hypertension.

Management Medical management of systemic scleroderma aims to slow disease progression and systemic involvement. Symptomatic management involves aspirin and NSAIDs (where these are not contraindicated) to reduce inflammation and pain.

Prognosis In mild limited systemic involvement there is 60–70% survival at 10 years after diagnosis. In more aggressive disease there is 20% survival at 10 years. The prognosis is worse in younger patients, African–American individuals, and those with pulmonary and renal involvement.

Crystal arthropathies

The crystal arthropathies are a group of disorders in which the deposition of crystals in joints leads to inflammation.

Two main types of crystal involved are sodium urate and calcium pyrophosphate. Neutrophils attack the deposited crystals and produce an inflammatory reaction.

Gout

Epidemiology Gout is more common in men, although some postmenopausal women may be affected. It affects 0.2% of Europeans. A third have a positive family history.

Aetiology In gout, hyperuricaemia results in the deposition of monosodium urate crystals in the joint.

The most common form is idiopathic (primary) gout. There tends to be a family history of the condition.

Secondary gout may occur as a result of:

- Increased production of uric acid, e.g. increased cell turnover in carcinomas, and leukaemia following chemotherapy, and in enzyme defects
- Impaired excretion, e.g. renal failure, chronic excessive alcohol consumption, hyperlipidaemia and diuretic therapy
- High dietary intake of purine, e.g. red meats.

Pathology Urate is a product of the breakdown of purines found in DNA (i.e. adenine, guanine) and is normally excreted in the urine.

Excess uric acid results in the deposition of crystals in:

- Joints, the most commonly affected being the metatarsophalangeal (MTP) joint in the big toe. The ankle joint may also be affected
- Soft tissues: this may lead to the formation of tophi (palpable masses), which develop at the extensor surfaces of the elbow joint or on the pinna of the ear
- The urinary tract, in the form of urate stones.

The deposition of crystals in the synovium and periarticular soft tissues causes an acute inflammatory reaction. Hyperuricaemia may be precipitated by alcohol, dietary excess, surgery, starvation or drugs, especially thiazide diuretics.

Chronic gouty arthritis occurs after recurrent attacks, with a progressive increase in the number of joints becoming involved. It is characterized by cartilage degeneration, synovial hyperplasia and secondary osteoarthritis.

Clinical features   Patients with gout present between the ages of 20 and 60 years, but most commonly in middle age.

An acute attack involves an extremely painful monoarthritis of sudden onset. The affected joint is oedematous, hot, red and exquisitely tender; more than one joint may be affected in certain cases.

Diagnosis   Serum uric acid is usually raised, but may also be normal in acute gout. Serum urea and creatinine levels should be checked for signs of renal impairment.

Synovial fluid demonstrates the presence of needle-shaped crystals, which are diagnostic. These crystals are negatively birefringent. Neutrophils are also found.

The presence of tophi on the earlobes or around joints may help in making the diagnosis.

Complications   Hyperuricaemia is genetically associated with an increased risk of hypertension and coronary artery disease. Renal disease can also occur.

Management   An acute attack of gout is treated with NSAIDs and cyclo-oxygenase 2 (COX2) inhibitors. Oral colchicine can be prescribed if NSAIDs are contraindicated.

Allopurinol, a drug that decreases uric acid synthesis, is used in long-term management. The patient should be advised to maintain a good fluid intake and avoid the precipitating factors described above; lifestyle modifications such as weight loss are advised for obese patients.

In persistent symptomatic disease, joint effusions can be aspirated, followed by steroid injections into the joint.

Prognosis   Attacks of gout may be infrequent, and treatment can reduce the extent of joint damage. However, renal complications are frequent.

Pseudogout

Pseudogout is an acute synovitis that may mimic gout. It is more common in elderly women. Its aetiology is unknown, but it may occur secondary to other conditions, including hyperparathyroidism, haemochromatosis and hypothyroidism, particularly in younger patients.

In pseudogout, calcium pyrophosphate crystals are deposited in articular cartilage and periarticular tissue. Inflammation results if the crystals are shed into the joint space.

Its presentation is similar to that of primary osteoarthritis. The knee is commonly affected, but it also affects the wrist, shoulder and ankle in a typically asymmetrical manner.

Analysis of synovial fluid aspirate shows characteristic brick-shaped crystals that are positively birefringent (compared to those found in gout, which are negatively birefringent). The white cell count may be raised. Serum calcium is usually normal.

The mainstay of treatment is rest, with NSAIDs and joint aspiration and steroid injection.

Arthritis associated with infection

Septic arthritis

Septic arthritis occurs where a joint becomes infected with pyogenic organisms.

Epidemiology   Infectious (septic) arthritis is an uncommon condition that usually affects children and young adults.

Aetiology   Infectious arthritis is usually caused by bacteria, most commonly Staphylococcus aureus, but also Streptococcus pyogenes, Neisseria gonorrhoea, Haemophilus influenzae and Gram-negative organisms. Tuberculous arthritis is now rare.

Predisposing factors include osteomyelitis in the bone adjacent to the joint, rheumatoid arthritis, immunosuppressive therapy, trauma or surgery to the joint, such as joint replacement. It can rarely arise as a complication of a viral infection, such as rubella or mumps.

Pathology   In infectious arthritis the infecting organism gains access to the joint:

- Haematogenously
- As a result of local trauma
- By direct spread from adjacent foci of infection, e.g. osteomyelitis.

Clinical features   Usually, only one joint is affected in infectious arthritis, the patient presenting with an acutely painful, swollen, erythematous, immobile joint and an associated fever. There are often systemic signs of sepsis, although these may be absent where the patient has rheumatoid arthritis or is on immunosuppressive treatment. The joint should be aspirated for culture if infection is suspected. Septic arthritis must be excluded in children who present with a painful joint because, unlike in adults, the disease causes devastating damage to the joint if left undiagnosed.

Diagnosis Where septic arthritis is suspected, the joint should be aspirated for culture, white cell count, Gram stain and crystal analysis. In infectious arthritis the synovial fluid is turbid and purulent, with a neutrophilia. Culture is positive. Patients need an X-ray to exclude trauma.

Blood samples should be taken for culture, full blood count and acute-phase reactants. X-rays will not be diagnostic in acute infection, but can be kept as a baseline for comparison in order to determine whether joint destruction has occurred.

Management Intravenous antibiotics should be started immediately where infectious arthritis is suspected. This is initially 'blind' broad-spectrum agents and is modified according to organism sensitivities when culture results are available. Generally, intravenous antibiotics should be given for 2 weeks, followed by 4 weeks of oral antibiotics.

Drainage of the joint is needed to remove debris. The joint should also be immobilized. In the acute stage, only NSAIDs or COX2 inhibitors can be given for pain relief.

Prognosis Infectious arthritis can be life-threatening and should be managed as an emergency, with immediate treatment.

Recovery can take anywhere from a few days to a few weeks.

DISORDERS AFFECTING SPECIFIC JOINTS

Disorders of the hand and wrist

De Quervain's tenosynovitis

De Quervain's tenosynovitis is inflammation of the fibrous sheath at the radial stylus that holds the tendon of the abductor pollicis longus in place as it passes over it. There is local tenderness at the site, with the pain exacerbated on flexing of the thumb. A palpable nodule can develop proximal to the wrist joint on the radial aspect.

De Quervain's tenosynovitis may be caused by overuse of the tendons, e.g. wringing out washing. Treatment is with rest, and hydrocortisone injection or surgical splitting of the tendon sheath may be required.

Tendon lesions

'Trigger finger'

'Trigger finger' or digital stenosing synovitis is thickening of the tendon sheaths, constricting the flexor tendons (Fig. 5.12). It affects the ring and middle fingers in adults and the thumb in children. Upon extension of the finger, the tendon has to move through a narrower space, causing difficulty in extending the finger and commonly causing a snapping noise to be elicited when extension does occur. The condition is treated with steroid injections.

'Mallet finger'

'Mallet finger' is also called 'baseball finger' (Fig. 5.12). The extensor tendon is damaged at its insertion into the distal phalanx so that the DIP joint cannot be fully extended. It is treated by splinting the finger with the joint fully extended.

'Dropped finger'

'Dropped finger' is caused by tendon rupture at the wrist, either directly or as a complication of

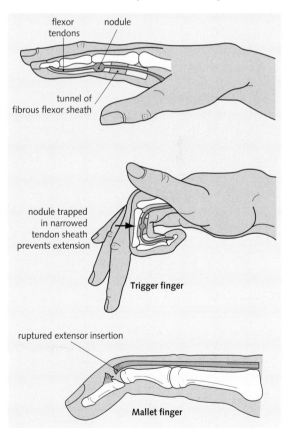

Fig. 5.12 'Trigger finger' and 'mallet finger' due to tendon injuries. See text for details.

rheumatoid arthritis, resulting in loss of finger extension at the MCP joint.

Ganglia

Ganglia are smooth, painless, unilocular swellings containing clear viscous fluid caused by a weakening or partial tear in a joint capsule. They appear as painless lumps around a joint or tendon sheath, most commonly on the dorsum of the wrist (Fig. 5.13). Treatment is not usually required as they do not generally cause problems. They can be surgically excised, although in half of cases they recur.

Dupuytren's contracture

In Dupuytren's contracture the palmar aponeurosis is fibrosed, becoming thickened and contracted, causing skin tethering (Fig. 5.14). The fingers gradually become flexed at the MCP and PIP joints, usually of the ring and little fingers. It is more common in Caucasian men. Predisposing factors include alcohol abuse, diabetes, a family history of the condition and Peyronie's disease (fibrosis of the corpus cavernosum).

Surgical release of the contracture is performed only in those who develop severe deformity of the fingers that interferes with their function.

Carpal tunnel syndrome

Aetiology Carpal tunnel syndrome is caused by compression of the median nerve as it passes through the canal beneath the flexor retinaculum sheath in the wrist. Compression can arise by enlargement or inflammation of the structures surrounding the nerve, such as the flexor retinaculum and flexor tendons, or from direct external pressure due to fractures and dislocations. It can occur in the last trimester of pregnancy, as well as in hypothyroidism and rheumatoid arthritis.

Clinical features Characteristic symptoms are paraesthesia and pain in the distribution of the median nerve of the hand (thumb, index, and middle and radial half of the ring finger), often waking the patient at night or occurring after repetitive movements. Later, wasting can develop in those muscles innervated by the median nerve, and sensation may be reduced in its cutaneous distribution.

Management Splints are used to hold the wrist in dorsiflexion overnight to relieve symptoms, and this can assist clinical diagnosis. Where symptoms persist, steroid injections into the carpal tunnel offer transient relief in over two-thirds of patients. Surgical decompression is used in persistent disease, or where it interferes with nerve conduction.

Carpal tunnel syndrome commonly occurs in rheumatoid arthritis, hypothyroidism, diabetes mellitus, acromegaly and gouty arthritis. Oedema of the flexor retinaculum causes compression, which can occur in the third trimester of pregnancy, as well as renal failure and congestive cardiac failure.

Fig. 5.13 Ganglion at the dorsal surface of the wrist. (Courtesy of Dr JH Klippel.)

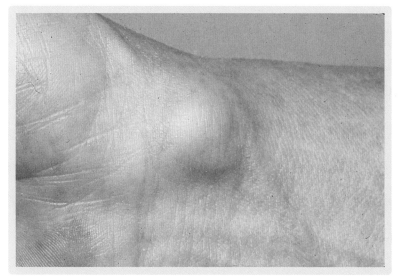

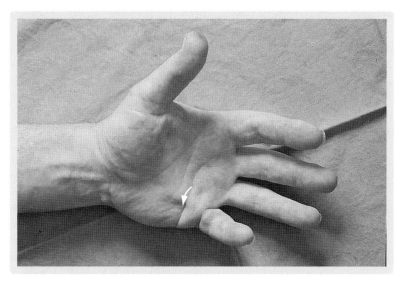

Fig. 5.14 Dupuytren's contracture of the palmar fascia. (Courtesy of Dr JH Klippel.)

Disorders of the elbow

Tennis elbow

Tennis elbow is inflammation (enthesitis) or microtrauma of the common extensor attachment at the lateral epicondyle (lateral epicondylitis). Despite the name, tennis elbow is not related to tennis. It is treated with rest, and a physiotherapy opinion can be sought. Steroid injections can help where pain is severe. It frequently settles spontaneously.

Golfer's elbow

Golfer's elbow is inflammation of the common flexor attachment at the medial epicondyle (medial epicondylitis). Despite its name, it is not related to golf. Patients are advised to rest the joint, and a physiotherapy opinion can be sought. Steroid injections can be used where pain is severe, but care should be taken to avoid the adjacent course of the ulnar nerve.

Olecranon bursitis

Olecranon bursitis occurs after trauma, sepsis, rheumatoid arthritis and gout. It involves a hot, painful swelling behind the olecranon. Movement is not usually uncomfortable or impaired, and it is only painful when pressure is applied to the bursa. It has also been called 'student's elbow' as excessive friction, for example from propping the elbows on books or desks for long periods, can cause olecranon bursitis. The joint must be aspirated and examined to exclude infection. Local steroid injections can relieve pain.

Cubitus valgus and cubitus varus

Cubitus valgus is when the 'carrying angle' of the elbow joint is greater than the normal 10° in men and 15° in women (Fig. 5.15). It is caused by malunion of a previous lateral condylar fracture or retarded lateral epiphyseal growth. There may be an association with Turner's syndrome. Complications include ulnar neuritis and osteoarthritis.

Cubitus varus is the opposite deformity, with a decreased carrying angle (see Fig. 5.15). Its most

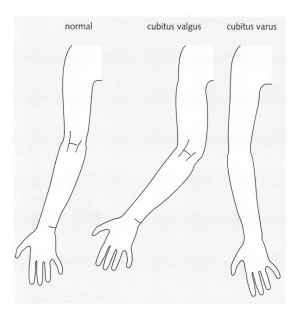

Fig. 5.15 Normal angle of the elbow, cubitus valgus and cubitus varus.

common cause is malunion of a supracondylar fracture. Both cubitus valgus and cubitus varus may be corrected by osteotomy.

Ulnar neuritis

Aetiology The ulnar nerve may be subjected to constriction (osteoarthritis, rheumatoid arthritis) or constant friction (for example in conditions such as cubitus valgus), as it lies in a groove behind the medial epicondyle. This can lead to nerve fibrosis and eventual ulnar neuropathy.

Complications In ulnar neuritis there is hand clumsiness, reduced sensation over the little finger and the ulnar side of the ring finger, and weakened small muscles of the hand innervated by the nerve.

Management Treatment of ulnar neuritis involves surgery to release the nerve and transpose it to the front of the elbow.

Loose bodies in the elbow joint

Loose bodies in the elbow joint may arise from osteochondral fractures, osteophytes of osteoarthritis, and other conditions such as synovial chondromatosis and osteochondritis dissecans. The bodies cause locking of the elbow as they become stuck between the bones, causing sharp pain and swelling, and are treated by surgical removal.

Disorders of the shoulder

Dislocation of the shoulder joint

A dislocated shoulder joint is a very common injury, usually occurring when the arm is forced back in external rotation and abduction, such as when falling on to an outstretched arm, e.g. when playing rugby. The joint may be displaced in different directions, but anterior displacement of the humeral head to below the coracoid process is the most common occurrence.

Complications Complications of a dislocated shoulder include damage to the circumflex axillary nerve and axillary artery as they run adjacent to the joint, as well as joint stiffness and recurrent dislocations.

Management A dislocated shoulder is treated by reducing the joint and immobilizing it for about 3 weeks.

Painful arc syndrome

In painful arc syndrome, shoulder abduction causes pain in the mid-ranges but not extremes of movement, i.e. between 60° and 120°. It is caused by degeneration, injury or inflammation of the rotator cuff, most commonly where the tendon of the supraspinatus muscle becomes inflamed and compressed between the greater tuberosity of the humerus and the acromion (known as impingement), or by partial tears of its tendon, producing pain and limiting movement (Fig. 5.16). It can also be caused by incomplete tears of the supraspinatus tendon, inflammation of the supraspinatus tendon (supraspinatus tendonitis) and inflammation of the subacromial bursa (subacromial bursitis).

The syndrome may be associated with supraspinatus tendon calcification (perhaps a variation of crystal arthropathy), rheumatoid arthritis or acromioclavicular joint osteoarthritis.

Management Painful arc syndrome is treated with anti-inflammatory agents such as NSAIDs, or steroid joint injections where this fails to control symptoms. Surgery can be considered in severe cases.

Rotator cuff tears

Rotator cuff tears are partial tears that often occur with supraspinatus tendonitis, leading to painful arc syndrome. Complete tears limit shoulder abduction, causing joint pain at the shoulder tip and upper arm, and tenderness under the acromion. The tears are usually in the supraspinatus tendon (although subscapularis and infraspinatus may be involved) and allow communication between the joint capsule and the subacromial bursa, seen on arthroscopy.

Aetiology Rotator cuff tears may be caused by age-related degeneration, trauma such as a fall, or sporting injuries.

Management Rotator cuff tears are treated by repairing the tendon. Better results are obtained in young people with less degeneration.

Adhesive capsulitis (frozen shoulder)

Adhesive capsulitis or 'frozen shoulder' is a common but poorly understood condition affecting the glenohumeral joint. It causes pain and limitation of all movements (to about half the normal range), but no changes are seen on X-ray.

Aetiology Adhesive capsulitis may follow a minor injury or be due to an autoimmune response to localized rotator cuff tissues. It causes pain and stiffness.

It may take months to heal.

Management Adhesive capsulitis is treated initially with NSAIDs, analgesics and gentle exercise. Joint manipulation is undertaken when the joint is stronger.

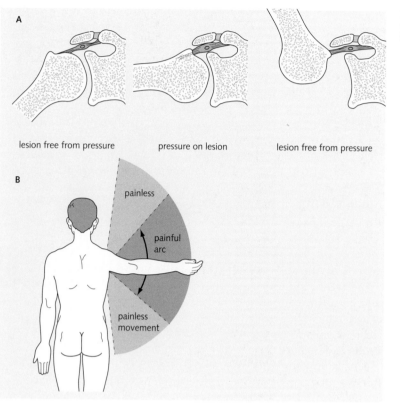

lesion free from pressure   pressure on lesion   lesion free from pressure

painless

painful arc

painless movement

Fig. 5.16 Mechanism and aetiology of painful arc syndrome. (A) Mechanical basis; (B) areas of pain.

Biceps rupture

In biceps rupture the patient often describes feeling something 'snap' during lifting, which is followed by an aching in the shoulder. A 'ball' appears in the anterior belly of the biceps muscle on elbow flexion, but function is unaffected.

Aetiology Biceps rupture may be caused by degenerative changes or trauma, such as a fall or injury.

Management As the function of the biceps remains intact during rupture, no treatment is required.

Biceps tendonitis

Biceps tendonitis is an uncommon condition in which the biceps tendon becomes inflamed. This is made worse on forced muscle contraction.

Management Biceps tendonitis is treated by hydrocortisone injection.

Pain referred to the shoulder

Pain may be referred to the shoulder via C5 to the deltoid, via C6, C7 and C8 to the superior border of the scapula, or via C3 from the diaphragm to the shoulder tip.

Referred pain may originate from the brachial plexus and roots (e.g. prolapsed cervical disc, herpes zoster, or the presence of a first cervical rib), upper arm, abdomen (e.g. cholecystitis, or a subphrenic abscess that creates diaphragmatic irritation), and infection within the thorax (e.g. angina, pleurisy) may contribute to referred pain.

> Pain is not always felt at the site of its origin, particularly with regard to a diseased organ. It can be felt at skin sites supplied by the spinal nerves that correspond to the afferent supply of the organ, and is called referred pain. A good example of this is the heart, whose sensory afferent fibres enter the spinal cord through the posterior roots of the upper four thoracic nerves. Consequently, pain is often reported on the medial upper arm. Another example is knee pathology, which can commonly cause pain to be referred to the hip.

Disorders of the hip

Coxa vara

Aetiology Coxa vara is a term that includes any condition in which the angle between the neck and the shaft of the femur is less than the normal 125° (Fig. 5.17). This leads to true shortening of the limb and a limping walk due to a Trendelenburg 'dip'.

The cause of coxa vara may be:

- Congenital
- A slipped upper femoral epiphysis
- Fracture (trochanteric with malunion, non-united fractures of the femoral neck)
- Bone softening (rickets, osteomalacia or Paget's disease of bone).

Developmental dysplasia of the hip (DDH)

DDH is a spectrum of hip instability ranging from a shallow acetabulum (acetabular dysplasia) to hip instability.

The true birth prevalence is 1.5 per 1000 births. Girls are eight times more likely to have DDH than boys, with the left hip more commonly involved than the right. Risk factors include a breech delivery, a family history or a neuromuscular disorder. It should be diagnosed and treated as soon as possible after birth so as to prevent delayed walking and abnormal gait. Consequently, all babies are routinely examined for signs of DDH as part of their neonatal baby check, although because of the broad spectrum of joint pathology 40% of cases are not detected. On examination, the child has limited abduction of the flexed hip. The femur may be shortened. Late presentation can be difficult to treat, and presents with asymmetrical skin folds around the hip, limited hip abduction, shortening of the leg, a limp or abnormal gait, and can be complicated by contractures.

Ultrasound is diagnostic. X-ray films are not useful until the femoral head becomes ossified after 5 months of age.

Management Ninety per cent of cases resolve spontaneously without active treatment. DDH is

There is an ongoing argument in favour of making ultrasound a routine test for newborn babies to screen for developmental dysplasia of the hip, as signs are not entirely specific to the condition and clinical detection is variable. The National Library for Health reports one study having determined ultrasound to have 88.5% sensitivity and 96.7% specificity. However, owing to the broad spectrum of pathophysiology, most cases resolve spontaneously, so there has not yet been an identified requirement for definitive diagnosis greater than that provided by newborn medical examination.

treated in various ways according to the age of the patient. Treatment is usually conservative, and may involve specialized slings to maintain the joint in abduction. In complicated cases, or those unresponsive to conservative treatment, joint reduction or osteotomy can be performed.

Perthes' disease

Perthes' disease develops as a result of ischaemia of the femoral head epiphysis in children between 5 and 10 years of age. It affects boys five times more than girls. It results in avascular necrosis, causing bone fragmentation with concurrent revascularization and new bone formation that takes over 18–36 months. It presents with a limp and hip pain, and occurs bilaterally in 10–20% of cases. There is narrowing of the joint space, sclerosis and flattening of the femoral head. The cause is unknown. In early disease that involves less than half of the epiphysis it is treated with bed rest and traction. With more severe involvement, management requires the maintenance of hip abduction with plaster casts. Surgical containment is necessary to treat severe cases.

Fig. 5.17 Normal femur and coxa vara.

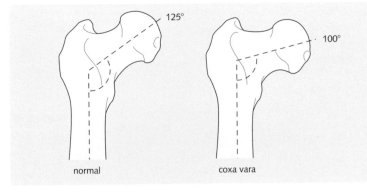

125°

100°

normal   coxa vara

The prognosis is good in children with less than half of the epiphysis involved. Where there is greater involvement there is an increased chance of the femoral head becoming deformed, with damage to the metaphysis. These patients are at increased risk of degenerative arthritis in later life.

Slipped upper femoral epiphysis (SUFE)

Aetiology SUFE usually affects adolescents between 10 and 15 years of age during the growth spurt. There is displacement of the upper epiphysis downward and backward from the femoral neck along the epiphyseal line (Fig. 5.18). In 20% of cases it occurs bilaterally. Slipped upper femoral epiphysis usually affects overweight individuals, and males are affected more often than females. There is limping and pain in the groin, which may be referred to the thigh or knee, with limited abduction and internal rotation of the hip.

Complications include avascular necrosis and coxa vara.

An X-ray film is usually diagnostic.

Management Slipped upper femoral epiphysis is treated surgically by pinning the femur into position,

and by corrective realignment in severe slips where the epiphyses have fused.

Transient synovitis

Transient synovitis is a common, short-lived condition of unknown aetiology that affects children between 2 and 12 years of age. It presents with a sudden onset of pain, limping and limited range of movement of the hip. It often occurs alongside or shortly after a viral infection. The child is usually afebrile. X-rays are normal. Septic arthritis must be excluded. Blood cultures, white cell count and acute-phase reactants are usually normal. A small joint effusion may be visible on ultrasound. No treatment is required, as transient synovitis usually improves spontaneously within a few days. The patient should be advised to take bed rest in the meantime.

Tuberculous arthritis

Aetiology Tuberculosis (TB) frequently affects the hip joint, causing pain, limping, limited movement and muscle spasm. X-rays show bone rarefaction (decreased density but normal volume) and erosion of articular cartilage and bone.

Management Tuberculous arthritis is treated by treating the underlying infection, with the administration of appropriate analgesia where required. If the joint has been destroyed, arthrodesis (joint fusion) is performed.

Pain referred to the hip

Pain may be referred to the hip from the spine (prolapsed disc, sacroiliac arthritis), the pelvis and lower abdomen (appendicular abscess, pyosalpinx, irritation of the obturator nerve or muscle spasm), or from thrombosis of the lower abdominal aorta and its main branches.

Disorders of the knee

Genu varum and genu valgum

Genu varum (bow legs) is bowing of the tibiae: the knees are wide apart, deviating away from the midline when the feet are together. It is common in children up to 3 years of age. No treatment is required as it resolves spontaneously. In genu valgum (knock-knees) the feet are wide apart, with the knees pointing toward the midline. It is common in children up to 7 years of age. Again, no treatment is required as it usually resolves spontaneously (Fig. 5.19). These conditions may occasionally occur secondary to

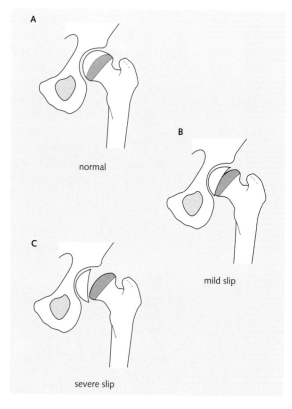

Fig. 5.18 (A) Normal femoral epiphysis; (B) mild; (C) severe slipped upper femoral epiphysis.

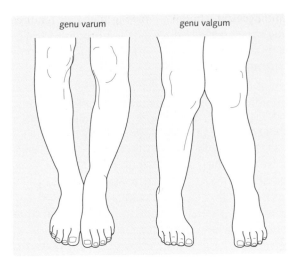

Fig. 5.19 Genu varum and genu valgum.

injury or disease (fractures, rheumatoid arthritis or osteoarthritis, rickets, osteomalacia and Paget's disease of bone).

Meniscal tears

The menisci are C-shaped fibrocartilage structures that are found between the femur and the tibia. They act as shock absorbers. Meniscal tears are common in young men.

Aetiology They are usually caused by a twisting injury, especially in sport.

Pathology The meniscus tears at the medial side more often than the lateral as it is less mobile (Fig. 5.20). The meniscus can tear in a number of different ways. Radial tears are common, causing the knee to click and give way. A 'bucket-handle' tear is when the tear extends over the width of the meniscus, the meniscus remaining attached at both ends. If the unattached torn portion flips over it can become trapped in the joint, preventing its full extension and causing the knee to lock.

Clinical features There is usually a history of injury, commonly during sport, especially on a twisting movement or change of direction. The knee can lock and become painful immediately after injury, or a gradual, chronic pain can develop and persist months after the injury, depending on the location of the tear.

Investigations are not usually reliable and the diagnosis is mostly clinical, with a thorough history and examination findings. On examination, joint

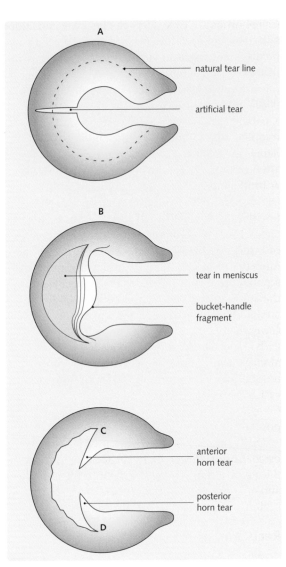

Fig. 5.20 Patterns of meniscal tears. (A) The natural tear line; (B) 'bucket-handle' tear (the most common type); (C) anterior horn tear; (D) posterior horn tear.

line tenderness can be elicited. There may be a joint effusion, locking of the knee or a meniscal cyst, which can be felt laterally.

Management Initial management is with RICE:

- Rest
- Ice
- Compression
- Elevation.

Patients should undergo physiotherapy.

Where they fail to heal, meniscal tears are treated by arthroscopic excision of the displaced tag.

Complications Tears deep in the knee are more avascular and therefore cannot heal. Torn tags can predispose to secondary osteoarthritis because of the irritation to the joint.

Meniscal cysts

Meniscal cysts occur where synovial fluid becomes trapped within a meniscal tear and cannot escape. Pain is often felt over the joint line.

Management Meniscal cysts are treated by arthroscopic excision.

Osteochondritis dissecans

Osteochondritis dissecans is local ischaemic necrosis of bone and articular cartilage. It affects the knee more than any other joint. Osteochondral fragments separate from the bone to produce loose bodies in the joint capsule. It commonly occurs in young adults. The cause of the condition is not known.

Clinical features There is pain arising after exercise, with intermittent swelling of the joint.

Management It usually heals spontaneously and requires no treatment. Attached fragments can be excised or pinned.

Complications Osteochondritis dissecans predisposes to arthritis.

Other causes of loose bodies in the knee include osteoarthritis (fewer than 10 bodies), fracture of the joint surface (fewer than three loose bodies) and synovial chondromatosis (more than 50 loose bodies).

Recurrent dislocation of the patella

Aetiology Dislocation can be habitual, usually in young women in whom the lateral femoral condyle is underdeveloped and/or there is laxity of the support ligaments. Recurrent dislocation of the patella tends to affect adolescent girls, often bilaterally.

Other predisposing factors include anatomical abnormalities of the patella and genu valgum deformity. It can also occur secondary to trauma, usually a blow to the side of the knee when the knee is in slight flexion.

Clinical features The patella displaces laterally when the knee is flexed. There is severe pain in the front of the knee, often with tenderness over the medial joint margin and an effusion. The patient cannot extend the joint and will be unable to bear weight on that leg.

Repeated dislocations can predispose to osteoarthritis.

Management Initial management requires reduction, with short-term immobilization. Physiotherapy is then required to strengthen the quadriceps muscle (especially the vastus medialis muscle). If this fails, the joint needs to be stabilized surgically.

Chondromalacia patellae

Aetiology There is softening of the articular cartilage of the patella. This is an important cause of anterior knee pain, especially in teenage girls.

Clinical features Pain is worse on climbing up and down stairs, and there may be joint effusion. The patient may feel aching around the patella after prolonged sitting. Diagnosis is clinical.

Management Chondromalacia patellae is treated with analgesics and physiotherapy to strengthen the vastus medialis muscle. Surgical correction is not appropriate.

Bursitis of the knee

This is also known as 'housemaid's knee'. Bursae can become inflamed because of infection, gout, trauma or repeated friction, giving rise to an erythematous, warm swelling or effusion.

There are a staggering 16 bursae around the knee. The most commonly affected are the prepatellar ('housemaid's knee'), infrapatellar ('vicar's knee'), and semimembranous bursae (which produces a popliteal cyst).

Infection and gout should be excluded by aspirating fluid and sending it for analysis. The patient should be advised to avoid activities that aggravate the problem, such as kneeling, which may be difficult for those employed in occupations that require kneeling.

Management Rest with NSAIDs and pain relief is usually adequate. Aspiration can relieve symptoms in some cases. Recurrent cases may require a surgical opinion.

A Baker's cyst is a herniation of the joint synovium posteroinferiorly (backwards and downwards). It should not be confused with a popliteal cyst, which is caused by an inflamed semimembranous bursa protruding into the popliteal fossa.

Disorders of the ankle and foot

Club foot (congenital talipes equinovarus)

Congenital club foot occurs in 1 in 1000 births, with boys affected twice as often as girls. The aetiology is unclear, although it is believed there is arrest of normal limb bud development *in utero*. The condition is also associated with spina bifida.

Features include:

- An inverted, supinated foot at the subtalar joint
- Adduction of the forefoot
- Inward rotation (varus) and plantarflexion (equinus) of the heel
- Wasting or underdevelopment of the calf muscles
- A high arch (cavus deformity).

Soft tissue contractures can develop on the medial side of the foot.

Management Congenital club foot is corrected by serial casting changed weekly for 3 months, effective while the ligaments are lax. In severe cases, corrective surgery is usually required but is delayed until the child is 6–9 months old. Most patients go on to lead a normal life.

Pes planus and pes cavus

Pes planus (flat foot) is a flattened longitudinal arch causing the medial border of the foot almost to touch the ground (Fig. 5.21). It is classified as flexible if the arch is flat only on weightbearing, or inflexible (or rigid) if it remains flat when not weightbearing, e.g. standing on tiptoe. It can be congenital or caused by underlying general joint laxity, muscle weakness or paralysis, or postural deformity. Often there are no symptoms, but there

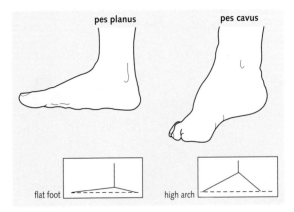

Fig. 5.21 Features of pes planus.

may be foot strain and osteoarthritis of the tarsal joints in later life. Rigid pes planus can be corrected by the use of orthotics.

In pes cavus (hollow foot) there is a high longitudinal arch, which may be congenital or associated with neurological disorders, e.g. Friedreich's ataxia, Charcot–Marie–Tooth disease and peroneal muscular atrophy, leading to weak intrinsic muscles (Fig. 5.21). It is classed as flexible if the height of the arch is reduced when the patient is not weightbearing, or rigid if it is not. There is a predisposition to complications caused by lack of shock absorption, such as stress fractures or metatarsalgia. The toes may become clawed and the metatarsal heads prominent, as they are bearing the weight of the body. Treatment is required if the foot becomes stiff or painful.

> A full neurological examination is required in a patient presenting with pes cavus, as it could be a result of a neuromuscular disorder that may yet be undiagnosed.

Hammer toes

In this condition the toes are flexed at the PIP joint and extended at the MTP joint (Fig. 5.22). The second toes are most commonly affected. The disorder is treated by lengthening the tendons and excising the MTP joint.

Claw toes

In claw toes, the toes are flexed at both the PIP and DIP joints and extended at the MTP joint (see Fig. 5.22). Claw toes occur in rheumatoid arthritis and after poliomyelitis, and are treated by a flexor–extensor transfer operation.

Mallet toes

In mallet toes there is damage to the extensor tendon at its insertion into the distal phalanx. The DIP joint cannot be extended fully. They are treated by placing a splint on the toe with the DIP joint fully extended (Fig. 5.22).

Hallux valgus

In hallux valgus (Fig. 5.23) the big toe deviates laterally at the MTP joint, which develops a protective bursa (bunion) where the shoe rubs.

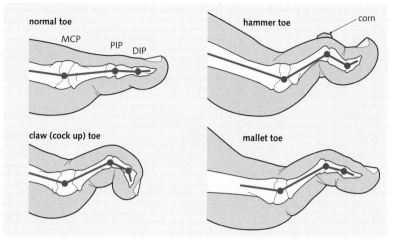

Fig. 5.22 Toe deformities: normal toe, 'claw toe', 'hammer toe' and 'mallet toe'.

This condition may lead to hammer toes, bursitis, metatarsalgia and secondary osteoarthritis of the MTP joint.

The wearing of high heels with pointed toes may contribute to this deformity; it is most often seen in elderly women.

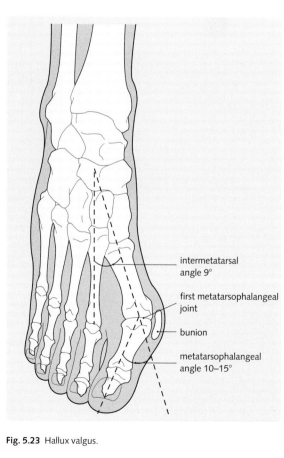

Fig. 5.23 Hallux valgus.

Hallux rigidus

Aetiology Joint stiffness in the big toe, or hallux rigidus, may be due to osteoarthritis of the MTP joint, trauma, osteochondritis dissecans in the head of the first metatarsal bone, or gout. There is pain on walking and limited movement.

Epidemiology Men are more commonly affected than women.

Management Treatment involves dealing with the underlying cause, only replacing the joint where necessary.

Forefoot pain (metatarsalgia)

Forefoot pain may be caused by foot or toe deformities (pes planus, pes cavus, hallux valgus, claw toes). It also occurs in rheumatoid arthritis, stress fractures and Morton's metatarsalgia (Fig. 5.24).

Stress fractures (march fractures)

Stress fractures occur in the shaft of the second (or third) metatarsals of young adults after excessive walking or marching. The fractures are treated by rest and wearing a plaster for 6 weeks during healing.

Morton's metatarsalgia (plantar digital neuritis)

Morton's metatarsalgia is pain produced by compression of an interdigital neuroma between the metatarsals, such as that produced by fashionable shoes. The pain radiates to the third and fourth toes. A compression test over the area of the neuroma is specific and diagnostic. Excision of the neuroma may be required.

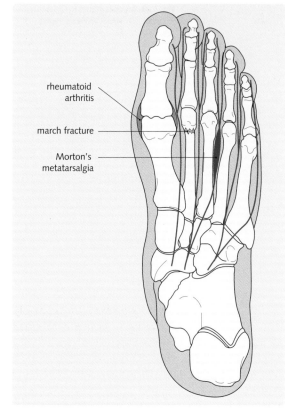

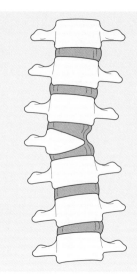

Fig. 5.25 Hemivertebra in the spine, producing scoliosis.

Fig. 5.24 Causes of forefoot pain.

Disorders of the back

Congenital abnormalities

Lumbarization is when S1 remains as a vertebra, and sacralization is fusion of the body of L5 with the sacrum. These are of no clinical consequence.

Hemivertebrae are congenital abnormalities where vertebrae are formed on one lateral side only (Fig. 5.25). The vertebral body is therefore wedge-shaped, causing the spine to angle laterally at this site and producing a degree of scoliosis.

Scoliosis

Scoliosis is the lateral curvature and rotation of the spine with subsequent rib rotation (Fig. 5.26).
Epidemiology It affects up to 2.5% of the population.
Aetiology The causes of scoliosis can be classified as:

- Congenital due to bony anomalies, e.g. hemivertebrae
- Idiopathic, seen in infants and adolescents

- Neuromuscular, e.g. polio, torsion, dystonia
- Secondary to another process, e.g. Duchenne muscular dystrophy, Friedreich's ataxia, osteogenesis imperfecta, sciatica or limb length discrepancy.

Clinical features The patient or their relatives/parents notice a deformity of the ribcage or spine, or a discrepancy in limb length. Pain is not commonly a feature, unless it is associated with an underlying condition causing secondary scoliosis, such as sciatica.
Complications The earlier the onset, the worse the resultant deformity and the greater the risk of progression. The resulting abnormal posture can cause pain. Severe deformity can cause impaired lung function.

Kyphosis

Kyphosis is a flexion deformity of the spine, with cervical and lumbar spine extension and thoracic spine flexion (Fig. 5.27). It can be progressive, eventually producing a hump.

Kyphosis can be caused by conditions affecting the structure of the spine, such as wedge fractures of the vertebrae (e.g. osteoporosis, metastatic carcinoma and TB), ankylosing spondylitis and developmental deficiencies. Congenital kyphosis is rare but serious, as it can rapidly produce cord compression and paraplegia.

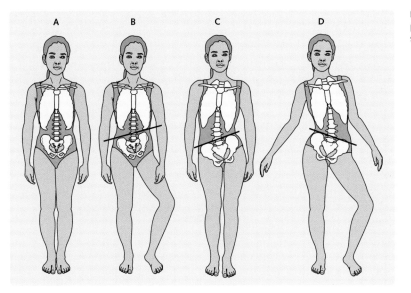

Fig. 5.26 Types of scoliosis. (A) Normal posture; (B) scoliosis due to sciatica; (C) short leg; (D) fixed deformity.

Lordosis

Lordosis is excessive anterior curvature of the spine, usually in the lumbar region (see Fig. 5.27). It may be caused by bad posture, be compensatory for hip deformities, or occur secondary to other conditions such as ankylosing spondylitis.

Disc prolapse

Disc prolapse usually occurs when the nucleus pulposus herniates posteriorly through a weak part of the annulus fibrosus and presses on a spinal nerve root, usually in the lumbar region (Fig. 5.28).

Epidemiology   Disc prolapse is common, with 3% of men and 1% of women suffering from sciatica secondary to a prolapsed disc. It commonly occurs in those between 35 and 55 years of age.

Pathology   The annulus through which herniation commonly occurs is thinner posterolaterally. The

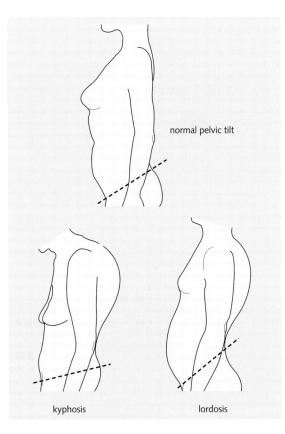

Fig. 5.27   Features of kyphosis and lordosis. Normal posture, kyphosis and lordosis.

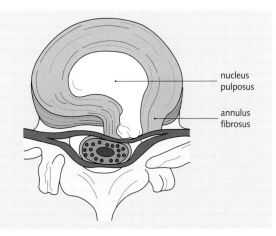

Fig. 5.28   Intervertebral disc prolapse.

herniated nucleus can press on adjacent spinal nerve roots, irritating them and producing pain along their peripheral distribution. Central prolapse of the disc can occur, compressing combined nerve roots, including those supplying the bladder and bowel and causing cauda equina syndrome. Disc prolapse can occur at any level, but most commonly at L4/L5 or L5/S1, compressing the sciatic nerve roots.

Clinical features Sudden pain can be felt in the lumbar region (lumbago) or, if there is compression of a nerve root, may radiate to the buttocks and legs (sciatica). There is limited flexion and extension.

In cauda equina syndrome there is bowel and bladder dysfunction and saddle anaesthesia. There is a loss of anal tone and decreased peripheral sensation.

Diagnosis X-rays should be performed to exclude bony pathology, and are normal. An MRI is a gold standard diagnostic test.

Management Disc prolapse is usually treated conservatively, with rest, analgesia and gentle physiotherapy; 70% of cases settle spontaneously. Surgery is indicated where the patient develops cauda equina syndrome, where symptoms do not settle after 6–8 weeks, are progressive or a neurological deficit develops.

Spondylolisthesis

In spondylolisthesis there is forward displacement of a vertebral body onto the one below, usually at L5/S1. The degree of slip can be graded on a scale of 1 to 4.

It presents with persistent back pain, and a 'step' can be palpated over the spine, with tenderness on palpation. Nerve root irritation can develop. A degree of kyphosis or scoliosis can also occur.

Spondylolisthesis is common, affecting 5% of the population, but most often patients remain asymptomatic.

Diagnosis An oblique X-ray can demonstrate a characteristic 'collar on Scottie dog' appearance, with a lateral X-ray showing the degree of slip. It can also be clearly seen on CT. An MRI scan is required if there is nerve root irritation.

Treatment The patient should be advised to rest and reduce their activities, given adequate analgesia and referred for physiotherapy. Surgery is indicated where pain is persistent or radiculopathy and deformity develop. Fusion and a bone graft can be performed.

Spinal stenosis

Spinal stenosis is narrowing of the spinal canal. It may be caused by degeneration and long-term osteoarthritis, and results in compression of the nerve roots.

Standing and walking lead to severe pain in the buttocks and thighs, as nerves and blood vessels are cramped, producing ischaemia of the spinal nerves they supply. The pain is referred down the legs to the calves and the feet. Pain is exacerbated by extending the spine and relieved by flexing it or by rest.

X-rays can reveal degenerative changes. CT and MRI scans reveal the degree of stenosis and nerve root involvement.

In mild disease, depending on the cause, weight loss, physiotherapy and NSAIDs may relieve symptoms. Severe symptoms may require surgical decompression. The condition tends to progress.

Back strain

Without an adequate warm-up, the muscles and ligaments of the lumbar spine can be strained during unaccustomed or sudden movements.

Back strain is treated by rest, analgesics, application of heat and gradual remobilization.

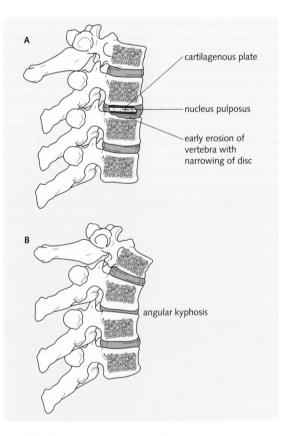

Fig. 5.29 Tuberculosis of the spine (Pott's disease) showing (A) erosion of vertebra; (B) subsequent collapse in front, resulting in angular curvature.

Tuberculosis in the back (Potts' disease)

Tuberculosis (TB) of the spine is called Pott's disease (Fig. 5.29). The spine is the most likely part of the skeleton to be affected by TB.

In Pott's disease the vertebral bodies collapse onto each other, creating a sharply angled 'gibbus' deformity. Local osteoporosis later gives rise to bone destruction, producing wedging of the vertebrae. There is also a risk of cord compression (Pott's paraplegia), abscess formation, chronic discharging sinus, and the spread of TB to other organs.

Pott's disease is treated with antituberculous chemotherapeutic drugs. The pus is surgically drained and any dead bone removed. The vertebrae may require fixation with bone grafting.

Pain referred to the back

Retroperitoneal disease in the abdomen (duodenal ulcer, pancreatic cancer, aneurysm) may cause back pain.

Period pain and sciatic pain also radiate to the back. A comprehensive systemic history and examination are essential to identify clinical signs that may distinguish factors in most cases, and to direct further investigations.

Skin 6

Objectives

By the end of this chapter you should be able to:

- Describe the layers of the epidermis and the associated stages of keratinocyte maturation
- Distinguish between lanugo, vellus and terminal hair
- Explain finger clubbing and list some important causes
- Differentiate between eccrine and apocrine sweat glands and list the functions of sweat.
- Understand the functions of the skin and the specific cells that carry out those functions
- Describe the different functions of Merkel cells, Meissner's corpuscles and Pacinian corpuscles
- Explain the functions and types of melanin
- Describe the four different types of hypersensitivity reaction

ORGANIZATION OF THE SKIN

The skin is the largest organ in the body, making up 16% of the body's weight, and has a surface area of ~1.8 m². It has an essential role in homoeostasis and protection from external influences. The skin is composed of three layers:

- The epidermis—stratified squamous epithelium
- The dermis—supportive connective tissue matrix
- The subcutaneous layer—loose connective tissue and fat.

The epidermis and dermis are derived from different embryonic components. The epidermis, developing from ectoderm, develops by the first month of gestation. The dermis develops from mesoderm and develops later, usually at around 11 weeks. By 17 weeks' gestation, the skin ridges that cause fingerprints have developed.

The composition of the three separate layers of the skin (see Fig. 1.3) is described below.

Epidermis

The epidermis is a stratified epithelium of ectodermal origin. It is generally around 0.1 mm thick, although it reaches depths of between 0.8 and 1.4 mm on the palms of the hands and soles of the feet. The epidermis is very cellular but avascular. It comprises four separate layers:

- Stratum basale (basal cell layer)
- Stratum spinosum (prickle cell layer)
- Stratum granulosum (granular cell layer)
- Stratum corneum (horny layer).

These four layers are formed by keratinocytes (the main cell type of the epidermis) that progress through their different stages of maturation to form the protein keratin (Fig. 6.1).

Some agents are sufficiently lipid soluble to be absorbed through the skin or mucous membranes and can be applied directly to the site where action is required. An example is steroids, which are used for many inflammatory skin conditions. However, caution with the dosage and frequency of application is required because appreciable absorption can occur, leading to systemic side effects.

Stratum basale

This layer is firmly anchored to the underlying basement membrane. It is composed of 90% basal

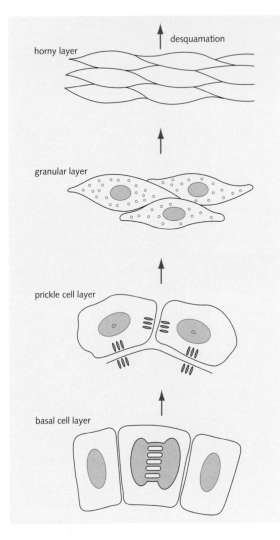

horny layer

desquamation

granular layer

prickle cell layer

basal cell layer

Fig. 6.1 The differing stages of keratinocyte maturation. (Adapted with permission from Gawkrodger DJ. Dermatology: an illustrated colour text, 2nd edn. Edinburgh: Churchill Livingstone, 1997.)

cells (keratinocytes), melanocytes (5–10%) and infrequent Merkel cells. Basal cells are the skin's stem cells, which divide to replace superficial keratinocytes shed at the epithelial surface. They are anchored to the basement membrane by hemidesmosomes.

Melanocytes synthesize melanin, which protects the basal cells by absorbing the energy of ultraviolet radiation and acting as a free-radical scavenger. Melanocytes originate from the neural crest and are most numerous on sites exposed to the sun. Merkel cells are specialized epithelial cells, which are sensitive to touch and stimulate sensory nerve fibres when they are physically stimulated. They also contain neuroendocrine vesicles that can be

visualized on electron microscopy. The stratum basale forms epidermal ridges that extend into the dermis, increasing contact between the two layers. These are highly developed in areas exposed to high levels of shearing stress, such as the hands and feet.

Stratum spinosum

As keratinocytes divide in the stratum basale, new daughter cells migrate upwards, forming the stratum spinosum. They are bound together by desmosomes. When seen under a light microscope, desmosomes form the 'prickles' that give the layer its name. This layer is around 8–10 cells thick. It also contains Langerhans' cells, which migrate from the bone marrow and bind penetrating environmental antigens, presenting them to lymphocytes in a mechanism participating in the systemic immune response.

Stratum granulosum

In this layer, keratinocytes produce keratohyalin and keratin granules. As the keratinocytes begin to mature, the cells flatten, lose their intracellular organelles and nuclei, and die. Disintegration of their intracellular content causes them to dehydrate, which results in the production of a tough, impermeable layer of keratin surrounded by keratohyalin.

Stratum corneum

This outer 'horny' layer contains 15–30 layers of keratinized, overlapping cells that lack nuclei, glued together tightly by desmosomes. The keratin provides flexibility and strength. The stratum corneum is water resistant, but not waterproof. Interstitial fluid is lost through the stratum corneum in the process of insensible perspiration.

Dermis

Lying beneath the epidermis, this layer varies greatly in thickness, ranging from 0.6 mm on the eyelids to 3 mm on the palms and soles. It consists of two layers: the superficial papillary layer and the underlying reticular layer.

The papillary layer contains capillaries and sensory nerves that supply the skin surface, embedded in loose connective tissue. This layer projects into the epidermis in papillae to form so-called rete ridges. The reticular layer contains bundles of collagen fibres that anchor the papillary layer to the underlying subcutaneous layer. In addition, the dermis contains mast cells and specialized nerve endings as well as vascular plexuses, hair follicles and sweat glands.

Subcutaneous layer

Situated directly beneath the dermis, the subcutaneous layer is made up of loose connective tissue and fat. It is important in maintaining the stability of the skin with relation to its underlying tissues and structures. Most fat cells in the body are housed within this layer, and these subcutaneous fat deposits are collectively referred to as adipose tissue. Adipose tissue helps to reduce heat loss, absorb blows to the body, and is an important energy reserve.

> Agents that can be delivered in transdermal patches include nicotine for smoking cessation and oestrogen in hormone replacement therapy. The drug is incorporated into a patch that is applied to a relatively thin skin area, providing a steady rate of drug delivery and thereby avoiding presystemic hepatic metabolism. However, such patches can cause cutaneous irritation, which can be minimized by varying the site of application.

SKIN PHYSIOLOGY

Keratinocytes, the basic building blocks of the skin, take around 15–30 days to mature fully as they rise from the basal layer to the stratum corneum; dividing cells in the stratum basale replicate every 200–400 h.

Dead corneocytes are shed from the horny layer around 2 weeks later. This cell turnover period of 28 days is dramatically shortened in disorders of keratinization, such as psoriasis.

Keratinocytes are also involved in the pathology of primary blistering skin disorders. Circulating autoantibodies bind to components within the intercellular epidermal substance and induce the release of proteolytic enzymes from the adjacent keratinocytes. These enzymes cause the loss of adhesion between cells and result in splits within the epidermis or at the dermoepidermal junction.

> In an average lifetime, the body sheds about 40 lb of skin

Nerves in the skin

The skin is responsible for the perception of touch and temperature, and is richly innervated. The densest concentrations of nerve endings are found in areas where sensation is most important: the hands, face and genitalia. Different types of sensory detectors are found in the skin (Fig. 6.2). Free sensory nerve endings are found within the dermis and epidermis, and detect pain, itch and temperature. They contain neuropeptide transmitters such as substance P. Corpuscular receptors, which are specialized for certain types of sensation, are also found in the dermis: these are Pacinian corpuscles, which detect pressure and vibration, and Meissner's

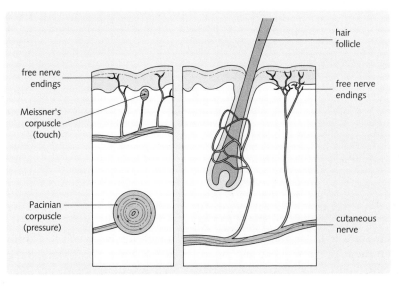

Fig. 6.2 The different types of nerve detector within the skin. (Adapted with permission from Gawkrodger DJ. Dermatology: an illustrated colour text, 2nd edn. Edinburgh: Churchill Livingstone, 1997.)

free nerve endings

Meissner's corpuscle (touch)

Pacinian corpuscle (pressure)

hair follicle

free nerve endings

cutaneous nerve

corpuscles, which are sensitive to touch and are found in the dermal papillae of the feet and hands. Merkel cells are derived embryologically from the neural crest and play a role in sensation by acting as mechanoreceptors. They are located in the basal layer of the epidermis.

The sensory nerve fibres that innervate the skin are both myelinated and non-myelinated, and their cell bodies are contained within the dorsal root ganglia.

Vessels in the skin

The skin has a rich blood supply, formed by two main plexuses that originate from larger vessels in the subcutaneous layer and localized to the reticular dermis.

The superficial vascular plexus runs in the upper reticular layer of the dermis, close to the papillary dermis, with capillaries running from it to the basement membrane at the dermoepidermal junction.

The deep vascular plexus runs in the lower reticular dermis, running close to the subcutaneous layer.

Blood vessels form arteriovenous anastomoses in the dermis, which are under sympathetic autonomic control. By controlling their dilatation, or contraction, they regulate blood flow, altering the level of direct heat loss through the skin. In this way they play a direct role in thermoregulation of the body (Fig. 6.3).

Lymphatic drainage of the skin occurs through lymphatic meshes that originate in the papillae and go on to become larger lymphatic vessels, which subsequently drain into regional lymph nodes.

A burn is an injury to the skin caused by heat, electricity, chemicals or radiation. A scald is an injury caused by hot fluids, often localized to one area.

FUNCTIONS OF THE SKIN

Skin performs several functions, including:

- Mechanical barrier to infections, toxins, antigens and external insults
- Contributing to thermoregulation
- Maintaining cutaneous immunity and coordinating wound-healing responses
- Synthesizing vitamin D within the epidermis on exposure to sunlight
- Protecting against excessive water absorption or loss
- Protecting, via skin pigmentation, against ultraviolet (UV) light
- Providing and mediating sensation, distinguishing between pain, touch, pressure and temperature modalities.

Keratinocyte function

The main function of keratinocytes is to produce the protein called keratin. The stages of keratinocyte maturation have been described. Each different stage of maturation produces different molecular weight keratins (e.g. 50, 55, 57 and 67 kDa), hence different keratins are found in each separate layer of the epidermis.

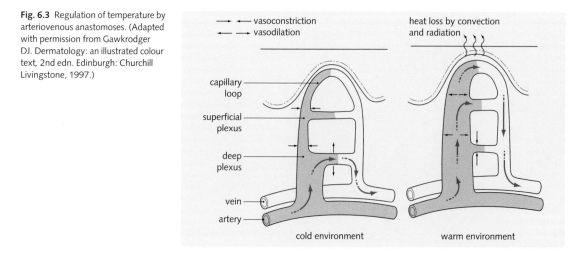

Fig. 6.3 Regulation of temperature by arteriovenous anastomoses. (Adapted with permission from Gawkrodger DJ. Dermatology: an illustrated colour text, 2nd edn. Edinburgh: Churchill Livingstone, 1997.)

Melanocyte function

Melanocytes are found within the basal layer of the epidermis. They produce melanin, a brown pigment that forms a protective cap over the nuclei of keratinocytes in the epidermis, protecting them from the UV rays of the sun. They are in the basal layer, in contact with the basement membrane. They have long dendritic processes that extend between keratinocytes. The number of melanocytes remains constant. In fact, it is their melanin-synthesizing activity that is responsible for skin colour across different races, not the number of melanocytes. Their level of activity is genetically determined. In addition, the amount of melanin in the skin can be temporarily increased in response to exposure to sunlight, as preformed melanin is photo-oxidized, stimulating melanocytes to produce more melanin, resulting in a 'tan'.

As well as absorbing the energy of UV radiation, melanin also acts as a free-radical scavenger and an energy sink. Melanin itself is produced from tyrosine (Fig. 6.4) and comes in two forms, eumelanin and phaeomelanin. Eumelanin, the more common form, produces a brown–black colour. Phaeomelanin produces a yellow–red coloration, the pigment in blonde and red-haired people. Most melanins are a mixture of the two different forms.

Fibroblast function

Fibroblasts produce and secrete the components of the extracellular matrix, an intricate meshwork of fibrous proteins embedded in a gel-like ground substance. The extracellular matrix holds the cells together, so the majority are not in direct physical contact with each other. Nutrients, waste products and other water-soluble materials diffuse through the matrix between the blood vessels and cells.

The main components of the extracellular matrix produced by fibroblasts are collagen, elastin and structural proteoglycans such as glycosaminoglycans (GAGs). Their functions are discussed in Chapter 1. Collagen is the major structural protein of the dermis, and makes up 70–80% of its dry weight. Four main types of collagen are found in the skin (Fig. 6.5).

The structure of collagen fibres provides tensile strength, conferring resistance to longitudinal stress. In disorders where there is pathology of the collagen, such as scurvy (a disease caused by vitamin C deficiency), tissues that rely on collagen for strength become fragile. In skin, the blood vessels are easily

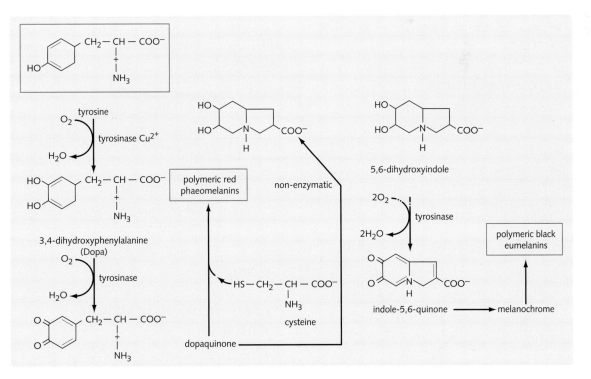

Fig. 6.4 Biosynthesis of melanin from tyrosine. (Adapted with permission from Gawkrodger DJ. Dermatology: an illustrated colour text, 2nd edn. Edinburgh: Churchill Livingstone, 1997.)

Fig. 6.5 Types of collagen found in the skin

Types of collagen	Location
type I	reticular dermis
type III	papillary dermis
types IV and VII	basement membrane structures

damaged and bleeding is very noticeable in the mucous membranes, especially in the gums.

Elastin is a rubber protein fibre that mediates the natural tissue stretch and recoil. In the skin, it maintains normal elasticity and flexibility.

The structural proteoglycans that make up the ground substance of the skin are mainly glycosaminoglycans; these provide turgor and maintain hydration of the skin.

Although other more sophisticated techniques are used to assess the size of a burn in hospital management, a burn can be quantified acutely using the 'rule of nines' comparing the proportion to the size of body areas: full arm 9%; front of torso 18%; back of torso 18%; full head 9%; full leg 18%; genitalia 1%; palm 1%.

Thermoregulation

Thermoregulation helps to maintain the body's core temperature at $37°C$ in different climatic conditions and during physical exertion. It is dependent on metabolic and physical factors. Evaporation of sweat from the skin surface aids cooling, and the diversion of blood between deep and superficial vascular plexuses also plays an important role in temperature regulation (see Fig. 6.3).

Immune functions of the skin

The skin provides a barrier to protect the body from invading organisms. Where it is broken or infiltrated there is activation of the natural defence mechanisms of the cutaneous immune system (Fig. 6.6).

Epidermal barrier

This physical structure provides an impenetrable barrier to most microorganisms that come into contact with it.

Cutaneous immunity

Langerhans' cells are the first line of defence against microorganisms penetrating the epidermis. Found predominantly in the stratum spinosum, these are dendritic cells from which cytoplasmic processes extend and interweave between keratinocytes. They can be distinguished histologically by Birbeck granules, a cell-specific cytoplasmic organelle. Langerhans' cells play an important role in the cutaneous immune response by binding an antigen and 'presenting' it to the immune system.

Mast cells

Mast cells are found within the dermis and are involved in the immediate (type I) hypersensitivity reaction. They can be recruited to sites of inflammation and infection within the dermis.

Keratinocytes

As well as producing keratin, keratinocytes also synthesize proinflammatory cytokines, such as interleukin-1 (IL-1), which are important messengers in the immune response. Keratinocytes can also express surface immune reactive molecules such as intercellular adhesion molecules (e.g. ICAM-1) and the gene products of major histocompatibility complex (MHC), such as class II antigens (e.g. HLA DR), which play an important role in immunological recognition (Fig. 6.7) and human allotransplantation.

Cytokines and eicosanoids

The cytokines include γ-interferon, IL-1, IL-2 and IL-3. Produced mainly by T lymphocytes, they are important mediators in the cutaneous immune response, binding to antigenic surface receptors and signalling to other cells involved in the immune response, recruiting them to attack the antigen. Eicosanoids are a class of oxygenated hydrophobic mediators, derived from arachidonic acid and produced by mast cells, macrophages and keratinocytes. They are non-specific inflammatory signalling mediators.

Hypersensitivity reactions of the skin

Hypersensitivity is an immune reaction to an innocuous molecule that the body recognizes as foreign, in which the adaptive immune response is exaggerated or inappropriate. An allergy is an antigen-

Fig. 6.6 Immune components of the skin

Type of defence	Different components	Action
structural	skin	impenetrable physical barrier to most outside organisms
	blood and lymphatic channels	provide transport network for cellular defence
cellular	langerhans cells	play important role in antigen presentation
	T lymphocytes	facilitate immune reactions, including cell destruction. Self-regulating through the action of suppressor T cells
	mast cells	facilitate inflammatory reaction of the skin
	keratinocytes	produce inflammatory cytokines; have the ability to express surface immune reactive molecules
systemic	skin-associated lymphoid tissue	as skin contains the above immune cells and structural defences, it can be classified as a fully functioning immunological unit
	cytokines and eicosanoids	cytokines are cell-mediation molecules produced by components of the cellular defence system; eicosanoids are non-specific inflammatory mediators produced by mast cells, macrophages and keratinocytes
	complement cascade	activation of the complement cascade initiates a variety of destructive mechanisms, including opsonization, lysis, chemotaxis and mast cell degranulation
	adhesion molecules	cellular binding e.g. T cells
immunogenetic	major histocompatibility complex (MHC)	facilitates immunological recognition of antigens. Located on HLA gene cluster; the appearance of specific HLA genes is associated with certain pathologies, e.g. ankylosing spondylitis is associated with HLA B27

specific inappropriate immune reaction to a normally harmless substance in the environment. There are four main types of hypersensitivity response, all of which are exhibited in the skin (Fig. 6.8). You should refer to a good immunology text book to refamiliarise yourself with the pathophysiology of inflammation and immunology.

Skin secretions

The components of sweat, sebum and epidermal lipids differ in content. Sweat is a watery isotonic liquid that is secreted at the skin's surface. It has a low pH of between 4 and 6.8, which makes the skin slightly acidic and discourages microbial growth. The minimum insensible loss through perspiration per day is 0.5 L and the maximum daily output is 10 L, which is limited by the body's ability to sweat 2 L/h. Men sweat more than women.

As well as lowering the skin's pH and cooling the skin, sweat hydrates the outer layers of the epidermis and aids the hands and feet in gripping.

Fig. 6.7 HLA antigens associated with skin diseases

Skin disease	HLA antigen
psoriasis	Cw6
Reiter's disease	B27
dermatitis herpetiformis	B8

Hormone production and the skin

The skin manufactures vitamin D in the dermis but is also affected by many other hormones (Fig. 6.9). See Chapter 4, and specifically Figure 4.12, for further reference.

Fig. 6.8 Hypersensitivity reactions of the skin

type I (intermediate)	Fc receptors bind immunoglobulin E(IgE) to the surface of mast cells; when an antigen is encountered, the IgE molecules cross-link. This action stimulates the release of inflammatory mediators such as histamine, prostaglandins and leukotrienes. The response occurs within minutes, although there is a delayed component present, and results in urticaria in the skin. Massivehistamine release can cause anaphylaxis. The most common allergens that provoke anallergic reaction are pollen grains, bee stings, penicillin, certain foods, moulds and house-dust mites.
type II (antibody-dependent cytotoxicity)	when antigens bind to target skin cells on the basement membrane, a reaction occurs whereby cytotoxic killer T cells or complement activation destroy the foreign body. The powerful effects of complement cascade activation include opsonization, lysis, mast cell degranulation, smooth muscle contraction and chemotaxis. Haemolytic anaemia and transfusion reactions are examples of type II hypersensitivity, as is the pathology involved in pemphigus: IgG antibodies, which are directed against keratinocyte surface antigens, result in lysis of the keratinocytes causing intra-epidermal splitting. This results in characteristic skin blisters of pemphigus.
type III (immune complex disease)	when antigens and antibodies bind in the blood, an immune complex is formed, which is deposited in the walls of small blood vessels such as those found in the skin. Although these complexes are usually removed by the reticuloendothelial system, a leucocytoclastic vasculitis can sometimes occur; vascular damage caused by complement activation and lysosomal enzymes released from polymorphs. This vasculitis is seen in systemic lupus erythematosus, dermatomyositis and microbial infections such as infective endocarditis.
type IV (cell-mediated or delayed)	pre-sensitized T cells come into secondary contact with the antigen after it has become bound to an antigen-presenting cell. The T cells release cytokines, which in turn activate other T cells and macrophages—the process takes some time and the damage to tissue is most pronounced after 48–72 hours. Disorders that contain a variant of type IV hypersensitivity in their pathology include allergic contact dermatitis, leprosy and tuberculosis.

Adapted with permission from Gawkrodger DJ. Dermatology: an illustrated colour text, 2nd edn. Edinburgh: Churchill Livingstone, 1997.

Adapted with permission from Gawkrodger DJ. Dermatology: an illustrated colour text, 2nd edn. Edinburgh: Churchill Livingstone, 1997.

Fig. 6.9 Hormones and the skin

Hormone	Site of production	Action on skin
corticosteroids	adrenal cortex	vasoconstriction, decreased mitosis of basal cells, anti-inflammatory role
androgens	adrenal cortex, gonads	stimulate growth of terminal hair, stimulate sebum production
oestrogens	adrenal cortex, ovaries	stimulate melanin production
melanocyte-stimulating hormone (MSH)	pituitary gland	stimulates melanin production
adrenocorticotrophic hormone (ACTH)	pituitary gland	stimulates melanin production
epidermal growth factors (EGF)	skin	stimulates cell differentiation, a role in calcium metabolism
vitamin D	skin	no effect on skin, plays a role in bone metabolism

DERIVATIVE STRUCTURES OF THE SKIN

Hair

In our now relatively bald state, humans no longer rely on hair to play a vital role in the conservation of heat. Although scalp hair does provide some protection against the harmful effects of ultraviolet radiation and minor injuries, the main role of hair today is as an organ of sexual attraction. There are approximately 5 million hairs on the body, 98% of which are located on the skin surface. Hair is found in varying densities over the entire surface of the body except for the vulval introitus, glans penis and the palms and soles. Hairs emerge from follicles, which are most densely distributed on the scalp and face.

Structure of the hair follicle

Follicles extend into the deep dermis or subcutis, and surround the developing hair fibre. Invaginating the base of the follicle is the hair papilla, a structure formed from connective tissue, which holds capillaries and nerves that supply the follicle. The hair bulb surrounds the papilla with epithelial cells. The epithelial wall of the follicle contains the germinative cells that produce the structural components of the hair. It is formed by two layers:

- An internal root sheath, found deep within the follicle, that surrounds the root. It does not extend up through the entire length of the follicle, but blends into the external root sheath
- An external root sheath, extending the entire length of the follicle. It is composed mostly of the same layers that form the superficial epidermis.

Arrectores pilorum are smooth muscle strands that extend from the papillary dermis to the base of the hair follicle. In response to cold, fear and emotion they contract and pull the hair erect, producing 'goosebumps'. This is thought to be a leftover from our evolution from mammals, in which this reflex increases the insulatory capabilities of the skin.

As a person ages, their hair can lose its natural colour and become grey, owing to depigmentation of the growing hairs. Melanocytes at the base of the hair follicles are responsible for producing pigment, and over time there is a reduction in melanin production, leading to a gradual loss of colour. Some genes have been implicated with the process of greying.

Structure of hair

Hair is produced by the division of an epithelial layer called the hair matrix (Fig. 6.10). The hair fibre consists of three layers:

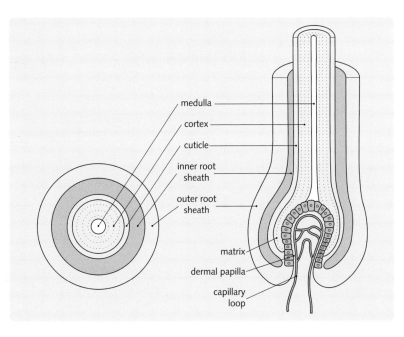

Fig. 6.10 Structure of hair follicle. (Adapted with permission from Gawkrodger DJ. Dermatology: an illustrated colour text, 2nd edn. Edinburgh: Churchill Livingstone, 1997.)

medulla
cortex
cuticle
inner root sheath
outer root sheath
matrix
dermal papilla
capillary loop

- The inner medulla, or core, which contains flexible keratin
- The outer cortex, which contains hard keratin that gives a hair its stiffness.
- The hair fibre is coated by a surface layer of keratin, termed the cuticle.

The length of a hair follicle can be seen to consist of two parts:

- The hair root—the lower part in which the hair is produced
- The hair shaft forms the upper part of the hair.

Classification of hair types

There are three types of hair:

- Lanugo hairs: these are formed at 20 weeks' gestation and are usually shed before the fetus is born. They can be seen in premature babies, and are fine and long. In adults, they only develop in certain pathological conditions
- Vellus hairs: the commonest hair type, covering most of the surface of the body. They are short, fine and light in colour
- Terminal hairs: these are thick and long. There are around 100 000 terminal hairs on the scalp, and they are also found in the eyebrows, eyelashes, pubic and axillary regions. They are also the hairs that compose the beard.

Stages of hair production

Hair growth is cyclical, with the normal rate being ~0.4 mm/day. During growth, the hair root remains firmly attached to the matrix. When growth is complete, the follicle becomes inactive and shrinks

and the attachment breaks down. As another growth cycle begins to produce a new hair, the old hair is pushed upwards and is eventually shed (Fig. 6.11)

Abrupt cessation of hair growth (anagen effluvium) occurs after ingestion of drugs such as cytotoxins, heparin and warfarin, carbimazole, colchicine and vitamin A. It may also follow ingestion of poisons such as thallium.

Hair colour is determined genetically by variations in pigment production by melanocytes in the hair bulb. It is also influenced by hormones and environmental factors.

Nails

Consisting of a dense plate of cells packed with hardened keratin between 0.3 and 0.5 mm thick, the nail is a remnant of the mammalian claw. Its function is to protect the tip of the finger and facilitate grasping.

Structure of the nail

The nail is composed of a nail plate, which originates from the nail matrix (or root) and overlies the nail bed (Fig. 6.12). Growth originates from the root, an epithelial fold that lies close to the periosteum of the tip of the bone. It is composed of dividing keratinocytes which mature and keratinize into the nail plate. Underneath the nail plate lies the nail bed; this structure produces a small amount of keratin. The pink appearance of the nail plate is

Fig. 6.11 Stages of hair development. (Adapted with permission from Gawkrodger DJ. Dermatology: an illustrated colour text, 2nd edn. Edinburgh: Churchill Livingstone, 1997.)

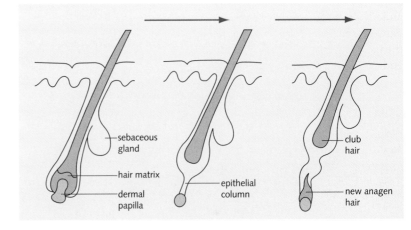

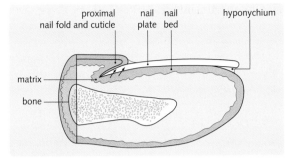

Fig. 6.12 Structure of the nail. (Adapted with permission from Gawkrodger DJ. Dermatology: an illustrated colour text, 2nd edn. Edinburgh: Churchill Livingstone, 1997.)

Fig. 6.13 Some causes of finger clubbing

respiratory	lung cancer, cystic fibrosis, idiopathic pulmonary fibrosis, pleural mesothelioma, bronchiectasis, pleural empyema and lung abscess
cardiac	cyanotic congenital heart disease, infective endocarditis
castrointestinal	ulcerative colitis, Crohn's disease, primary biliary cirrhosis, cirrhosis of the liver

(Adapted with permission from Kumar PJ, Clarke ML. Principles of clinical medicine, 2nd edn. London: Baillière Tindall, 1990.)

caused by dermal capillaries that underlie the nail and which are obscured from view near the root by the white lunula at the base of the nail. The thickened epidermis that underlies the free margin of the nail at the proximal end is called the hyponychium. A portion of epithelium extends up from the nail root to form the protective cuticle.

The nail is bound at the base by the proximal nail fold, and on either side by the lateral nail folds.

Nail growth

Fingernails grow at 0.1 mm/day; the toenails grow more slowly. Any pathological process that disturbs nail growth can leave visible clinical signs in the nail. Systemic illness may lead to transverse grooves in the nail called Beau's lines, which indicate an interruption to the growth of the nail matrix. Cytotoxic drugs cause black transverse bands in the nail, heavy metal poisoning causes white transverse bands, and trauma to the nail matrix can cause white spots within the nail or splinter haemorrhages.

Clubbing of the nails is caused by many disorders (Fig. 6.13); the nail matrix increases in vascularity and feels fluctuant. In addition, the normal angle between the base of the nail and the nail fold is lost, the nail curvature increases in all directions, and the end of the finger may expand.

Injuries to the nail bed usually heal well, although the patient should be advised that there may be permanent deformity of the nail. New nail growth can take months, and even then it can take years for the affected nail to regain its proper shape.

Glands of the skin

There are two types of exocrine gland in the skin:

- Sebaceous glands
- Sweat glands.

Sebaceous glands

Derived from epidermal cells, sebaceous glands are closely associated with hair follicles and produce an oily sebum (Fig. 6.14). Sebum is a mixture of triglycerides, cholesterol, proteins and electrolytes. It flows into the hair follicles and travels to the surface of the skin, where it oils both the hair and the keratinized surface of the skin to help protect them from dehydration and cracking. The secretions are bactericidal (toxic to bacteria). Sebaceous glands are sensitive to androgens and become active at puberty. They are most numerous over the scalp, face, chest and back. They are not present on hairless skin.

The normal pH of facial skin is about 5.5. As soaps are alkaline, they can produce irritant contact dermatitis in susceptible individuals, such as those with sensitive skin or those who suffer atopic conditions. Allergic contact dermatitis is commonly caused by perfumes or preservatives found in cosmetics such as moisturizers and hair dyes.

Sweat glands

These glands are located within the dermis and are present over the whole of the body surface—there are an estimated 2.5 million of them. They are composed

Fig. 6.14 Location of sebaceous and sweat glands

Type of gland	Location
sebaceous	associated with hair follicles; found on scalp, face, chest and back. Absent from hairless skin
eccrine sweat	widely distributed, but most numerous on palms, soles, axillae and forehead
apocrine sweat	open into hair follicles; profuse around axillae, perineum and areolae

(Adapted with permission from Kumar PJ, Clarke ML. Principles of clinical medicine, 3rd edn. London: Baillière Tindall, 1990.)

of coiled tubes that secrete a watery substance, and are divided into two different types (Fig. 6. 14):

- Eccrine
- Apocrine.

Eccrine glands

Eccrine glands occur as downgrowths of epidermis around the 16th week of gestation. They are found all over the skin, especially in the palms, soles, axillae and forehead, but not in mucous membranes. They release their secretions directly onto the skin surface. Eccrine glands are under psychological and thermal control and are innervated by sympathetic (cholinergic) nerve fibres. They produce sweat as part of the body's thermoregulatory process, thereby cooling the skin. It is also a means by which electrolytes and some drugs are excreted. Sweat is chiefly composed of water, but also contains sodium chloride, urea, fatty acids and organic nutrients.

Apocrine glands

These are large sweat glands, the ducts of which empty into the hair follicles. They are present in the axillae, anogenital region, areolae and eyelids. They become active at puberty and produce a sticky, odourless, protein-rich secretion that gives out a characteristic odour when modified by skin bacteria. They are surrounded by myoepithelial cells, whose contractions cause the glands to discharge into the hair follicle. These glands are under the control of sympathetic (adrenergic) nerve fibres and circulating hormones. The apocrine glands are a phylogenetic remnant of the mammalian sexual scent gland. Wax in the ears is produced by a modified version of the same gland.

The slightly acidic pH of the skin (between 6 and 7) is maintained by sebum, sweat, and the intercellular lipids of the stratum corneum. This lower pH level discourages microbial growth on the skin surface.

Disorders of the skin

Objectives

By the end of this chapter you should be able to:

- Differentiate between vesicles, bullae and pustules
- List the five different types of psoriasis and describe the differences between them
- Describe the topical treatments for eczema
- Describe the pathways through which histamine is released in urticaria
- List the physical features of Reiter's disease
- Name some conditions aggravated by sunlight
- List the staphylococcal infections that affect the skin
- Describe the course of an infection with *Herpes simplex*
- List the factors that predispose to *Candida albicans* infection
- Describe the treatments available for scabies
- Describe the different types of naevi and their distribution
- List the risk factors for malignant melanoma
- Discuss the differences between basal cell and squamous cell carcinoma
- List the causes of hirsutism
- Explain Raynaud's phenomenon
- Describe the differing pathologies of leg ulcers
- List the cutaneous forms of malnutrition
- Name skin changes in pregnancy.

TERMINOLOGY OF SKIN DISORDERS

Dermatologists use very specific terms to describe skin disorders. They can manifest locally as lesions, or in a more widespread pattern of involvement as eruptions (rashes). These terms are split into macroscopic and microscopic.

Macroscopic appearances

Macule (Fig. 7.1A)

A flat, circumscribed lesion; an area of colour or textural change. Macules are seen in vitiligo (hypopigmentation), freckles (hyperpigmentation) and capillary haemangioma (red/purple).

Papule (Fig. 7.1B)

A solid, circumscribed, palpable elevation of skin less than 5 mm in diameter. They can appear in various forms: e.g. dome shaped (xanthomas), flat topped (lichen planus).

Nodule (Fig. 7.1C)

An elevation more than 5 mm in diameter that may be either solid or oedematous. Nodules are seen in rheumatoid arthritis, and a dermatofibroma is another example of this type of lesion.

Plaque (Fig. 7.1D)

A plaque is an extended, flat-topped lesion, a palpable elevation of skin (measuring no more than 5 mm in elevation but generally more than 2 cm in diameter). Plaques are commonly seen in psoriasis and mycosis fungoides (cutaneous T-cell lymphoma).

Blister (Fig. 7.1E)

A lesion of any size, filled with clear fluid, that forms because of cleavage of the epidermis. It may be a result of constant abrasion of the skin, or as part of a pathological process. The cleavage may be intraepidermal or at the dermoepidermal junction.

Vesicle (Fig. 7.1 F)

Less than 5 mm in diameter, a vesicle is a skin blister filled with clear fluid. Vesicles may be subepidermal or intraepidermal, and may be single or grouped.

Pustule (Fig. 7.1G)

Similar to a vesicle, a pustule is filled with a visible collection of yellowish pus. This may indicate infection. A furuncle is an example of an infected pustule; the pustules that appear in psoriasis are sterile.

Bulla (Fig. 7.1H)

A bulla is a large, fluid-filled blister more than 5 mm in diameter. They occur typically in primary blistering disorders such as bullous pemphigoid, and sometimes in cardiac failure (oedema blisters).

Wheal (Fig. 7.1I)

Wheals are transitory, itchy, raised, discoloured papules or plaques of oedema. They are usually a sign of urticaria or angio-oedema.

Scale (Fig. 7.1J)

Scales are abnormal flat flakes on the skin surface that indicate disordered keratinocyte maturation and keratinization. They vary in appearance, from large white or brown polygonal, like fish scales in ichthyosis, to thick silvery layers in psoriasis.

Lichenification

This is chronic thickening of the epidermis with prominent skin markings, caused by continual rubbing or scratching.

Excoriation

Superficial scratch marks.

Onycholysis

Onycholysis is the separation of the nail plate from the nail bed. Subungual hyperkeratosis subsequently occurs, with the nail plate becoming thickened, crumbly and yellow. It is a feature of many disorders, including psoriasis, fungal infections and trauma.

Petechiae

Petechiae are small, round, flat red spots caused by haemorrhage into the skin or the mucous membranes. They can coalesce to form a purpuric rash.

Purpura

This is a skin rash caused by haemorrhage into the skin from capillaries. It can develop as a result of fragility or damage of the capillaries or an abnormally low blood platelet count.

Microscopic appearances

Hyperkeratosis

This is thickening (hypertrophy) of the surface layer of the epidermis (stratum corneum).

Parakeratosis

Parakeratosis is a pathological process where the nuclei of the cells in the stratum corneum persist. It is seen in disease states such as psoriasis.

Acanthosis

This is thickening (hypertrophy) of the stratum spinosum of the epidermis. It can be regular or irregular.

Dyskeratosis

This term describes a process in which keratinocytes mature early, becoming keratinized before they reach the surface of the skin.

Acantholysis

This is a pathological process where the prickle cells of the stratum spinosum separate, leading to atrophy of the epidermis. Acantholysis is seen in diseases such as pemphigus vulgaris and keratosis follicularis.

Papillomatosis

Accentuated undulating configuration of the demoepidermal junction often seen in psoriasis.

Spongiosis

This is an inflammatory intercellular oedema of the epidermis.

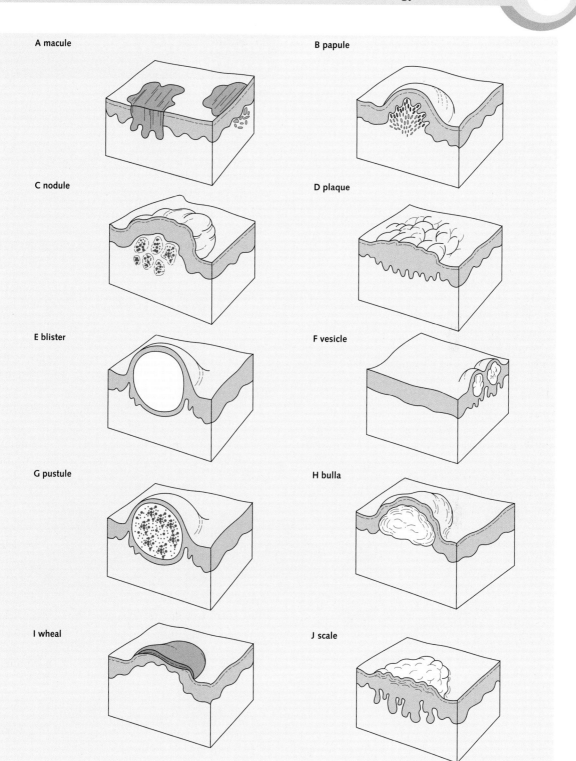

A macule

B papule

C nodule

D plaque

E blister

F vesicle

G pustule

H bulla

I wheal

J scale

Fig. 7.1 (**A**) Macule; (**B**) papule; (**C**) nodule; (**D**) plaque; (**E**) blister; (**F**) vesicle; (**G**) pustule; (**H**) bulla; (**I**) wheal; (**J**) scale. (Adapted with permission from Gawkrodger DJ. Dermatology: an illustrated colour text, 2nd edn. Edinburgh: Churchill Livingstone, 1997.)

Exocytosis

This term is used in pathology to describe the migration of inflammatory cells into the epidermis.

Erosion

A destructive lesion of the skin that causes a superficial discontinuity confined to the epidermis, and that heals without scarring.

Ulceration

The formation of a surface defect of the skin (by sloughing of inflammatory, necrotic tissue or trauma).

A Mongolian (blue) spot is a dark brown to blue pigmentation of the sacral area that is present at birth in most babies of east Asian and African descent, as well as some Caucasians. They can also be present in infants of mixed race. It is of no clinical significance and usually fades by 6 years of age.

INFLAMMATION AND SKIN ERUPTIONS

Psoriasis

Psoriasis is an immune-mediated hyperproliferative disorder that involves the skin. It is a chronic inflammatory dermatosis that presents with well-demarcated, silvery-scaled erythematous plaques.

Classification of types

There are six different clinical variants of psoriasis: plaque, flexural, palmoplantar pustulosis, guttate, scalp and acrodermatitis of Hallopeau, the last being extremely rare and therefore not covered in this text (Fig. 7.2).

Plaque psoriasis

This is the most common type, affecting 80–90% of those with psoriasis. Plaques are well-defined, red, raised lesions topped with silvery-white scales and are usually seen over the extensor surfaces of the limbs, especially the elbows (Fig. 7.3) and knees, over the scalp and at the hairline. Plaques can be large or small and may itch, although itching is not a cardinal

Fig. 7.2 Distribution of the different types of psoriasis.

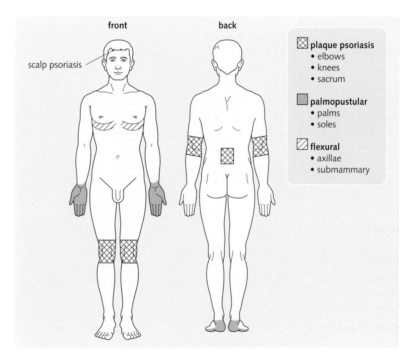

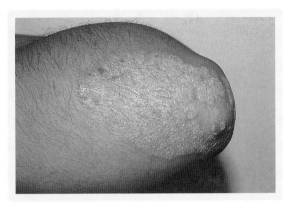

Fig. 7.3 Plaque psoriasis.

feature of plaque psoriasis. Nail involvement can occur, manifesting as pitting and separation from the nail bed (onycholysis). Psoriatic arthropathy can also develop.

Flexural psoriasis
The lesions in flexural psoriasis are clearly demarcated, pink lesions that lack scales. The sites normally affected are the skin folds, especially the groin, perianal regions and genital skin. Less commonly the inframammary skin folds and the umbilicus may be affected. Flexural psoriasis is aggravated by sweat and friction, and there is a risk of secondary infection.

Pustular psoriasis
This can occur in localized (palmoplantar) or generalized forms.

Generalized pustular psoriasis, the most severe form of erythrodermic psoriasis, is a severe systemic variant in which sterile pustules and scaling develop over the trunk and limbs. It causes widespread inflammation with malaise, pyrexia and circulatory disturbance. It can be lethal, as the skin loses its ability to maintain efficient thermoregulation and fluid balance. It can develop spontaneously, or occasionally as a complication of potent corticosteroid therapy (especially when high-dose systemic steroids are rapidly withdrawn). Management is similar to that for burn patients, as the disruption to the skin's functions must be minimized and controlled.

Palmoplantar psoriasis is limited to sterile pustule formation on the palms and soles without systemic symptoms. It is more common in cigarette smokers, typically middle-aged women, some of whom also have classic plaque psoriasis elsewhere.

Guttate psoriasis
Guttate psoriasis is characterized by multiple small, oval, 'raindrop-like' lesions that appear on large body areas such as the trunk, scalp and limbs. It frequently develops after a streptococcal throat infection, and is more common in children and young adults.

Scalp
Scalp lesions can be the only clinical manifestation of psoriasis. Hyperkeratotic plaques can be seen at the hair margin; the scales appear thicker and are better demarcated than in simple dandruff.

Epidemiology
Two per cent of people living in temperate climates are affected by psoriasis. The male:female ratio is 1:1. The disease commonly presents in the second and third decades where there is a positive family history, though onset may occur at any age, with a late-onset peak between 50 and 60 years of age. It is rare in children.

Aetiology
The cause is unknown, although it is believed to have a strong genetic link, with identical twin studies showing high concordance, and a third of patients showing a family history. It is associated with several HLA-specific antigens, particularly HLA-Cw6. Trigger factors include drugs such as β-blockers, lithium and antimalarials, as well as streptococcal infection, local trauma and stress. It is not contagious.

Pathology
Pathological features of psoriasis to note are:

- Accentuated, deepened rete ridges
- Incomplete maturation of keratinocytes through the epidermal layers, resulting in abnormal keratin production (parakeratosis), creating silvery scales on the skin surface
- Active, psoriatic skin has a cell turnover rate 20–30 times faster than that of normal skin, and this results in an abnormally thin epidermis only 2–3 cells thick. Where this is associated with dilated blood vessels in the upper dermis it can result in erythema, or bleeding spots (Auspitz sign), caused when scales become cut or are dislodged
- Polymorphs migrating through the dilated vessels can aggregate to form sterile pustules (Fig. 7.4)

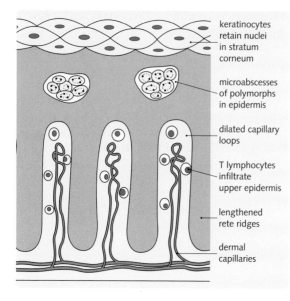

keratinocytes retain nuclei in stratum corneum

microabscesses of polymorphs in epidermis

dilated capillary loops

T lymphocytes infiltrate upper epidermis

lengthened rete ridges

dermal capillaries

Fig. 7.4 Histological changes in psoriasis.

- Trauma to the upper layers of the skin, such as a scratch or a surgical incision, may lead to the formation of psoriatic skin at the site of damage: this is known as the Koebner phenomenon.
- Sunlight aggravates psoriasis in a minority of individuals, although for most it is beneficial.

Complications

Erythroderma
Erythroderma is a term used to describe any inflammatory dermatosis that involves more than 90% of the skin surface. It requires prompt intensive hospital management, as its systemic complications can be fatal. Erythrodermic psoriasis can be precipitated by the withdrawal of systemic steroid treatment or an intercurrent drug eruption.

Psoriatic arthritis
Around 5% of patients with psoriasis develop joint disease. This most commonly manifests as a distal arthritis that causes swelling of toes and digits (called dactylitis), but a rheumatoid-like arthritis may also develop, with a similar polyarthritic pattern.

Severe psoriasis may cause arthritis mutilans, a destructive arthritis that erodes the small bones, especially of the hands and feet, leading to progressive deformity. In addition, patients with psoriasis who are HLA B27 positive may develop spondylosis or sacroiliitis.

Nail involvement
The nails become involved in up to half of patients with psoriasis. Nail changes in psoriasis include:

- Nail plate pitting
- Separation of the nail plate from the underlying nail bed (onychloysis)
- Discoloration of the nail
- Subungal hyperkeratosis.

Sometimes nail changes can precede cutaneous disease.

Bacterial infection
Psoriatic plaques can occasionally become infected, although this is uncommon.

Management
The treatment objective is to control the progression of the disease and control its symptoms.

Localised, topical therapy is usually the first line of treatment, with systemic therapy used for psoriasis that is not responsive to topical treatment, is life-threatening in severity, or which significantly reduces the patient's quality of life.

Topical
Emollients are often prescribed, as they hydrate the dry scaly skin.

First-line therapy involves:

- Vitamin D analogues
- Topical steroids
- Coal-tar-based products
- Dithranol.

Vitamin D analogues These act by inhibiting cell proliferation and promoting keratinocyte differentiation, thereby reversing some of the structural abnormalities of the skin present in psoriasis.

Topical corticosteroids Topical steroids should only be used for stubborn plaques, symptomatic disease, or for treating plaques on the face, genitalia or flexures, as the steroids are non-irritant compared to other agents. Their use must be carefully monitored, as the side effects of steroid usage include:

- Atrophy (thinning) of the skin
- Induction of acne or perioral dermatitis
- Precipitation of unstable psoriasis upon treatment withdrawal
- Allergic contact dermatitis
- Infection (fungal, bacterial or viral) precipitated by steroid treatment

- Reduced efficacy after prolonged use (tachyphylaxis)
- Systemic effects of steroidal treatment—growth retardation, a cushingoid appearance, and endocrine effects caused by systemic absorption of steroid.

Topical steroids are available as creams, ointment, lotion and gels (for the scalp).

Tar-based preparations   These are distilled from coal tar. Often used in combination with ultraviolet (UV) B (UVB) exposure or dithranol (see below), the tar preparations appear to work by altering the DNA synthesis of the skin.

Dithranol   is applied as a paste and retards skin mitosis. However, despite being effective, it is problematic as dithranol is messy and smelly. It can also irritate normal skin adjacent to the treatment area, so protective measures are required.

Salicylic acid ointment   can be used as an adjunct to other therapies, especially for psoriatic lesions associated with thick layers of scale.

Systemic therapy

Methotrexate   This drug acts by inhibiting cell mitosis. It is usually administered orally, although it can be given intramuscularly or intravenously. Normal liver, kidney and marrow function must be established before the treatment begins, and monitored carefully throughout the course. The most serious side effects of methotrexate include hepatic fibrosis and cirrhosis. A therapeutic response is usually observed within 2–4 weeks.

Retinoids   Oral retinoids such as acitretin, a vitamin A analogue, can be used to treat both plaque and pustular psoriasis. It can be used alone or combined with UVB or PUVA therapy. Acitretin is teratogenic, so premenopausal women must use contraception from 1 month before beginning treatment and for 3 years after stopping the course, because of the long half-life of the drug.

Immunosuppressants   such as ciclosporin clear psoriasis when taken in high doses. Ciclosporin is nephrotoxic, however, and renal function should be carefully monitored throughout the course. The long-term side effects of ciclosporin are not yet fully clear, but there may be a small increase in the occurrence of certain malignancies, particularly lymphoma.

Eczema and dermatitis

The terms eczema and dermatitis are used interchangeably to describe the same non-infective inflammatory condition. There are several different forms of eczema.

Atopic eczema

Aetiology

Atopic eczema commonly occurs in patients with a past medical or family history of atopic disease such as asthma and hay fever, and affects 10–15% of children in Europe; 65% of patients have an atopic family history, and the majority of those likely to present with atopy will do so in the first year of life. In half of patients, the disorder will remit by the age of 15 years.

Pathogenesis

The pathophysiology of atopic eczema is not fully understood. Underlying genetic factors such as variants in the filaggrin gene contribute to a state in which inflammation is caused by high levels of circulating IgE antibodies, coupled with abnormal T-cell activation in reaction to commonly encountered allergens, such as house-dust mites, and exacerbating factors such as chemicals and stress. The resulting inflammation is pruritic, and affects both the dermis and the epidermis (Fig. 7.5).

Clinical features

Atopic eczema can present in a variety of different ways, but most commonly with general skin dryness or itching (pruritus) with itchy, red, scaly patches on the flexor creases of the body. In the first 6 months of life it can present as a symmetrical erythematous eruption affecting the face, trunk and limbs (Fig. 7.6). As the child reaches 2 years, the eruption increasingly affects the flexures (Fig. 7.7). Acute eczematous lesions are vesicular and can weep. Dry skin, excoriations and lichenification (thickening of the skin, with accentuated crease marks) all occur, and these are aggravated by the child scratching or rubbing the affected skin (the itch–scratch cycle). The pruritus often causes difficulty with sleep. The skin often feels rough to the touch owing to the dryness of eczema, and in eczema patients fish-like scaling of the skin can sometimes occur without inflammation (ichthyosis vulgaris). Atopic eczema can also involve the nail beds, causing ridging or pitting.

Diagnosis is usually clinical, although allergen sensitivity tests, such as skin prick testing or RAST (radioallergosorbent assay) tests, can sometimes be helpful. Blood eosinophilia is often seen.

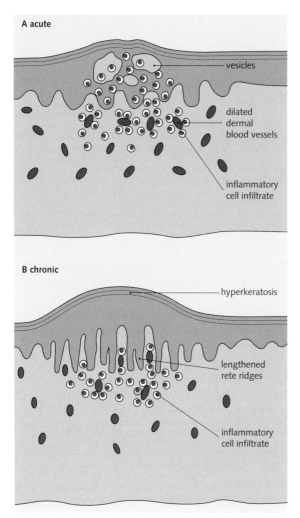

Fig. 7.5 Histological changes in eczema. (Adapted with permission from Gawkrodger DJ. Dermatology: an illustrated colour text, 2nd edn. Edinburgh: Churchill Livingstone, 1997.)

Fig. 7.6 Atopic eczema.

Complications

Eczematous areas are prone to secondary infection. Bacterial colonization is common with *Staphylococcus aureus* and occasionally streptococci. Viral infections can occur, e.g. *Herpes simplex,* which in atopic patients can develop into the severe condition eczema herpeticum.

Management

Conservative management Educating the patients and their family is very important in the management of atopic eczema. Various lifestyle changes can lessen skin irritation: loose-fitting cotton clothing, avoiding heat and known irritants (e.g. wool, and occupational irritants or allergens), filing the nails to limit scratching. If pet hair is thought to aggravate the disease care should be taken to minimize contact. Efforts to reduce the presence of house-dust mites can sometimes be helpful. Dietary changes are rarely helpful unless there is a history of reaction to specific foods.

Both local and national support groups exist for patients with atopic eczema; details of both should be made available to the patient.

In children, it should be made clear to the patient that the condition improves in the majority of cases and often remits by the teenage years.

Topical therapy Topical therapy controls atopic eczema in most patients, usually with a combination of emollients (moisturizers), alternatives to soap (e.g. aqueous cream) and topical steroids.

Emollients Aqueous cream, emulsifying ointment and bath-oil emollients moisturize the skin, hydrating the surface layers and reducing pruritus.

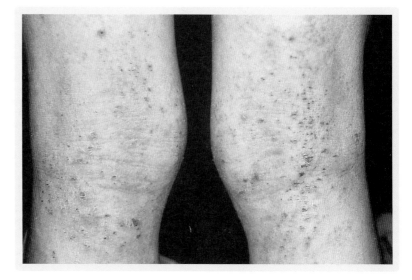

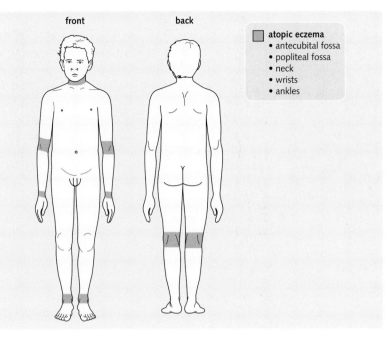

Fig. 7.7 Distribution of eczema.

front   back

atopic eczema
- antecubital fossa
- popliteal fossa
- neck
- wrists
- ankles

Fig. 7.7 Distribution of eczema.

Topical steroids Topical steroids of different potencies are used, depending on the body site being treated. The mildest is 1% hydrocortisone, which is usually sufficient for the face and flexures, where the skin can easily become atrophic with the use of stronger steroids. For other body sites, potent steroids such as betamethasone (Betnovate) preparations are often needed.

Medicated bandages Bandages may be useful in excoriated or lichenified eczema, improving the absorption of topical medication and providing a barrier against scratching. With exudative eczema, non-medicated wet wraps may help.

Antibiotics and antiseptics These are used to treat the infective complications of eczema (usually bacterial, with *Staphylococcus aureus*).

Systemic therapy Antihistamines Sedative antihistamines, e.g. hydroxyzine, given at night may help reduce scratching in severe cases.

Oral antibiotics and antiviral agents Flucloxacillin given four times daily (qds) is used to treat secondary staphylococcal infection, and penicillin V qds for streptococcal infections. Aciclovir is used to manage eczema herpeticum and in severe cases may need to be given intravenously as inpatient therapy.

Second-line treatments Severe eczema unresponsive to treatment can be treated by a course of PUVA or a 12-week course of ciclosporin or azathioprine. However, these are associated with significant side effects and require careful monitoring.

Contact dermatitis

Eczema precipitated by an environmental agent is termed contact dermatitis. Clinically similar to atopic eczema, it is caused by repeated exposure to a chemical irritant or an allergen. Irritant dermatitis is a major cause of morbidity in industry (Fig. 7.8). It is caused by wet work, detergents, and a wide range of other products. Atopic patients are more prone to the development of contact dermatitis.

An unusual or localized site of presentation may raise suspicion of contact dermatitis and of possible causative factors (Fig. 7.9).

Whereas irritant dermatitis is more likely with intensive or repeated exposure to the causative factors, allergic dermatitis can result from brief exposure even to very small traces of the allergen concerned. The commonest causes of allergic contact dermatitis include nickel, latex, perfume and plants. The most common of these is nickel, which affects one in 10 women and one in 100 men. Patch testing is useful if a suspected allergen is involved, and management is based largely on avoiding it once identified. Topical steroids are the second line of treatment.

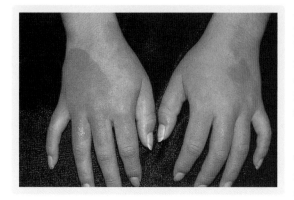

Fig. 7.8 Contact dermatitis.

Other forms of dermatitis

The other forms of dermatitis are listed in Fig. 7.10.

Urticaria and angioedema

These two conditions are associated with acute oedema. Urticaria, often known as nettle rash or hives, is a common condition characterized by the development of transient, itchy swellings (or wheals) that are caused by extravascular plasma leakage. Angio-oedema is a more widespread collection of extravascular fluid that involves the dermis and subcutis.

Aetiology

In most cases the condition is idiopathic. It is believed to have an autoimmune component and is commoner in atopic individuals. It can also occur as a reaction to bacterial or viral infections, drug or food allergies, and sometimes in response to cold, stress or heat.

Pathology

The lesions arise from the release of inflammatory mediators such as histamine from mast cell degranulation, causing dermal capillaries to become leaky. This release can be mediated through autoantibodies against IgE receptors of mast cells in those with a genetic susceptibility (a form of type 1 hypersensitivity reaction). It can also occur in response to some drugs, or through blockage of the prostaglandin pathway (caused by drugs such as aspirin and NSAIDs).

Clinical features

Urticaria is classified as acute if it lasts less than 6 weeks, and chronic if it lasts longer than this. Itchy, red wheals rapidly appear and disappear on the skin, usually within 24 hours, leaving no residual mark. The lesions vary in size, shape and number. Severe urticaria may be accompanied by soft tissue swelling (angio-oedema), especially of the tongue and lips. Dermographism (wheals induced by firm stroking of

Fig. 7.9 Distribution of contact dermatitis. (Note that medical ointments and creams may cause rashes wherever applied.) (Adapted with permission from Gawkrodger DJ. Dermatology: an illustrated colour text, 2nd edn. Edinburgh: Churchill Livingstone, 1997.)

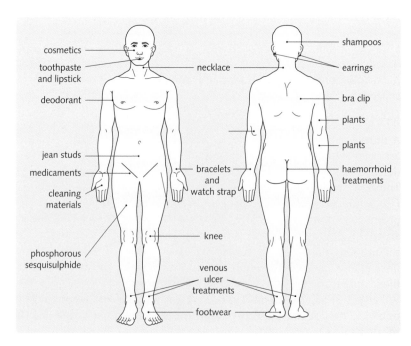

cosmetics

toothpaste
and lipstick

deodorant

jean studs

medicaments

cleaning
materials

phosphorous
sesquisulphide

necklace

bracelets
and
watch strap

knee

venous
ulcer
treatments

footwear

shampoos

earrings

bra clip

plants

plants

haemorrhoid
treatments

Fig. 7.10 Endogenous forms of dermatitis

Type of dermatitis	Comments
seborrhoeic dermatitis	disease of adults; *Pityrosporum ovale* plays an important role; dry, persistent redness and scaling seen on face; pruritus ani and chronic otitis externa are common symptoms
venous dermatitis of legs	feature of chronic venous insufficiency in legs; caused by venous hypertension in deep veins owing to valve incompetence
hand dermatitis	includes pompholyx, a vesicular pattern of dermatitis; may also be caused by discoid dermatitis, primary irritant hand dermatitis, allergic contact dermatitis and hyperkeratotic eczema
asteatotic dermatitis	seen mainly in the elderly, particularly in the winter, and usually on the legs; consists of fine scaling, minor erythema and superficial fissuring
neurodermatitis	localized lichenification seen in adult women on occipital scalp, nape, neck and arms; lesions are well-defined ovoid or elongated plaques; hyperpigmentation is common; itching intermittent and intense
discoid dermatitis	multiple, well-defined discoid lesions with prominent oedema; may be atopic, or may be precipitated by emotional stress
generalized exfoliative dermatitis	also known as erythroderma; skin is erythematous, oedematous and scaly; may be complicated by reversible loss of body hair

the skin) can be demonstrated, and cold urticaria can be induced by applying ice to the skin for 1 minute. Often no underlying cause is found, and the disorder usually resolves spontaneously within a few months. A careful and thorough history can sometimes suggest the causative factor.

Management

A thorough history is necessary, but investigations are rarely required. Hereditary angio-oedema can be detected by a low serum level of C_1 esterase inhibitor. The mainstay of treatment is oral antihistamines (H_1 blockers such as cetirizine) and avoidance of provoking factors. Severe acute angio-oedema causing acute anaphylactic shock or airways obstruction requires immediate treatment with a subcutaneous injection of adrenaline and systemic steroids—this is life saving.

Patients should be advised to not take aspirin or opiate-containing agents as they can stimulate mast cell degranulation.

Lichenoid eruptions
Lichen planus

This is a fairly common, itchy inflammatory dermatosis. It can occur anywhere, but is most common on the flexor surfaces of the wrists and lower legs. It presents as pruritic, papular, flat polygonal lesions, which may coalesce to form small plaques (Fig. 7.11). A white lace-like pattern may form on the top of plaques (Wickham's striae). Lichen planus may also present as annular, atrophic or hypertrophic lesions. Mucosal involvement is common, particularly around the mouth, but also around the genitalia, causing white plaques or ulcers, which may be painful. Severe forms of the disease can affect the nails, causing dystrophy. Most patients recover spontaneously within 18 months. Hypertrophic and atrophic disease are generally more persistent, and ulcerative mucosal disease is premalignant. Although the disease is self-limiting, symptomatic treatment involves the use of potent

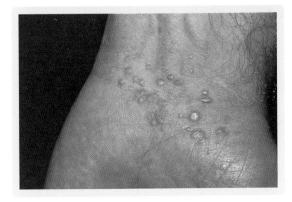

Fig. 7.11 Lichen planus.

topical steroids, or, in resistant cases, systemic steroids and immunosuppressive agents.

Lichen sclerosus et atrophicus

This uncommon disorder is characterized by well-defined white, macular, atrophic lesions that particularly affect the genital region. Lichen sclerosus is an autoimmune-associated disorder that more commonly affects females than males. Individuals can be affected at any age. Where there is clinical doubt, a biopsy of the lesion may be taken to confirm the diagnosis. Management of genital lichen sclerosus is symptomatic, involving potent topical steroids, with an antiseptic or antibiotic if necessary. Extragenital lichen sclerosus does not always require treatment. The condition can disappear of its own accord some years after presentation. Long-term disease can result in scarring and deformity of the genital area, causing complications such as phimosis, anal fissuring, and fusion of the labia minora.

Papulosquamous eruptions

Pityriasis rosea

Pityriasis rosea is typically preceded by a single erythematous oval macule (herald patch) which appears 4–14 days before a generalized eruption of multiple, smaller plaques over the trunk, upper arms and thighs. The rash is symmetrical and may follow the distribution of the dermatomes, forming a 'Christmas tree' pattern.

Individual lesions can appear as oval, pink patches which are slightly raised around the edges (medallion plaques) and may have a fine collar of scales, or as maculopapules (Fig. 7.12). It commonly affects

young adults and adolescents. Clearance usually takes 1–2 months and recurrence is very uncommon. The aetiology of the disease is unclear, but the eruption is thought to be a response to a viral infection. It is a self-limiting condition. Lesions may be pruritic; the itch can be relieved by a mildly or moderately potent topical steroid.

Pityriasis versicolor

Previously known as tinea versicolor, this disorder is caused by *Pityrosporum* yeasts. It presents as brown or pinkish macules that coalesce to form larger, superficially scaly lesions. Eruption sites include the neck, shoulders, upper arms and upper trunk.

Pityriasis versicolor mostly affects young adults and is more common in tropical climates. On microscopy, skin scrapings demonstrate the spores and short, rod-like hyphae—the so-called 'grapes and bananas' appearance. Treatment involves applying 2.5% selenium sulphide shampoo, or a topical imidazole cream. Oral itraconazole can be used for resistant cases. When proliferative yeasts are cleared, persistent hypopigmented areas may remain at the site of previous inflammatory lesions. Hypopigmentation usually clears, but this may take several months.

Reiter's disease

This term is used to describe a collection, or triad, of physical signs, which include a seronegative arthritis, urethritis and iritis/conjunctivitis. It affects HLA B27-positive men, and usually follows a non-gonococcal urethritis or enteritis. Skin lesions that may occur in Reiter's disease include brown aseptic abscesses

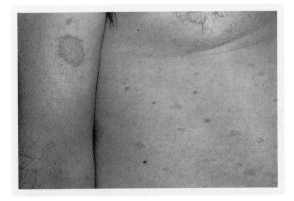

Fig. 7.12 Pityriasis rosea.

(keratoderma blennorrhagicum) forming on the palms and soles and a painless penile rash (circinate balanitis). Arthropathy and nail involvement may be severe. Management includes treating the initial infection, anti-inflammatory analgesia for the arthropathy, and topical steroids for skin lesions.

Parapsoriasis

Known also as chronic superficial dermatitis, this is an eruption of pink, oval or round plaques that are topped by scales. The lesions may be premalignant. They appear in mid to late adulthood and are usually sited on the abdomen, buttocks or thighs. Some lesions progress to malignant cutaneous T-cell lymphoma (mycosis fungoides), although the majority remain benign. Biopsy is necessary to detect premalignant plaques; treatment is with topical steroids for benign parapsoriasis, and ultraviolet phototherapy (PUVA or UVB) for premalignant plaques.

Photodermatoses

Idiopathic causes

Polymorphic light eruption

This is the most common of the photodermatoses in temperate climates and occurs most commonly in young women. A pruritic rash develops hours after the skin has been exposed to the sun. Lesions can be urticarial papules, plaques or vesicles that can persist for hours to days. The condition begins to manifest in spring, but improves during the summer as prolonged exposure to the sun hardens the skin, desensitizing it. Sunscreen is an effective protective measure in mild cases. In more severe cases a course of ultraviolet phototherapy in the spring can often desensitize or harden the skin, so that a patient will not suffer light-induced problems during the summer months.

Chronic actinic dermatitis

Known also as photosensitive eczema, this is a rare disorder that typically affects men in mid to late adulthood. It is characterized by the development of thickened, lichenified plaques on sun-exposed skin, and there may be a previous history of eczema. Diagnosis is made by specialist monochromator light testing. It is managed by avoiding sunlight, and by the use of emollients and protective sunscreen. Treatment with topical steroids can be effective in mild cases. If the dermatitis is resistant to these measures, oral steroids or azathioprine may be necessary. A combination of PUVA and steroids can help to desensitize the skin.

Solar urticaria and actinic prurigo

In solar urticaria, skin wheals appear within minutes of exposure to sunlight and clear within 1–2 hours. With actinic prurigo, sun-induced papules and lichenified nodules first appear in childhood and may resolve by adolescence. Both conditions are rare.

Other non-idiopathic causes

Other photodermatoses include:

- Porphyria—a metabolite accumulation due to enzyme insufficiency
- Pellagra—nicotinic acid deficiency
- Genetic—e.g. xeroderma pigmentosum
- Drug-induced photosensitivity—e.g. nifedipine, thiazides, angiotensin-converting enzyme inhibitors and NSAIDs
- Systemic lupus erythematosus (SLE).

Effects of sunlight on other dermatological conditions

Sunlight aggravates the following conditions:

- SLE
- Herpes simplex, especially cold sores
- Rosacea
- Psoriasis (a minority)
- Vitiligo.

It benefits the following conditions:

- Acne
- Psoriasis
- Parapsoriasis
- Pityriasis rosea
- Atopic eczema.

Sunlight consists of the ultraviolet (UV) rays A and B (UVA, UVB). Both can damage DNA and cause skin cancer, but UVA has the greatest ageing effects on the skin; UVB stimulates vitamin D production. Sunblock products have a numerical sun protection factor (SPF) rating for protection against UVB and a star rating for UVA protection. Products with only UBV protection should be avoided.

INFECTIONS AND INFESTATIONS

The normal skin microflora

Normal bacterial flora resident on the skin include staphylococci, micrococci, corynebacteria and propionibacteria, and these prevent pathogenic organisms from residing on the skin. In addition to bacteria, other microorganisms present in healthy skin include yeasts and mites. The numbers of microorganisms vary depending on the site (e.g. forearm versus moist environs of axillae) and the individual.

Bacterial infections

Diseases caused by overgrowth of normal flora

Erythrasma

Colonization with *Corynebacterium minutissimum* can lead to this dry, orange–brown rash that usually affects the flexural creases such as the toe webs or axillae. The affected skin will fluoresce coral pink under Wood's light. Erythrasma clears when treated with topical or oral antibiotics, including erythromycin or tetracyclines.

Pitted keratolysis

This is a proliferation of corynebacteria that frequently involves the soles of the feet, exacerbated by tight-fitting footwear and excessive sweating. It may lead to small, punched-out lesions, a foul-smelling odour, and discoloured and pitted nails. Improved hygiene will limit the problem. Topical antimicrobials, e.g. clindamycin, 1:10 000 aqueous potassium permanganate foot soaks, and antiperspirants, such as aluminium chloride, may help.

Staphylococcal infections

Impetigo

Impetigo is a highly contagious skin disease that most commonly affects schoolchildren. It is usually caused by staphylococci, but group A streptococci can also cause this clinical picture, so skin swabs should be taken to determine the cause and guide treatment. It presents as superficial exudative lesions that develop a characteristic yellow crust (Fig. 7.13). The lesions spread rapidly. Occasionally the bacteria produce toxins that cause the lesions to blister (bullous impetigo). The lesions may complicate other skin disorders such as atopic eczema and herpes simplex. Management involves topical fusidic acid and antiseptics applied to localized disease. Children should be kept off school for 1 week after the lesions first crust, and picking of the lesions should be discouraged. If the infection becomes widespread, systemic antibiotics are necessary. With

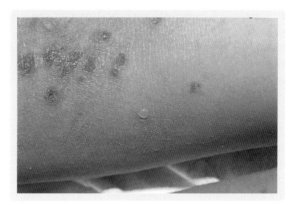

Fig. 7.13 Impetigo.

the most serious form of impetigo, that caused by *Streptococcus pyogenes*, oral penicillin is given to prevent glomerulonephritic complications.

Ecthyma

Ecthyma is an uncommon disease resulting from cutaneous infection with *Staph. aureus* or streptococci. It presents as round, well-demarcated ulcerative lesions, usually on the legs. After treatment with systemic antibiotics the ulcers crust over and scar upon healing. The disease is associated with poor hygiene and states of malnutrition, and is more commonly seen in developing countries, and in the Western world among IV drug users and immunosuppressed patients.

Folliculitis

Folliculitis is an inflammation of the hair follicle that presents with itchy or tender papules or pustules. It is often caused by infection with *Staph. aureus*. The pustules have erythematous edges and often contain an emerging hair shaft. Management is with topical antiseptics and antibiotics, or systemic antibiotics; to prevent recurrence the patient should be educated about improved hygiene.

Streptococcal infections

Erysipelas

Presenting with localized erythema, swelling and tenderness, erysipelas is an acute infection of the dermis and the upper subcutaneous layer, usually caused by streptococci. The inflammation is well defined and may have palpable borders. It occurs with general malaise and flu-like symptoms. The clinical picture in erysipelas overlaps with that of cellulitis. The eruptions usually clear within

2–3 weeks of treatment with oral or intravenous penicillin to prevent haematogenous systemic spread and streptococcal septicaemia. Penicillin can also be used prophylactically in recurrent cases; these lead to lymphatic damage and irreversible oedema.

Cellulitis

This is an infection of the deep subcutaneous layer of the skin, usually by streptococci. The area becomes erythematous, hot and tender to the touch, and the infection can spread rapidly (Fig. 7.14). Patients are systemically unwell and pyrexial. Infection can arise from breaks in the skin barrier, such as IV catheters, wounds, surgical incisions or leg ulcers, and injection sites in IV drug users. Broad-spectrum antibiotic cover should be initiated as soon as possible until the results of blood cultures yield the organism and its antibiotic sensitivities. Any identified underlying cause should be treated. It is common practice to draw around the site of erythema on the skin, as this allows monitoring of any spread and response to treatment.

Necrotizing fasciitis

This serious infection may occur after minor trauma; it must be treated immediately to prevent serious skin necrosis in the affected area and death. The infection is characterized by a high fever and an ill-defined erythema that usually occurs on the leg. High-dose IV antibiotics and surgical debridement of the necrotic tissue are required.

Mycobacterial infections

Lupus vulgaris

This condition, which is now very rare in the Western world, is the most common type of cutaneous TB. It arises as a postprimary infection and usually begins in childhood. Painless, red–brown nodules form, which scar and heal slowly. They can coalesce to form larger, erythematous plaques, which are most commonly seen on the head and neck. Complications include the destruction of deeper skin tissues and the increased risk of developing squamous cell carcinoma in chronic lesions. A biopsy will aid the diagnosis and the Mantoux test is positive. Treatment is that for the eradication of TB.

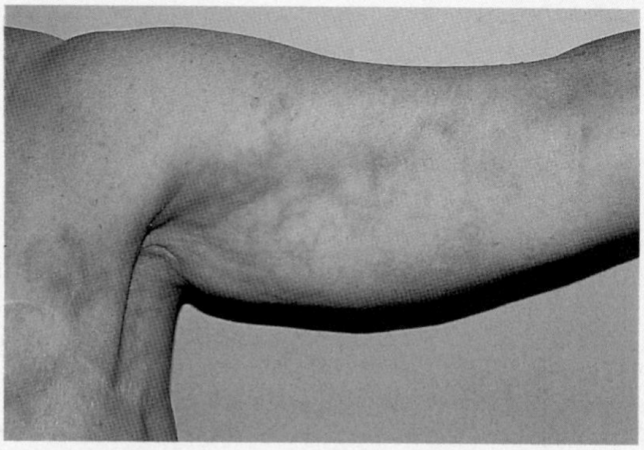

Scrofuloderma

This is an infection that occurs on the skin overlying a lymph node infected with TB, or an affected bone or joint. A dull red nodule develops, which ulcerates and can lead to fistulae, granulation, scarring and discharge.

Warty tuberculosis

This results from the inoculation of TB into the skin of previously infected patients. It forms warty plaques on cold erythematous areas, commonly of the hands, knees and buttocks. The condition is now extremely rare in the Western world, but is still common in developing countries.

Spirochaetal infections

Secondary syphilis

The secondary stage of syphilis begins 1–3 months after the primary chancre, and is characterized by pink or copper-coloured papules that appear on the trunk, palms, limbs and soles. The papules resolve spontaneously in 1–3 months without treatment.

Yaws/bejel/pinta

These non-venereal treponemal infections are endemic in tropical developing countries. In all three serology is positive for syphilis, and the infection may be treated with penicillin.

Lyme disease

This condition is caused by *Borrelia burgdorferi* and is spread by tick bites. Lyme disease is characterized by a slowly expanding erythematous ring at the site of the initial bite. Complications include arthritis, neurological pathology and cardiac sequelae. Treatment is with penicillin or tetracycline.

Other bacterial infections

Anthrax

Primarily a disease of animals, anthrax causes haemorrhagic bullae at the site of inoculation. The lesions are accompanied by oedema and fever. The diagnosis is made by culture of blister fluid and

Fig. 7.14 Cellulitis.

the disease is treated by intramuscular injections of penicillin or intravenous tetracycline (followed by an oral course).

Gram-negative infections

Gram-negative bacilli, such as *Pseudomonas aeruginosa*, may secondarily infect skin wounds such as leg ulcers. They may also cause nail discoloration, folliculitis and, occasionally, cellulitis (see Fig. 7.14).

Viral infections

Viral warts

Viral warts are benign overgrowths (tumours) of cutaneous squamous epithelium caused by infection with human papillomavirus (HPV). The virus spreads through direct or indirect contact (e.g. feet in swimming baths) and through sexual contact. There are over 70 HPV subtypes, responsible for lesions including warts of the hands, the plantar surfaces of the feet and the anogenital region. Certain HPV types have a much increased risk of associated malignancy (e.g. carcinoma of the cervix).

Common warts appear as dome-shaped papules with a rough surface (Fig. 7.15). They spread by direct contact and commonly develop in children and young adults. At least 50% of common warts resolve spontaneously without scarring. Treatment includes paring, and topical keratolytic agents such as salicylic acid; cryotherapy and cautery can also be considered. Genital warts are treated by cryotherapy, topical podophyllin or curettage and cautery. A more recent topical therapy is the immune response modifier imiquimod. It is important to screen patients presenting with genital warts for other STDs, along with their partners.

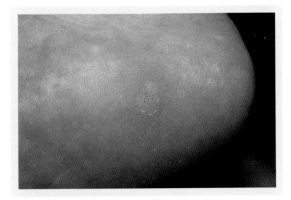

Fig. 7.15 Simple viral wart.

Scalded skin syndrome

This is a serious condition, usually caused by toxins released from specific strains of staphylococci. It usually affects infants, and causes severe erythema and the shedding of large sheets of epidermis from the body. The disorder responds well to prompt treatment with flucloxacillin or erythromycin, although a drug-induced adult variant of the condition (toxic epidermal necrolysis) is often fatal.

Molluscum contagiosum

Caused by a poxvirus, molluscum contagiosum mainly affects children. The lesions appear as multiple pearly-pink papules a few millimetres in diameter, with a central punctum. They commonly occur on the face, neck and trunk but can occur on any site of the body, including the genitalia. They tend to occur in crops over a 6–12-month period. They resolve spontaneously, although trauma such as squeezing or scratching the lesions can help stimulate a host response and speed up recovery. Cryotherapy can be considered in older children but may cause significant scarring.

Herpes simplex

The *Herpes simplex* virus has two genomic subtypes that cause different types of (primary) infection. Type 1 primary infection is spread by direct contact, commonly causing a subclinical infection but occasionally causing painful blisters of the face and gums (gingivostomatitis).

Type 2 primary infection occurs after sexual contact in young adults, with lesions in the genital region. If the primary infection occurs in women more than 36 weeks pregnant, caesarian section is required to minimize the risk of vertical transmission to the baby during labour, as neonatal infection is associated with severe neurological sequelae.

After the primary infection has subsided the virus can become latent, residing in dorsal root ganglia. Recurrent attacks lead to lesions at a similar site each time, and are commoner in immunosuppressed patients. The vesicular eruption may be preceded by a tingling or burning sensation, crusts form within 1–2 days, and the lesions clear after about a week.

Primary herpes simplex virus manifestations and painful genital lesions can be treated with oral aciclovir. Treatment of recurrent cold sores is with antiviral drugs such as aciclovir or famciclovir. Those suffering from genital herpes can also use famciclovir. Barrier contraception should be used by those infected, and sexual intercourse should be avoided altogether during symptomatic episodes.

Herpes zoster

Otherwise known as shingles, this infection occurs as a result of reactivation of the varicella zoster virus (VZV) following a previous infection, commonly 'chickenpox' in childhood. Following prodromal paraesthesia and tingling, painful vesicular eruptions occur in crops following a dermatomal distribution, accompanied by local lymphadenopathy. The thoracic dermatomes are most often involved (Fig. 7.16).

Complications include persistent pain (postherpetic neuralgia). Involvement of the ophthalmic division of the trigeminal nerve results in ocular disease and corneal ulcers. The disease is most severe in older patients.

Treatment is with analgesia, and if secondary bacterial infection occurs topical antiseptic or antibiotic is necessary. Oral aciclovir can be given in severe cases and in the immunosuppressed.

Fungal infections

Fungal skin infections are called mycoses. Fungi are saprophytic organisms present throughout the environment. Three groups of pathogenic fungi are:

- Dermatophytes
- Candida albicans
- Pityrosporum.

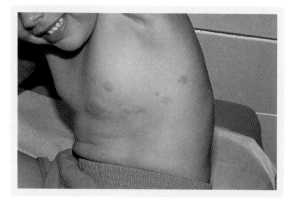

Fig. 7.16 Herpes zoster.

Dermatophyte infections

These fungi reproduce by producing spores, causing a 'ringworm'-type (tinea) rash. The usual sites of dermatophyte infection are the nails, hair and stratum corneum. Three different types of dermatophyte cause tinea in humans: *Microsporum*, *Trichophyton* and *Epidermophyton*. All are spread by direct contact from infected humans or animals.

Microsporum

Infecting skin and hair, *Microsporum* organisms fluoresce under Wood's light. They usually cause infection during childhood. Along with *Trichophyton* they cause tinea capitis (ringworm of the scalp). Two *Microsporum* organisms are responsible: *M. audouinii*, which spreads from child to child, creating epidemics in schools, and *M. canis*, which is passed on from family pets, mainly kittens and puppies.

Trichotophyton

Trichophyton organisms cause many types of tinea; this type of dermatophyte cannot be detected by Wood's light and diagnosis requires examination of skin scrapings under microscopy. The commonest example is *T. rubrum*, which causes tinea cruris (ringworm of the groin), tinea pedis (ringworm of the foot), tinea barbae (beard), and tinea facei (glabrous skin of the face) as well as infection of the hands (tinea manuum), feet (tinea pedis) and nails (tinea unguium).

Epidermophyton

Epidermophyton causes tinea cruris (ringworm of the groin) and tinea pedis (ringworm of the foot).

Treatment

Localized or flexural ringworm is effectively treated with a 2-week course of topical antifungal cream.

Widespread ringworm, such as tinea pedis and capitis, requires a 2-month course of oral antifungal therapy in adults.

Tinea unguium is more resistant to treatment and often requires: oral antifungal treatment given for 3 months or more.

Candida albicans infections

Candida albicans is a yeast organism normally resident in the mouth and gastrointestinal tract. It is an opportunistic pathogen, colonizing and causing infection where the possibility arises. Risk factors that predispose to an increased risk of *Candida albicans* infection include:

- Pregnancy
- Oral contraceptive pill
- Wide spectrum antibiotics
- Corticosteroid treatment
- Immunosuppressive drugs
- Diabetes mellitus
- HIV infection
- Poor hygiene
- Humid environment.

Flexural areas provide a warm, moist environment ideal for candidal growth. Infection creates red, ragged edges with small pustules or papules (satellite lesions) (Fig. 7.17). It can affect the genital, oral mucocutaneous tissue and nails, either alone or as part of a systemic infection.

Candida can colonize the mucosa of the mouth, oesophagus and genital tract, producing superficial, white pseudomembranous lesions, commonly in those taking broad-spectrum antibiotics or those who are immunosuppressed.

Management involves improved hygiene, and removing any predisposing factors, such as stopping systemic antibiotics, if appropriate.

Topical therapy includes nystatin and imidazoles. Amphotericin, nystatin and miconazole lozenges are used for oral candida. Systemic therapy includes oral itraconazole and fluconazole, and can be also be used in candida nail infection. Vaginal candida can be treated by a single dose of clotrimazole or econazole given intravaginally as a pessary.

Pityrosporum

Pityrosporum yeast forms part of the skin's normal flora. It can colonize the scalp, flexural creases and the upper trunk in an opportunistic manner. It is responsible for the conditions pityriasis versicolor and pityrosporum folliculitis. Pityrosporum proliferates exuberantly in seborrhoeic dermatitis.

Infestations
Insect bites

Insect bites can cause a chemical, irritant or immune-mediated response in the skin, caused by the introduction of foreign material. Depending on the type of bite, the lesion can present as anything from itchy wheals to a large bulla. Lesions are identified as insect bites by their pattern—often grouped into clusters (papular urticaria) and may be tracking up a limb. Secondary infection of the lesions may occur, requiring antibiotic treatment.

Management involves elimination of the source of the insects (bedbugs, cat fleas, etc.). Symptoms may be alleviated with antipruritic agents.

Insect bites can cause an allergic or irritant reaction to foreign material introduced by the insect. They commonly become pruritic, and scratching can cause secondary bacterial infection. Hydrocortisone cream or calamine lotion can help relieve the itching.

Pediculosis (lice)

Lice infestations are of three types: from the pubic louse (phthiriasis pubis), the body louse (pediculosis corporis) and the head louse (pediculosis capitis) (Fig. 7.18). Head lice often cause epidemics in schoolchildren: they are spread by direct contact, encouraged by overcrowding. The lice lay their eggs (nits) on hair. Lice cause itching and excoriation of the scalp.

Body lice are found in conditions of poverty and poor hygiene. They are commonly found on clothing, rather than being visible on the skin. They are spread on infested clothing or bedding.

Pubic lice are generally found in young adults and are spread through sexual contact. Infestation causes nocturnal itching, the resulting excoriation leading to an increased risk of secondary infection.

Management involves treatment with malathion, permethrin or phenothrin lotions, depending on the type of infestation. A nit comb can to help to remove head lice and their eggs.

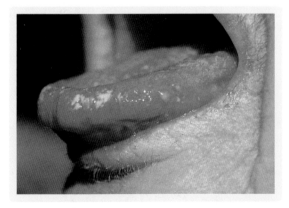

Fig. 7.17 *Candida albicans.*

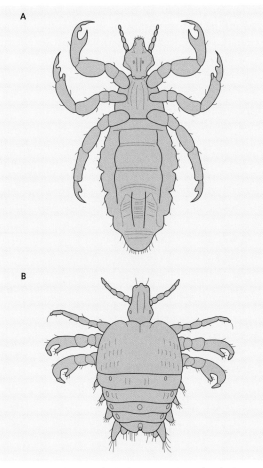

Fig. 7.18 (**A**) Body louse (*Pediculus humanus*). (**B**) Female pubic louse. (Adapted with permission from Gawkrodger DJ. Dermatology: an illustrated colour text, 2nd edn. Edinburgh: Churchill Livingstone, 1997.)

Scabies

Scabies is caused by *Sarcoptes scabiei*, a mite (Fig. 7.19) that can only survive on human skin. There are 300 million cases worldwide each year, more commonly in poorer countries with social overcrowding. Scabies infestation develops as a chronic, pruritic and highly contagious disease. The female mite burrows into the skin at a rate of 2 mm a day, laying eggs as she goes. After 3 days the eggs hatch, maturing after 2 weeks. The mites mate; the males die and the females continue the cycle.

The skin takes 4–6 weeks to react to the infestation, so the infection may be spread by direct contact before the problem is recognized. Once the hypersensitivity reaction occurs, scratching reduces the mite population down to 12 or fewer.

Clinical symptoms include itchy, red papules occurring anywhere except on the face. There may be excoriations caused by itching, and scaly burrows, measuring up to 1 cm in length (Fig. 7.20). Burrows can be found on the wrists and ankles, around the nipples and the umbilicus, in the webs of the fingers and toes, and on the genitalia. Itching is usually most intense at night. Excoriations can predispose to secondary bacterial infection. The diagnosis can be confirmed by taking skin scrapings of a lesion to look for mites or their eggs.

In immunosuppressed patients, proliferation of the scabies mite leads to the formation of large, hyperkeratotic, encrusted eruptions that carry large numbers of mites. This is known as 'Norwegian scabies' and is an extremely contagious form of infestation that requires vigorous treatment and strict barrier nursing procedures. Management includes contact tracing and the use of a topical scabicide, e.g. malathion or 5% permethrin lotion, to treat infected patients and contacts.

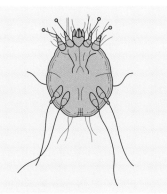

Fig. 7.19 Female scabies mite. (Adapted with permission from Gawkrodger DJ. Dermatology: an illustrated colour text, 2nd edn. Edinburgh: Churchill Livingstone, 1997.)

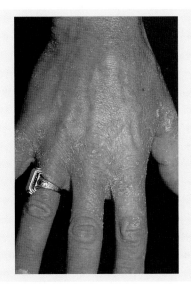

Fig. 7.20 Scabies infestation.

159

Children diagnosed with scabies should be excluded from school until 24 hours after treatment.

Tropical skin infections and infestations

Although not endemic in the West, tropical skin diseases can be seen in visitors and immigrants, and an awareness of the diseases listed below is useful in western medicine.

Leprosy

Caused by the acid-fast bacillus *Mycobacterium leprae*, leprosy is spread via nasal droplets and incubates for several years. Depending on the response of the host's cell-mediated immune system to the bacillus, the patient will develop either localized tuberculoid leprosy, where there is a strong cell-mediated immune response, or lepromatous leprosy, a serious systemic disease associated with a weak cell-mediated immune response. Tuberculoid leprosy affects the nerves, causing anaesthesia and muscle atrophy, as well as the skin, causing a hypopigmented, well-demarcated, single plaque, commonly on the face. Lepromatous leprosy affects all organs but affects the skin first, causing multiple symmetrical macules, papules, nodules and plaques on the face (leonine facies), arms, legs and buttocks.

Treatment lasts between 6 months and 2 years, and involves multidrug regimens because of increased resistance of the bacillus.

Leishmaniasis

This disease is caused by a protozoon transmitted to humans through the bite of sandflies. There are three types of leishmaniasis: cutaneous (endemic to the dry deserts around the Mediterranean), American (endemic to South and Central American tropics) and visceral (endemic to India).

Filariasis

Caused by the nematode worm *Wuchereria bancrofti*, filariasis is characterized by gross oedema of the legs and scrotum, termed 'elephantiasis'. It is treated with diethylcarbamazine.

Larva migrans

This is seen in holidaymakers returning from tropical beaches, where they may have been infested with a hookworm larva. These larvae emerge from eggs present in the faeces of infested cats and dogs; they penetrate the skin and migrate in a serpentiginous fashion, causing intensely itchy red burrows. The disease is self-limiting as the larvae die within a few weeks, but may be successfully treated with topical 10% thiabendazole cream, or oral albendazole, when symptomatic.

Onchocerciasis

Caused by *Onchocerca volvulus*, this filarial infestation is common in Africa and South America where the organisms are transmitted through gnat bites. The adult worm may grow up to 7 cm long, with microfilariae found in the dermis and, more seriously, in the eye, causing blindness.

Granulomatous nodules are present on the skin, following an itchy, papular eruption. Onchocerciasis can be treated with a single dose of ivermectin, followed by repeated doses at 6-month intervals until the worm has been eradicated.

Tumours of the skin

Benign tumours

Epidermal tumours

Seborrhoeic wart   Otherwise known as a basal cell papilloma, seborrhoeic warts are benign overgrowths of the basal cell layer of the epidermis of unknown aetiology. They are common in the elderly or the middle-aged (Fig. 7.21).

The lesions appear to be stuck onto the skin, with an irregular, greasy-looking surface, and well-defined margins. They can be flesh-coloured, brown or black in colour and vary in size and number. They are found on the trunk and face. They can be treated by liquid nitrogen cryotherapy, curettage or shave biopsy.

Skin tags   Skin tags are benign, pedunculated fibroepithelial polyps, commonly found on the neck, axillae, groin and eyelids of middle-aged to elderly patients. They are usually only removed for cosmetic reasons. The stalk of the polyp is cut or cauterized and the lesion removed. Skin tags can also be removed by cryotherapy.

Epidermoid cysts   These cystic swellings are filled with keratin and form a central punctum. They arise from the epidermis. They can occur at any site, and are firm lesions, up to about 3 cm in diameter. They can occasionally rupture, causing inflammation of

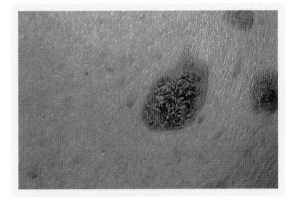

Fig. 7.21 Seborrhoeic warts.

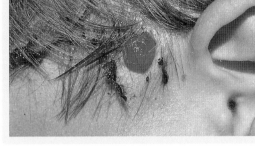

Fig. 7.22 Pyogenic granuloma.

the site. Excision will clear the lesion. They were previously known as sebaceous cysts. Pilar cysts are similar, arising on the scalp, although they lack a central punctum. They can have a familial tendency.

Milia   These are small (1–2 mm), keratin-filled white cysts usually found around the eyelids or on the cheeks. They can appear at any age, and may follow the healing of subepidermal blisters. They can be successfully excised using a sterile needle.

Dermal tumours

Dermatofibroma   Typically asymptomatic, dermatofibromas present as firm, purplish nodules that may or may not be pigmented. They usually occur on the legs, and are more common in women than men. If the diagnosis is in doubt, an excisional biopsy should be performed.

Pyogenic granuloma   This is a benign overgrowth of blood vessels, actually neither pyogenic nor granulomatous, which presents as a rapidly growing, bright-red papule or nodule, often on the fingers or lips (Fig. 7.22). The lesion, which develops rapidly over a few weeks, is pedunculated, friable and bleeds easily. Pyogenic granuloma is treated by curettage or excision. The excised material is examined histologically to exclude an amelanotic malignant melanoma.

Keloid   A keloid is a smooth, hard lesion caused by excessive collagen production, commonly after an injurious assault to the skin such as surgery or trauma. Unlike normal skin scarring, a keloid persists, often progressing beyond the limit of the

original injury. They most commonly develop on the upper back, chest, ear lobes and chin.

Keloids are more common in the Afro-Caribbean population. Management involves steroid injections into the lesion.

Campbell-de-Morgan spot   Also known as cherry angiomas, these are benign angiomas which present as bright-red/purple pinpoint papules, becoming increasingly prevalent with age. They are found mostly on the trunk. No treatment is required.

Lipoma   Lipomas present as soft subcutaneous masses on the trunk, neck and upper extremities. The fatty nodules may be multiple and are sometimes painful, in which case they can be removed by excision.

Naevi

Melanocytic naevi

Aetiology   Commonly known as 'moles', melanocytic naevi are benign overgrowths of melanocytes and are present in most white-skinned people. The number of naevi appears to be influenced by a genetic component. Most melanocytic naevi develop during childhood and adolescence. Pregnancy or excessive sun exposure may cause the development of further naevi in later life.

Skin changes that commonly occur during pregnancy are increased pigmentation, greater prominence of existing melanocytic naevi and the development of abdominal striae and spider naevi.

Pathology Naevus cells are thought to derive from melanocytes (Fig. 7.23) Naevi start with a proliferation of naevus cells at the dermoepidermal junction, forming brown macules (junctional naevi). Continued proliferation of naevus cells deeper into the dermis causes the mole to rise above the skin's surface, forming a compound naevus, with even pigmentation and a well-demarcated border. Eventually they may lose their pigmentation and develop into intradermal (cellular) naevi.

Complications Dysplastic naevi, which change size, shape or colour, and those that itch, become inflamed or encrusted must be examined and biopsied, as such alterations may be a sign of malignant melanoma.

Management Naevi displaying suspicious features should be biopsied and/or excised and sent for histology. Otherwise excision is rarely required, unless for cosmetic reasons. However, in this instance the patient should be counselled that excision could leave a scar and create cosmetic issues of its own.

Vascular naevi

These naevi are often present at birth. Most are derived from superficial capillary networks; larger angiomas are caused by deeper, multivascular plexuses.

Port-wine stain Also known as capillary haemangioma, this is a large, irregular, flat, red–purple macule arising as a result of abnormal dilatation of dermal capillaries. This lesion commonly affects the face asymmetrically. It does not resolve or improve, but in later life may become darker, thicker and nodular. If it occurs near the orbital region, ophthalmic function should be examined as there is an increased risk of glaucoma. Laser therapy can be very effective.

Salmon patch The most common vascular naevus, this lesion presents in half of all newborns. Pink patches on the upper eyelid often clear rapidly, but those at the back of the neck—'stork-marks'—may persist.

Strawberry naevus Also known as a capillary cavernous haemangioma, strawberry naevi affect about 1% of infants. They usually develop soon after birth as a red, lumpy nodule, growing to a maximum size at 1 year. The naevus begins to involute at about 2 years, and usually resolves by the age of 7 years. Strawberry naevi can occur anywhere on the skin. Management is usually simple reassurance to the parents.

Epidermal naevi These linear lesions are warty and pigmented, presenting at birth or in early childhood.

Fig.7.23 Clinical features of pigmented naevi	
Type of naevus	**Clinical features**
congenital	present at birth; usually greater than 1 cm in diameter; can become prominent and hairy; vary from light brown to black; 5% carry risk of malignancy
junctional	flat macules up to 1 cm in size; round or oval; light to dark brown in colour; usually found on palms, soles and genitalia
intradermal	dome-shaped papule or nodule; seen on face and neck; may or may not be pigmented
compound	macules usually smaller than 1 cm; vary in pigmentation; occur anywhere; larger lesions may develop warty surface
Spitz	firm, red–brown nodule; usually occur in children on face; growth initially rapid; dermal vessels are dilated
blue	usually solitary; blue in colour; common on hands and feet
halo (Sutton's)	seen on trunk of adolescents and children; indicative of destruction of naevi cells by body's defence system; white halo of pigmentation surrounds existing naevus; there is an association with vitiligo
Becker's	rare; unilateral lesion in adolescent males; hyperpigmented, becoming hairy; found on back and chest; non-melanocytic

They can range from a few centimetres long to involving the whole of a limb, and may recur after excision. A scalp variant, naevus sebaceous, should be removed as it may become neoplastic.

Malignant epidermal tumours

Malignant melanoma

Epidemiology

Melanoma is a malignant tumour of melanocytes (Fig. 7.24). It is the most lethal of the skin tumours as it metastasizes early. Childhood exposure to excessive amounts of sun, as well as intermittent sun exposure and sunburn, is thought to be associated with the development of melanomas. The incidence is 10–20 cases per 100 000 population per year in the UK, and is increasing. The male:female ratio is 1:1.5. Melanoma is commoner in older people, but also affects the young. Melanomas tend to develop on areas exposed to the sun. The back is the most common site in men and the leg in women.

Clinical features

Many melanomas develop at the site of a pre-existing melanocytic naevus. Individuals with multiple melanocytic naevi, a previous history of malignant melanoma, a family history of melanoma and those with a fair complexion (especially people with red hair and blue eyes) who burn easily in the sun are also at increased risk. The criteria used for diagnosis can be easily remembered as ABCDE:

- Asymmetry of a mole
- Border irregularity
- Colour variegation
- Diameter > 6 mm
- Elevation.

The patient may also report the lesion itching and bleeding.

Pathology

There are four main variants of malignant melanoma (Fig. 7.25).

The excised lesion is analysed and scored according to its:

- Thickness (Breslow)
- Depth (Clark's level)
- Mitotic rate.

The results from these can used to predict the prognosis. The prognosis relates to the depth of tumour (Fig. 7.26).

Management

Malignant melanomas are treated by wide surgical excision with a margin of healthy skin excised alongside the tumour, the extent of which is determined from the Breslow thickness. Patients are closely followed to detect recurrence, which may occur locally or through metastases. Public heath education about the disease and its association with sun exposure can help to reduce excessive sun exposure in the future and the incidence of disease.

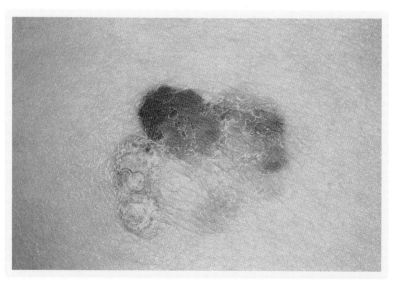

Fig. 7.24 Malignant melanoma.

Fig. 7.25 Main variants of malignant melanoma

Variant	Percentage of new UK cases	Clinical features
superficial spreading melanoma	50	occurs commonly in women; mainly on lower leg; macular; variable pigmentation; can regress; large, flat; grows laterally before it invades vertically
lentigo maligna melanoma	15	develops in pre-existing lentigo maligna (macular lesion arising in elderly or on sun-damaged skin); most common on face
acral lentiginous melanoma	10	affects palms, soles and nail beds; often diagnosed late so has poor survival rates; most common melanoma in Asian populations
nodular melanoma	25	commonly occurs in men; usually arises on trunk; non-pigmented nodule that grows rapidly, bleeds and ulcerates; most aggressive type; can mimic pyogenic granuloma

Basal cell carcinoma

Otherwise known as rodent ulcer, basal cell carcinoma is the most common type of skin malignancy. It arises from basal keratinocytes in the epidermis, and is most common in middle to late life.

Aetiology

Basal cell carcinoma is most commonly caused by excessive sun exposure, but can also result from chronic scarring. There is also some evidence of genetic predisposition. Fair-skinned individuals are most at risk, and the incidence is greater in men than in women.

Fig.7.26 Melanoma prognosis and tumour depth

Depth of tumour (mm)	5-year survival rate (%)
< 1.49	93
1.5–3.49	67
> 3.5	38

Pathology

The tumour is composed of basophilic cells, which bud down from the epidermis to invade the dermis. They often invade in a lobular fashion (Fig. 7.27).

Clinical features

The lesions tend to arise on sun-exposed areas of the face, such as the nose, eyelids and temple. They present as telangiectatic papules or nodules that can ulcerate. They usually grow slowly and are locally invasive. Owing to their slow growth, lesions may have been present for 2 or more years before the patient presents (Fig. 7.28). They almost never metastasize.

Management

If possible, complete excision is the best treatment. This can be difficult if lesions are around the eye or nasolabial folds. Radiotherapy can also be used. Cryosurgery may also be used on superficial trunk lesions.

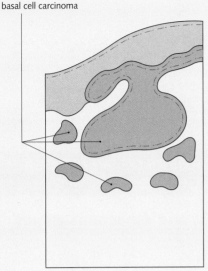

Fig. 7.27 Histopathology of basal cell carcinoma. (Adapted with permission from Gawkrodger DJ. Dermatology: an illustrated colour text, 2nd edn. Edinburgh: Churchill Livingstone, 1997.)

Squamous cell carcinoma

Aetiology

These arise from epidermal keratinocytes and usually develop in an area of damaged skin. The risk factors for squamous cell carcinoma (SCC) include:

- Chronic sun exposure causing actinic damage
- Irradiation
- Chronic ulceration/scarring.

The lesions usually occur in later life, and are more common in men than women. The tumour may metastasize if left untreated.

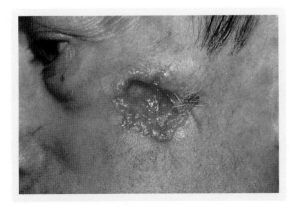

Fig. 7.28 Basal cell carcinoma.

Pathology

Cytology reveals keratinocytes, with a disordered and growth pattern and nuclear abnormalities (Fig. 7.29).

Clinical features

The lesions, which are usually found on sun-exposed sites, are keratotic nodules or plaques (Fig. 7.30). They often begin as small papules that can progress to ulcerated, crusted lesions.

Management

Surgical excision is the first line of management. Radiotherapy can also be used, although SCCs are relatively resistant to it compared to basal cell carcinomas. When metastasis occurs, regional lymph nodes are the most likely site for spread.

Premalignant epidermal tumours

Intraepidermal carcinoma (Bowen's disease)

Bowen's disease is a form of intraepidermal carcinoma (squamous carcinoma in situ) that can rarely become invasive. This form of cancer is commonest in elderly women. It usually presents on sun-exposed areas as a single scaly red patch or plaque with an irregular border, resembling psoriasis. The lesions gradually increase in size over time. They can be treated with topical 5-fluorouracil, cryotherapy or curettage.

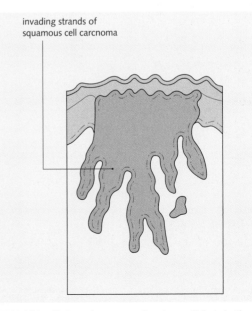

Fig. 7.29 Histopathology of squamous cell carcinoma. (Adapted with permission from Gawkrodger DJ. Dermatology: an illustrated colour text, 2nd edn. Edinburgh: Churchill Livingstone, 1997.)

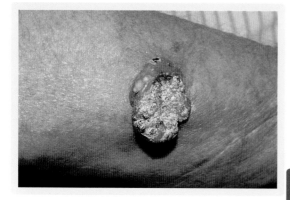
Fig. 7.30 Squamous cell carcinoma.

Keratoacanthoma

This is a rapidly growing tumour that arises in sun-exposed areas. It forms a dome-shaped papule, that can necrose and ulcerate, and grows to 2–3 cm in width. The lesion resembles a squamous cell carcinoma, but histologically is differentiated by a more symmetrical pattern. It may resolve spontaneously within a few months, but does scar. However, it is best to excise it in order to exclude squamous cell carcinoma and reduce scarring.

Cutaneous T-cell lymphoma

Also known as mycosis fungoides, this rare tumour is due to a lymphoma that develops in normal skin. It grows slowly, often following a relatively benign course. It presents insidiously with scaly plaques that are similar to those present in psoriasis or eczema, often developing on the buttocks. The lesions can come and go over years. Occasionally, nodules and ulcers develop within the plaques, and systemic disease results in spread of the tumour to lymph nodes and organs. It is diagnosed by skin biopsy. Early disease can be treated with topical steroids or PUVA to control plaque development. Advanced disease requires radiotherapy, chemotherapy and immunotherapy.

Kaposi's sarcoma

Kaposi's sarcoma is a multicentric tumour that arises from vascular and lymphatic endothelium and presents as purple nodules or plaques. The classic form mainly affects elderly men, with lesions developing on the lower limbs. The endemic form of the disease has a widespread cutaneous and lymphatic involvement with associated oedema, and affects men from central African countries. Kaposi's sarcoma can occur in immunosuppressed patients, notably those infected with HIV, following an aggressive course with systemic involvement of the skin, bowels, mouth and lungs.

All three forms can result from infection with herpesvirus 8.

Treatment of advanced disease requires radiotherapy, chemotherapy or immunotherapy.

DISORDERS OF SPECIFIC SKIN STRUCTURES

Sweat and sebaceous glands
Acne vulgaris
Pathology

Acne is one of the most common diseases of the skin. It can cause various lesions that result from chronic inflammation of the pilosebaceous apparatus, and affects chiefly those areas rich in sebaceous glands, mainly the face, shoulders and trunk. It commonly presents around puberty, and so appears in women earlier than in men, although both sexes are equally affected. Acne is essentially caused by excessive production of sebum, hyperkeratosis and blockage of the pilosebaceous duct, allowing colonization with *Propionibacterium acnes* to occur. This can lead to a release of inflammatory cytokines that results in inflammation of the lesions.

Clinical features

Lesions Comedones Comedones are either open or closed. Open comedones are dilated pores with a plug of keratin that contains melanin. Closed comedones are small cream-coloured papules (whiteheads).

Other lesions Comedones progress to inflammatory papules, pustules and cysts (Fig. 7.31). Cysts are the most destructive lesions as they leave scars that may be 'ice-pick', keloidal or atrophic. The skin may also be excessively greasy (seborrhoea).

Complications

Lesions can rupture, causing deep dermal inflammation and scarring in the long term. Although acne itself is a relatively harmless disease, the psychological effects it has on young patients cannot be overestimated. Patients severely devalue their own self-image because of the disorder. Upon remission or successful treatment,

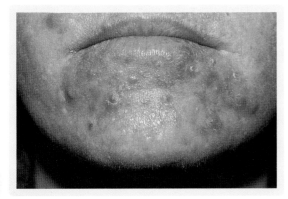

Fig. 7.31   Papulopustular acne.

Phototherapy is controlled exposure to light of a certain wavelength for a specific period of time. Different wavelengths and exposure times are used therapeutically in some skin conditions. For example, in acne vulgaris, blue light at 440nm activates porphyrin rings in the *Propionibacterium acnes* bacterium, creating free radicals that damage and subsequently kill the organism.

the psychological symptoms of acne usually improve. The disease tends to improve spontaneously over some years, although in some cases it can persist into adulthood.

Management
There are a variety of treatments for acne, listed in Figure 7.32. The patient should be advised to avoid picking the lesions and to wash the affected areas regularly to reduce greasiness.

Rosacea
Rosacea is a common, erythematous, inflammatory rash that affects the face. It can occur at any age, although it is most common in middle age. The aetiology is unknown; histology shows dilated dermal blood vessels, sebaceous gland enlargement and inflammatory cell changes.

Clinical features
The first sign of rosacea is facial flushing, which precedes the telangiectasia (dilated blood vessels), and papules and pustules on the nose, cheeks and forehead (Fig. 7.33). It occurs most commonly in middle age, although all age groups can be affected. Alcohol, sunlight, long-term topical steroid therapy and fluctuations in temperature can worsen the flushing.

Fig. 7.32 Treatment of acne vulgaris	
Treatment	**Comments**
benzoyl peroxide cream	eradicates *P. acnes*; bleaches clothes; may cause irritation and contact allergies
tretinoin	treats comedones before they evolve, but may cause irritation
antibiotics	first-line: tetracycline; second-line: erythromycin and trimethoprim; anitibiotics are suppressive, not curative; they are thought to affect lipase-producing bacteria present in pilosebaceous follicles
anti-androgens	used in combination with an oestrogen in women only; anti-androgen suppresses sebum production
retinoids	isotretinoin reduces sebum production, inhibits *P. acnes* and is anti-inflammatory: women must not be pregnant and must take oral contraceptive pill throughout 6-month course as retinoids are teratogenic; side effects can be severe
triamcinolone acetonide	steroid injected into acne cyst to aid healing
non-drug therapies	excision, cryotherapy, removal of comedones using an extractor

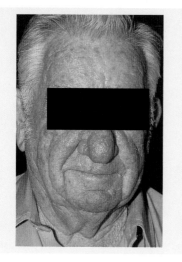

Fig. 7.33 Rosacea.

Complications

Complications include keratitis and hypertrophy of the sebaceous glands of the nose (rhinophyma), causing disfiguration. Blepharitis and conjunctivitis may also occur. Progressive disease can result in permanent facial erythema.

Management

Management aims to clear acute flares and slow disease progression. Long-term topical antibiotics such as metronidazole gel or clindamycin can be used. Topical steroid therapy should be avoided. If the rosacea proves resistant to these measures, oral antibiotics and isotretinoin can be used. Treatment improves the lesions but not the flushing or erythema. Plastic surgery can be used to correct rhinophyma.

Perioral dermatitis

This is a common perioral rash that tends to occur as a side effect of topical steroids. It presents as papules and pustules around the mouth and chin, with erythema and scaling. After withdrawing steroid therapy it is treated effectively with a 1–2-month course of low-dose oral tetracycline.

Others

Hidradenitis suppurativa

This term describes chronic inflammation of the apocrine sweat glands. Nodules, abscesses, cysts and sinuses develop in the axillae, groin and perineum, and may result in permanent scarring. Treatment depends on the severity of the condition and includes topical antiseptics, systemic antibiotics and excision of the affected glands.

Hyperhidrosis

Hyperhidrosis is excessive sweating caused by eccrine gland overactivity of unknown aetiology. It is exacerbated by heightened emotion. Aluminium chloride in alcohol is often used, applied to affected areas to reduce sweating.

Hair disorders

Alopecia

Classification

Hair loss or alopecia has a wide range of causes. It can be classified as:

- *Non-scarring* Hair loss with the scalp appearing normal. This may be androgen dependent (androgenetic alopecia), where the follicles are slowly converted from terminal to vellus hairs, and causes male pattern baldness (Fig. 7.34), being present to some degree in 80% of men by the age of 70 years. Androgenetic alopecia can also occur in women, but is usually less severe than in men.
- *Diffuse non-scarring alopecia* can also be caused by metabolic disorders such as hypothyroidism, iron or zinc deficiency. Telogen effluvium (e.g. following pregnancy) can result in diffuse non-scarring alopecia, as can the ingestion of certain drugs such as heparin and warfarin.
- *Localized non-scarring* Patchy hair loss may be caused by infection, especially tinea capitis, trauma or alopecia areata. In severe cases of alopecia areata complete hair loss can result. Alopecia areata is characterized by pathognomonic 'exclamation mark' hairs – short hairs with broken, splayed ends.
- *Scarring (cicatricial) alopecia* Scarring results from the permanent destruction of hair follicles, which can occur with burns, irradiation, infection such as shingles, kerion (occurring in tinea capitis) or tertiary syphilis, lichen planus, discoid lupus erythematosus and pseudopelade, a term used to describe the end-stage of an idiopathic destructive inflammatory process in the scalp.

Excess hair

Hirsutism

Hirsutism describes a male pattern of hair growth in a female. It can be idiopathic, presenting with

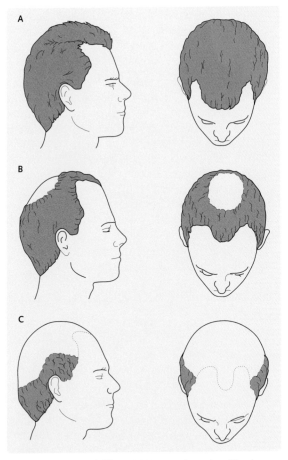

Fig. 7.34 Male pattern baldness. (**A**) Bitemporal recession; (**B**) vertex involvement; (**C**) most severe pattern of male baldness. (Adapted with permission from Gawkrodger DJ. Dermatology: an illustrated colour text, 2nd edn. Edinburgh: Churchill Livingstone, 1997.)

Cause of hirsutism	Example of disease
endocrine	acromegaly
	Cushing's syndrome
	virilizing tumours
	congenital adrenal hyperplasia
ovarian	polycystic ovaries
iatrogenic	excess androgens
	excess progesterones
idiopathic	end-organ hypersensitivity to androgens

Fig. 7.35 Other causes of hirsutism

Hypertrichosis

This term describes excessive growth of terminal hairs at any site of the body. It can occur in anorexia nervosa, with drugs such as ciclosporin or minoxidil, and rarely as a sign of underlying malignancy.

Hypertrichosis lanuginosa acquisita is the development of lanugo hairs associated with malignancy. These patients usually have metastatic disease at the time of diagnosis and hence a poor prognosis. It is most associated with lung, colorectal and breast carcinoma.

Others
Dandruff

The normal scalp is layered with fine scales of keratin; dandruff is simply a physiological exaggeration of the normal exfoliative process. Certain conditions (e.g. seborrhoeic dermatitis and psoriasis) can produce severe scaling of the scalp that may be mistaken for dandruff.

Tinea capitis

Tinea capitis is a fungal infection of the scalp (sometimes called ringworm) that may cause alopecia. It is commoner in children, especially those of Afro-Carribbean origin. Its incidence is slowly decreasing in developed countries, with the majority of UK cases caused by *Trichophyton tonsurans*. It is spread by close contact. Mild disease may imitate simple dandruff. Characteristically there are circular, scaly patches with hair loss and pustule formation.

terminal hair development in the beard area and around the nipples, or more frequently drug induced. Other causes are listed in Fig.7.35. A full endocrine assessment is required if the woman has other features of virilization, such as a deep voice, clitoromegaly, dysmenorrhoea and acne. Sensitivity is required, as the condition is often very distressing to the patient.

Skin and hair changes that occur in anorexia nervosa include the development of lanugo hair, soft vellus hairs over the body, in particular over the face and volar forearms. There may be a loss of hair from the scalp, as well as brittle nails, dry skin and a grey tinge to the skin.

Nail disorders

Congenital disease

Nail–patella syndrome

Inherited in an autosomal dominant fashion, nail–patella syndrome is a disorder in which the nails and patella are rudimentary or absent. There may be other skeletal anomalies. Thirty per cent of sufferers develop glomerulonephritis.

Trauma

Subungual haematoma

These lesions occur when the nail has been subjected to trauma. However, the possibility of a malignant cause such as a melanoma should always be considered where a subungual haematoma persists over time.

Splinter haemorrhages

These are commonly due to trauma. However, they may be indicative of infective endocarditis, so a full and thorough systemic examination should be performed to look for other features.

Ingrown toenails

Ingrown toenails are nails that have become embedded in the lateral nail folds, sometimes forming inflamed or pus-filled ulcerations. This produces intense pain and discomfort.

Two factors contribute to ingrown toenails: ill-fitting shoes predispose to physical pressure and subsequent deformity of the nails. Also, if toenails are not trimmed carefully, spicules of nail are left which can damage the nail fold. The nail of the great toe is most often involved.

Ingrown toenails can be prevented by good nail-cutting technique, and are treated by inserting gauze under the ingrowing edges of the nail to separate them from the skin fold. If this does not work, or they recur, removal of the nail and portions of its germinal matrix may be required.

> Other factors that can cause ingrown toenails are physical trauma to the nail bed, such as stubbing the toe or sports injuries, and abnormalities of the nail bed, which can lead to the nail growing in an irregular fashion.

Onychogryphosis

Chronic trauma predisposes to onychogryphosis, a condition in which the toenails become grossly thickened and hardened, and can progress to cause lateral curvature of the nails. It particularly affects the great toe. Psoriasis and fungal infection can also cause onychogryphosis. It is usually treated by chiropody.

Brittle nails

These are commonly caused by heavy exposure to detergents and water, but may also be caused by iron deficiency, hypothyroidism and digital ischaemia.

Undergrowing toenails (subungual exostosis)

Undergrowing toenails have a bony outgrowth (exostosis) from the dorsal surface of the distal phalanx that pushes the nail upwards. They are treated by excision of the exostosis.

Nail involvement in skin disease

Psoriasis

Psoriatic nail involvement includes:

- Pitting
- Thickening
- Onycholysis
- Discoloration
- Subungual hyperkeratosis.

Alopecia areata

Nail involvement can manifest as fine pitting and roughened nail surfaces.

Eczema

Nail features of eczema include:

- Coarse pitting
- Transverse ridging.

Lichen planus

In lichen planus there can be thinning of the nail plate, the development of longitudinal grooves, adhesions between the nail fold and the nail bed, or ultimately loss of the nail.

Infections

Tinea unguium (onychomycosis)

Fungal infection of the nails commonly presents as an uneven discoloration, spreading from the distal or lateral edge to involve the whole nail. As a result, the nail becomes thickened, yellow and crumbly, and subungual hyperkeratosis can be seen (Fig. 7.36). Crumbly white material can be found beneath the

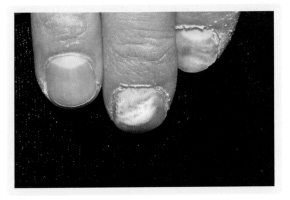

Fig. 7.36 Fungal infection of the nails.

nail and collected for diagnostic tests. Treatment is with oral terbinafine or itraconazole. Advanced infection can destroy the nail plate.

Chronic paronychia

This is often seen in wet-workers. The nail becomes boggy, the cuticle detaches, and pressure on the nail will cause pus to be extruded. Secondary involvement of the nail matrix can result in abnormal ridging of the nail, and the nail plate can become secondarily infected.

Management involves avoiding wet work by wearing rubber gloves, antiseptics, and antifungal creams such as clotrimazole.

Acute bacterial paronychia

Bacterial infection, usually staphylococcal, can arise at the junction of the posterior and lateral nail folds, with pus formation. Management requires oral antibiotics and sometimes drainage.

Tumours of the nails
Viral warts

Periungual warts are common. Treatment is the same as for warts elsewhere.

Periungual fibromas

These occur as a complication of tuberous sclerosis and are characterized by flesh-coloured papular tumours around the nails. They can be surgically removed.

Digital mucous cysts

These are found adjacent to the proximal fingernail fold; they contain mucin, a thick clear fluid, and

are fluctuant. They can be treated with cryotherapy, steroid injection or excision.

Malignant melanoma

If a pigmented streak appears in the nail, biopsy must be performed to exclude a malignant melanoma. Biopsies must also be performed on all atypical or ulcerating lesions around the nail fold.

Nail changes in systemic disease

Nails often show non-specific changes in systemic disease, the most important of which is clubbing. Discoloration, koilonychia, onycholysis, pitting and ridging are also important signs of systemic disease (Fig. 7.37).

Vascular and lymphatic disorders
Disorders of cutaneous blood vessels
Definitions

- *Erythema:* redness of the skin caused by vasodilatation. It may be localized or generalized.
- *Flushing:* sudden onset of erythema owing to vasodilatation. It is caused by a number of factors, including emotion (blushing), the menopause, certain foods and drugs, rosacea, carcinoid syndrome and phaeochromocytoma.
- *Telangiectasia:* abnormal visible dilatation of dermal blood vessels. This can result from skin atrophy, excessive oestrogen levels, connective tissue disease, rosacea and venous disease, or they may be congenital. The lesions can be treated by cautery, hyfrecation and laser ablation.

> Telangiectases are visibly dilated venules, and spider naevi are visibly dilated arterioles. They can occur in a state of oestrogen excess, and so can be present in pregnancy and in those taking the contraceptive pill. They can also occur in liver disease, as the liver's ability to break down oestrogen is impaired, resulting in raised oestrogen levels. In men this can also result in hypogonadism and gynaecomastia.

- *Purpura:* this describes a discoloration of the skin caused by the extravasation of blood cells. It can be caused by a number of factors, including vessel wall defects, defective dermal support, clotting defects or idiopathic pigmented purpura.

Fig. 7.37 Nail changes in systemic disease

Nail change	Causes
Beau's lines (tranverse grooves)	severe systemic illness
brittle nails	iron deficiency, hypothryoidism, loss of blood supply to nails, exposure to water and chemicals
colour change	drugs, cyanosis, infection, trauma, renal failure, tobacco staining, psoriasis
clubbing	bronchial carcinoma, fibrosing alveolitis, asbestosis, infective endocarditis, congenital cyanotic defects, inflammatory bowel disease, thyrotoxicosis, biliary cirrhosis
koilonychia (spoon-shaped nail)	iron-deficiency anaemia, lichen planus, chemical exposure
nail-fold telangiectasia (dilated capillaries)	connective tissue disorders
onycholysis (separation of nail from bed)	psoriasis, fungal infection, trauma, thyrotoxicosis, drugs (tetracyclines)
pitting	psoriasis, eczema, alopecia areata, lichen planus
ridging (transverse and longitudinal)	eczema, psoriasis, lichen planus

Raynaud's phenomenon

This is caused by paroxysmal spasm of the arteries supplying the fingers and toes, and mainly affects women. The resulting ischaemia causes the fingers to turn white and then blue, owing to cyanosis caused by pooled, deoxygenated blood in capillaries. They finally turn red, due to reactive hyperaemia as reperfusion ensues. There is associated numbness and paraesthesia. It is usually brought on by cold and relieved by warmth. The duration of attacks is variable, and between attacks the digits and their blood supply are normal. In persistent cases trophic changes can occur. Where the phenomenon occurs alone without any underlying disorder it is known as Raynaud's disease. Other causes of Raynaud's phenomenon include:

- Connective tissue disease
- Hyperviscosity of blood, e.g. cryoglobulinaemia, polycythaemia
- Vasoconstriction caused by the use of vibrating tools
- Toxins and drugs, particularly β-blockers.

As the phenomenon is often precipitated by cold, patients are advised to keep their hands warm and to avoid circumstances and occupations in which they are exposed to cold for prolonged periods. They should avoid smoking and β-blockers should be stopped. Nifedipine and diltiazem may also help.

Livedo reticularis

This is cyanosis occurring in a marble pattern on the skin. It is caused by reduced arteriolar flow and poor skin circulation. Reversible livedo is usually induced by cold and is seen in children, whereas fixed livedo is usually caused by vasculitis and requires further investigation.

Chilblains

These are painful, pink–purple inflamed swellings on the fingers, toes and ears, which are cold to the touch. The lesions may last for weeks and may be complicated by ulceration. Chilblains are much less common since the introduction of central heating.

Lymphatic disorders and the skin
Lymphoedema

Lymphoedema is a chronic, non-pitting oedema that affects the limbs, caused by a disruption of lymphatic drainage of the affected limb. It can be classified as a primary or secondary disorder.

Primary lymphoedema is caused by a genetic deficiency of lymphatic vessels and usually presents in adolescence. Secondary lymphoedema is usually due to obstruction to lymphatic drainage, recurrent infection (e.g. cellulitis), or damage from surgery or radiotherapy.

In chronic cases the skin can become dimpled and thickened. Lymphoedematous areas are at increased risk of infection, and where there is recurrent infection long-term antibiotic prophylaxis is required to prevent further damage.

Lymphangitis

Lymphangitis is an inflammation of lymphatic vessels, most frequently seen as a complication of infection such as cellulitis. It causes a tender red line that extends proximally from a focus of infection. It is treated with intravenous antibiotics. It can also be seen as a complication of malignancy permeating lymphatic channels.

Leg ulcers

Aetiology

Leg ulcers can be caused by venous disease, arterial disease, vasculitis or neuropathies (Fig. 7.38). The most common type in the Western world are venous ulcers. These affect 1% of the adult population and are twice as common in women as in men.

Pathology

Venous ulcers   These are caused by valvular incompetence in the perforating veins of the legs. This causes chronic venous hypertension, which leads to increased permeability. As a result, fibrin seeps through the vessel walls and is deposited adjacent to the capillaries. This interferes with oxygen and nutrient exchange, and ultimately leads to ulceration. Ulcers usually present in middle age and later life. Risk factors for the development of venous ulcers include obesity and previous deep vein thrombosis (DVT). The first

signs are a feeling of heaviness in the legs caused by oedema. There may be an associated discoloration of the skin, pain, venous eczema, and fibrosis of the dermis and subcutis (lipodermatosclerosis). Minor trauma can be enough to provoke ulceration in predisposed individuals. Ulcers usually affect the area between the lateral and medial malleoli (Fig. 7.39). Ulcers are initially exudative, but may then enter a granulomatous, healing phase, which can take many weeks or months; some larger venous ulcers never heal. On healing, dermal fibrosis can cause the affected area to be irreversibly disfigured.

With appropriate treatment, 80% can heal within 26 weeks. Treatment requires compression bandages and elevation of the leg to reduce venous pressure. However, it is vital that Doppler studies are performed to exclude arterial disease before compression therapy is used. Supportive treatments include antibiotics for secondary infection and analgesia for pain.

Arterial ulcers   Arterial disease affecting the leg leads to ischaemia and cyanosis, increasing the likelihood of arterial ulcers developing. These are painful lesions that appear well demarcated and 'punched out', and form on the foot or mid-shin of a cold, pale limb. There may be reduced or absent arterial pulses in the foot and hair loss from the leg. There may be a history of cardiovascular risk factors, in particular high blood pressure, intermittent claudication, ischaemic heart disease (IHD) or smoking. Doppler ultrasound confirms the diagnosis. Treatment requires maintenance of a high standard of hygiene around the

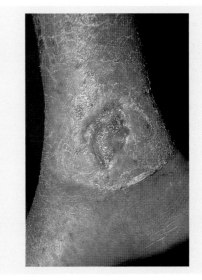

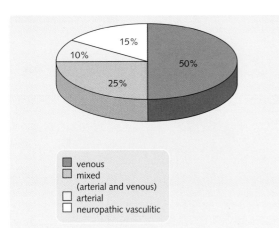

venous
mixed
(arterial and venous)
arterial
neuropathic vasculitic

Fig. 7.38 Percentages of leg ulcers caused by venous disease, arterial disease, vasculitic disease or neuropathy.

Fig. 7.39 Venous ulcer.

wound and appropriate analgesia. Surgery may be required to improve arterial flow.

Neuropathic ulcers These tend to occur on pressure areas of the foot owing to repeated, physical trauma, usually in those with neurological dysfunction that affects the patient's perception of pain or trauma. They particularly occur in diabetics with peripheral neuropathy. Optimal healing conditions require keeping the ulcer clean and minimizing further trauma.

Complications

Poor management of ulcers may cause them to enlarge and deepen, reducing the chances of them healing successfully. Complications include secondary infection, lymphoedema and contact dermatitis (sensitivity to topical medications). Rarely, malignant change to squamous cell carcinoma can occur with venous ulcers.

Management

Underlying risk and causative factors, such as obesity, cardiac failure, anaemia and arthritis, should be addressed. Elevation, exercise and a healthy, balanced diet should be advised to encourage normal blood flow.

Topical therapy includes antiseptics and desloughing agents. Hydrocolloid or gel dressings used with compression bandages increase granulation and promote healing of the ulcer.

Appropriate analgesia should be provided. Antibiotics should be used to treat secondary infection. Surgery is only helpful in younger patients and/or cases resistant to treatment, and in patients without significant comorbidity, such as cardiac failure.

Vasculitis and reactive erythemas

Vasculitis

This term refers to inflammation of the blood vessels. It can be caused by drugs, infection or connective tissue disease, but most cases appear to be idiopathic. Circulating immune complexes lodge in vessel walls and activate complement, causing damage to the vessel walls. This causes characteristic, palpable, often painful purpura at sites of vessel involvement. Vasculitis may be confined to the skin. However, it can also be a multisystem disorder affecting the vessels of the joints, kidneys, lungs, gut and nervous system (Fig. 7.40). There is often pyrexia and arthralgia. Cutaneous vasculitis can resolve spontaneously. General measures to alleviate symptoms include leg elevation, support stockings and analgesia. Systemic steroids and immunosuppressive agents are needed in some cases to control the disease process.

Erythema multiforme

This is an immune-mediated hypersensitivity reaction caused by infection, usually with *Herpes simplex* virus or *Mycoplasma*, or adverse drug reactions. It is characterized by target lesions consisting of erythematous rings that may blister. The rash occurs symmetrically, often involving the hands and feet. The mucous membranes may also be involved. Management is by treatment of the underlying cause.

Erythema nodosum

This is an inflammation of the dermis and subcutaneous tissues. It causes painful red–blue nodules on the calves and shins. It is more common

Fig.7.40 Types of vasculitis	
	Clinical features
Henoch–Schönlein purpura	cutaneous signs accompanied by arthritis, abdominal pain and haematuria; it often follows a streptococcal infection and mainly affects children
nodular vasculitis	painful subcutaneous nodules are found on the lower legs
polyarteritis nodosa	an uncommon necrotizing vasculitis that affects middle-aged men; subcutaneous nodules develop, together with hypertension, renal failure and neuropathy
Wegener's granulomatosis	a rare and potentially fatal vasculitis; malaise, lung involvement and glomerulonephritis are accompanied by cutaneous vasculitis in 50% of patients
giant cell arteritis	affects the elderly, who present with scalp tenderness owing to temporal artery involvement, which can cause scalp necrosis; prednisolone should be given, or sight may be lost

in females and younger adults. Circulating immune complexes play an important role in the pathology. The causes of erythema nodosum include infection, drugs, inflammatory bowel disease and sarcoidosis. Arthralgia and fever often accompany the nodules. The condition usually clears spontaneously over 1–2 months. Treatment includes NSAIDs, elastic bandaging or hosiery and bed rest.

Sweet's disease

Sweet's disease is an acute, febrile neutrophilic dermatosis, which is characterized by annular red plaques on the face and limbs. The lesions are accompanied by fever and a raised neutrophil count. The disease often occurs in patients with an underlying malignancy, particularly leukaemias and lymphomas. Treatment with prednisolone is usually effective.

DISORDERS OF PIGMENTATION

Hypopigmentation
Vitiligo
Aetiology
This is a common disorder, probably autoimmune in aetiology, that leads to macules of pigment loss on the skin with no preceding symptoms (Fig. 7.41). It affects around 0.5% of the population and about 30% of patients have a positive family history. It is associated with pernicious anaemia, thyroid disease and Addison's disease. The onset is usually in childhood or early adulthood, and it affects both sexes equally.

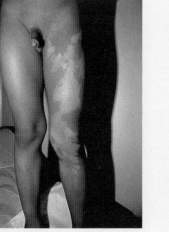

Fig. 7.41 Vitiligo.

Clinical features
The well-defined macules are usually symmetrical, and frequently affect the hands, wrists, face and neck, and the genitalia. The hair may also be depigmented. Vitiligo lesions may be precipitated by trauma and exacerbated by sun exposure. Repigmentation can occur spontaneously, but rarely occurs in chronic lesions.

Complications
As melanocytes are absent from lesions, care must be taken when skin is exposed to the sun as patients can burn easily.

Management
Camouflage cosmetics often prove unsatisfactory. Sunscreens must be used to protect lesions and prevent burning. Potent topical steroids and UV phototherapy may help to induce repigmentation. When vitiligo is nearly universal and very noticeable, it is worth considering inducing depigmentation of the remaining normal skin using 20% hydroquinone ointment.

Albinism

Albinism is a rare autosomal recessive disorder, with a prevalence of 1:20 000. Melanocytes fail to synthesize melanin, leading to a lack of pigment in the skin. The skin is universally pale, the hair is white and the eye lacks pigmentation, with the iris appearing pink. Patients suffer from photophobia, nystagmus and poor sight. As the body has no protection against UV rays, the sun should be strictly avoided as the risk of skin cancer is greatly increased; obsessive sun protection is necessary in circumstances where exposure is unavoidable.

Phenylketonuria

This is an autosomal recessive metabolic defect. The enzyme that converts phenylalanine into tyrosine is defective, leading to the accumulation of metabolites in the brain. If left untreated, mental retardation and choreoathetosis occur. The hair and skin are fair because melanin synthesis is impaired, and atopic eczema commonly develops. Management requires a diet with minimal phenylalanine content.

Hyperpigmentation
Freckles and lentigines

Freckles are small, light-brown macules in sun-exposed areas that darken with prolonged UV exposure. On stimulation by UV light the synthesis of melanin is increased without affecting the number of melanocytes. Freckles are common and are frequently seen on the face in the summer months. Lentigines are brown macules that do not darken in the sun. However, they contain an increased number of melanocytes. No treatment is required, although they may respond to cryotherapy if removal is desired.

Chloasma

Induced by pregnancy or by taking the oral contraceptive pill, chloasma is a symmetrical facial pigmentation that often involves the forehead. It sometimes improves spontaneously, although sunscreens and camouflage cosmetics may help.

Drug-induced pigmentation

Pigmentation is a side effect of certain drugs such as phenothiazines, minocycline, amiodarone, clofazimine, chlorpromazine and antimalarials.

Other causes

Peutz–Jeghers syndrome is an autosomal dominant condition that causes lentigines to form around the lips and mouth, in association with benign small bowel polyps. Addison's disease leads to new melanocyte production through the production of excess adrenocorticotrophic hormone, resulting in pigmentation on the buccal mucosa, palmar creases, scars and flexures.

BLISTERING DISORDERS

Pemphigus

Pathology

This is a potentially fatal disease in which autoantibodies develop against a desmosomal protein, desmoglein 3, that holds cells together. It affects both sexes equally, and usually presents between youth and middle age. Circulating IgG autoantibodies bind to the skin's intracellular matrix, inducing the release of proteolytic enzymes from adjacent keratinocytes. This subsequently results in thin-walled, fragile blisters. Pemphigus is often associated with other autoimmune disorders.

Clinical features

The disease presents in half of patients as an eruption of shallow mucosal blisters, especially in the mouth. Further flaccid lesions can follow several months later on the face and trunk. Blisters are sore and invariably rupture, so patients often present with red, weeping skin erosions rather than blisters. This is in contrast to pemphigoid, where the blister walls are thicker and more robust. Lesions can be extended under gentle pressure (Nikolsky's sign). Diagnosis is by skin biopsy, immunofluorescence and the detection of serum autoantibodies, which can subsequently be measured and used to monitor disease activity.

Management

High-dose oral steroids are given to control the blistering, often for long periods, in which case they are used in conjunction with steroid-sparing immunosuppressant drugs such as azathioprine. Both the disease and the treatments can produce significant morbidity and occasional mortality.

Pemphigoid

Pemphigoid usually affects older people, in particular those over 60. It is characterized by a chronic eruption of large, tense-walled blisters, often associated with or preceded by widespread pruritus (Fig. 7.42).

Pathology

The pathology is similar to that of pemphigus, with autoantibodies produced against BP-1 antigen in hemidesmosomes. However, the autoantibodies are deposited at the basement membrane, resulting in a subepidermal split through the membrane. Serum autoantibodies are present in 70% of patients. Pemphigoid is diagnosed through skin biopsy and immunofluorescence.

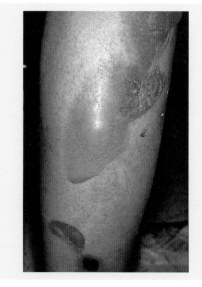

Fig. 7.42 Bullous pemphigoid.

Clinical features

Pemphigoid has three different patterns (Fig. 7.43).

Management

Oral prednisolone is prescribed at a lower dose than for pemphigus, and steroid-sparing agents such as azathioprine may also be used. The disease is self-limiting in half of all cases and is easier to control than pemphigus. Treatment can often be stopped after 2 years.

Dermatitis herpetiformis

Pathology

Dermatitis herpetiformis is an uncommon blistering disorder associated with gluten-sensitive enteropathy (coeliac disease). It causes a symmetrical eruption of intensely pruritic blisters.

Clinical features

The first sign of dermatitis herpetiformis is usually small, itchy vesicles that erupt on the scalp, elbows, knees and buttocks. They can present as crusted erosions (the blisters are frequently scratched off). Although small-bowel pathology is often present, gastrointestinal symptoms are uncommon. Dermatitis herpetiformis is diagnosed on skin biopsy and immunofluorescence. The condition responds to a gluten-free diet, which should always be implemented and maintained. Oral dapsone can control the skin disease, but treatment can be withdrawn when a gluten-free diet has been successfully established.

INHERITED DISORDERS OF THE SKIN

The ichthyoses

The ichthyoses are a group of rare disorders characterized by excessive amounts of dry, scaly skin. The classification of ichthyoses is listed in Figure 7.44.

Management

Regular use of emollients and moisturizing creams is the mainstay of treatment. Neonatal ichthyoses must be managed in a paediatric intensive care unit, as fluid losses may be huge and thermoregulation is disturbed.

Keratoderma

This disorder is characterized by gross hyperkeratosis of the palms and soles, creating papular or nodular raised lesions. It can develop in association with other conditions, such as reactive arthritis, or it may be inherited. The typical diffuse pattern of hyperkeratosis is known as tylosis; in rare cases it is; associated with oesophageal carcinoma. Keratoderma is treated with keratolytics such as salicylic acid ointment or urea cream.

Epidermolysis bullosa

This describes a rare group of disorders in which there are genetic abnormalities of structural skin proteins, resulting in fragile skin. Minor injury or trauma induces blistering. The disease ranges in severity from simple epidermolysis bullosa (the most common type), which features blisters limited to the hands and feet, to junctional epidermolysis bullosa, a potentially fatal disorder where large blisters develop or areas of skin are absent at birth. Dystrophic epidermolysis bullosa causes severe blistering and deformity of the nails. There are two patterns of inheritance, autosomal dominant and autosomal recessive. Autosomal dominant forms follows a milder course than the recessive form, in which joint contractures and fusion of digits may occur. The disease is best managed in a specialized centre, and management relies on the avoidance of trauma and secondary infection.

Fig. 7.43 Clinical patterns of pemphigoid	
Type of pemphigoid	Clinical features
bullous	large, tense, itchy blisters that usually affect elderly patients; limbs, hands, feet commonly affected; 10% of patients have oral lesions; may occur on reddened or urticarial skin, may be localized to a single site (see Fig. 7.42)
cicatricial	predominantly affects mucosal surfaces, especially ocular and oral mucosa; causes scarring
pemphigoid (herpes) gestationis	bullous lesions that are associated with pregnancy; clears after delivery but may recur in subsequent pregnancies

Fig.7.44 Classification of ichthyoses

Type of ichthyosis	Mode of inheritance	Incidence	Clinical features
ichthyosis vulgaris	autosomal dominant	1 : 250 births	disorder of epidermal cornification; onset between 1 and 4 years; granular layer is reduced or absent; dry skin with white scales on back and extensor surface of limbs; palmar and plantar markings are increased
X-linked ichthyosis	X-linked	1 : 7000 births	onset is early; scales are dark and widespread, with face, neck and scalp all involved; caused by deficiency of steroid sulphatase
bullous ichthyosiform erythroderma/ epidermolytic hyperkeratosis	autosomal dominant	1 : 100 000	presents at birth; skin is red, moist and eroded in parts; erythema eventually replaced by scales; flexures particularly affected; hyperkeratosis develops in childhood
non-bullous ichthyosiform erythroderma	autosomal dominant	1 : 100 000	presents at birth; collodion baby (newborn with tight, shiny skin causing feeding difficulties and ectropion); progresses to reddening and thickening of skin with fine, white scales; acanthosis is present

Neurofibromatosis

Neurofibromatosis is a condition characterized by multiple neurofibromas and associated skin pigmentary abnormalities. Two forms are recognized: NF1 (von Recklinghausen's peripheral neurofibromatosis) and NF2 (bilateral acoustic central neurofibromatosis).

NF1 is common and is inherited in an autosomal dominant fashion, affecting 1 in 3000 births. Skin involvement includes:

- *Café-au-lait* spots—flat, coffee-coloured skin patches that appear within the first year of life, progressively increasing in size and number. Six or more macules more than 2.5 cm in diameter are diagnostic
- Freckling in the axillae, groin, base of neck and under the breasts, developing by the age of 10
- Fleshy skin tags
- Deep, soft dermal tumours, which may become pedunculated and may itch. Nodular neurofibromata are firm, well-demarcated nodules stemming from the nerve trunks that may become numb when they are pressed. Lisch nodules—pigmented hamartomas in the iris—can be visualized using a slit lamp.

Potential complications include the development of malignancy (neurofibrosarcoma). Genetic counselling is an important part of management. Excision of some tumours may be required, depending on the site, the individual and their circumstances.

Tuberous sclerosis

This rare disorder is an autosomal dominant condition that varies in severity. It is characterized by hamartomas developing in organs and bone. Cutaneous features include:

- Ash-leaf patches—ovoid or elongated hypopigmented macules that fluoresce under Wood's light, presenting in infancy
- Adenoma sebaceum—an acne-like eruption of reddish papules or fibromas around the nose, presenting in late childhood and adolescence
- Periungual fibromata—fibrous pink nodules which arise from the nail bed
- Shagreen patches—firm, fleshy plaques sited on the trunk.

In addition to cutaneous features, there may be mental retardation and epilepsy.

Management is supportive, and involves genetic counselling and support groups.

Xeroderma pigmentosum

Caused by defective repair of UV-damaged DNA, this condition is characterized by photosensitivity that begins in infancy. The persistent damaged skin results in the development of skin tumours, from which patients can die as young as 30 years of age. Affected patients must avoid sunlight. The condition is very rare, and is autosomal recessive in inheritance.

Pseudoxanthoma elasticum

Pseudoxanthoma elasticum describes a group of disorders caused by abnormalities in elastin and collagen. It is characterized by loose, wrinkled skin that bears papules and is most often found in the flexures of the neck. The disorder is inherited in an autosomal recessive manner.

CONNECTIVE TISSUE DISORDERS

Systemic lupus erythematosus

Systemic lupus erythematosus (SLE) is an inflammatory multisystem disorder, a widespread vasculitis that affects the skin as well as the joints, kidneys, lungs and nervous system.

Aetiology

The aetiology is unclear. Ninety per cent of patients with SLE have circulating antinuclear antibodies detectable in their serum. SLE is associated with HLA B8 and DR3.

Pathology

There is a dysregulated immune response to cellular antigens that come to be expressed on the surface of apoptosing cells, resulting in the formation of antibody–antigen immune complexes within the blood vessels that are deposited in the basement membrane of the skin and the kidneys. Immune complexes, immunoglobulins and complement are deposited at the junction of the epidermis and dermis in the lesions (and in sun-exposed skin in SLE); these can be viewed by direct immunofluorescence. Patients develop annular lesions, which show epidermal atrophy, hyperkeratosis and basal layer degeneration. In SLE, lesions are accompanied by dermal oedema, inflammation, and occasionally vasculitis.

Clinical features

Skin involvement occurs in 75% of patients with SLE, the site and the nature depending on the variant of the disease. Involvement includes:

- An erythematous butterfly rash present on the face and the bridge of the nose
- Photosensitivity
- Annular lesions with a well-defined erythematous margin, becoming atropic and scaly, and associated follicular keratin plugs

- Diffuse alopecia
- Vasculitic lesions
- Purpura and urticaria.

Other systemic features (Fig. 7.45) must also be present for a diagnosis of SLE to be made.

In discoid lupus erythematosus the discoid lesions appear on the face, scalp or hands.

Palmar and plantar rashes and skin pigmentation can occur. Raynaud's phenomenon is common.

Complications

In addition to the systemic features listed in Figure 7.45, healed lesions can leave scarring and may lead to alopecia and hypopigmentation in pigmented skin.

Management

Patients should be advised to minimize sun exposure and sunscreen should be used to protect photosensitive skin. Active disease requires therapy with topical or oral steroids, or immunosuppressants.

Scleroderma

Scleroderma is a chronic multisystem inflammatory disease characterized by tightening, immobility, thickening and induration of the skin, especially over the fingers, limbs, trunk and face, and sometimes in a generalized distribution. There is excessive production of types I and III collagen that is

Fig. 7.45 Systemic features of systemic lupus erythematosus

System	Clinical features
musculoskeletal	arthritis
	tenosynovitis
cardiovascular	pericarditis
	endocarditis
respiratory	pneumonitis
	effusion
	infarction
central nervous system	psychosis
renal	glomerulonephritis
blood	anaemia
	thrombocytopenia

deposited in the microvasculature supplying the skin, as well as that supplying all the organs of the body. This results in inflammation and progressive fibrosis, and microvascular occlusion.

Scleroderma can be classified into localized and generalized according to the level of cutaneous and systemic involvement (also known as systemic sclerosis) (Fig. 7.46).

Localized scleroderma/morphoea

Localized scleroderma involves the skin, and possibly the bones and muscles underlying it, but spares the internal organs. Localized lesions may occur in a patchy or linear distribution and are often known as morphoea.

In linear scleroderma (morphoea) there is asymmetrical thickening of the skin that also affects the underlying bones and muscles, and can become severe enough to limit the range of movement of the area. It commonly affects the arms, legs and forehead.

In patchy morphoea, pale, indurated plaques develop a purple halo around them, leading to hairless and atrophic areas of skin. The disease may resolve spontaneously. It most commonly affects children and young adults.

Systemic sclerosis (generalized scleroderma)

In addition to skin and blood vessel involvement, the internal organs can also be involved in the disease. Cutaneous involvement includes:

- Raynaud's phenomenon: this occurs in almost all cases, and is the first manifestation of the disease in three-quarters of cases

- Resorption of finger pulps
- Tight, waxy and stiff skin on the fingers, forearms and calves, producing flexion deformities
- Perioral furrowing (microstomia) and characteristic 'beak-like' nose
- Telangiectasia.

It can be classified according to the pattern of involvement into CREST syndrome, limited systemic sclerosis and diffuse systemic sclerosis.

CREST is characterized by the presence of two or more of the following:

- Calcium deposition, usually in the fingers
- Raynaud's phenomenon
- (O)esophageal motility loss
- Sclerodactyly (deformity of fingertips, with loss of finger pulps and bone deformity)
- Telangiectasia, commonly over the fingers, face and buccal mucosa.

In limited systemic sclerosis skin involvement is limited to the hands, face and neck, whereas diffuse systemic sclerosis involves the skin above the level of the wrists.

Systemic features, such as renal involvement, can be severe and may be fatal.

Management

Management aims to reduce morbidity and complications and is based mainly on education and support. Corticosteroids and immunosuppressants can be used to suppress the immune response. Collagen cross-link inhibitors can help to reduce the level of collagen formation. Oral vasodilators, e.g calcium channel blockers such as nifedipine, may aid Raynaud's phenomenon. Physiotherapy and skin lubricants can help to slow contracture development.

Dermatomyositis

Dermatomyositis is a rare disorder of unknown aetiology characterized by inflammation of the striated muscle. Cutaneous involvement distinguishes it from polymyositis and can cause:

- Lilac blue (heliotrope) discoloration around the eyelids, cheeks and forehead, with or without periorbital oedema
- Blue–red papules or linear lesions on the extensor surfaces of joints and fingers
- Pigmentation

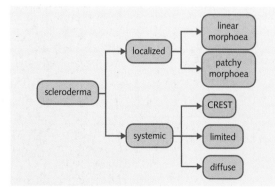

Fig. 7.46 Classification of scleroderma.

- Nail-fold telangiectasia
- Photosensitivity
- Contractures.

Dermatomyositis can occur in association with malignancy. Further information can be found in Chapter 2.

SKIN MANIFESTATIONS OF SYSTEMIC DISEASE

Skin signs of endocrine and metabolic disease

Diabetes mellitus

Cutaneous features of diabetes mellitus include:

- Candidal or bacterial infection, caused by poorly controlled blood sugar levels
- Ulcers—caused by neuropathy or arteriopathy of the feet
- Eruptive xanthomas—associated with secondary hyperlipidaemia.
  Diabetics are specifically affected by:
- Diabetic dermatopathy—flat-topped pigmented scars on the shins that are associated with diabetic microangiopathy
- Necrobiosis lipoidica—yellow–red atrophic plaques on the shins that are prone to ulceration
- Granuloma annulare—annular lesions found often on the hands and feet which tend to fade within a year.

Thyroid disease

Cutaneous signs of thyroid disease are listed in Figure 7.47.

Hyperlipidaemia

Hyperlipidaemia can manifest with xanthomas caused by lipid deposition in the skin. These can occur over tendons, around the eyes, in palmar creases, on extensor surfaces and on the buttocks. All patients with xanthomas should be investigated for hyperlipidaemia. The xanthomas are controlled by treating the underlying hyperlipidaemia.

Fig. 7.47 Cutaneous signs of thyroid disease

Thyrotoxicosis	Myxoedema
skin becomes soft and pink	alopecia
hyperhidrosis	coarse and thickened hair
alopecia	skin becomes dry, yellow and firm
pigmentation	asteatotic eczema
onycholysis	xanthomas
clubbing (Graves')	
pretibial myxoedema (Graves')	
palmar erythema	

Skin signs of nutritional deficiency and gastrointestinal disease

Malnutrition

Different forms of malnutrition lead to varying skin manifestations (Fig. 7.48).

Inflammatory bowel disease

The skin changes in Crohn's disease and ulcerative colitis are shown in Figure 7.49.

Skin signs of malignancy

Acanthosis nigricans

This is an uncommon condition associated with malignancy. It is characterized by thickening and pigmentation of the skin around the flexures and

Fig. 7.48 Cutaneous signs of malnutrition

Deficiency	Disease	Cutaneous signs
protein	kwashiorkor	altered pigmentation; desquamation; ulcers (with brown/red hair in Afro-Caribbeans)
vitamin C	scurvy	purpura; swollen, bleeding gums; indurated (woody) oedema
nicotinic acid	pellagra	scaly dermatitis; pigmentation
iron		alopecia; koilonychia; pruritus; angular cheilitis

Fig. 7.49 Skin changes in inflammatory bowel disease

Inflammatory bowel disease	Cutaneous signs
Crohn's disease	perianal abscesses; sinuses fistulae; erythema nodosum; Sweet's disease; pyoderma gangrenosum; aphthous stomatitis; glossitis
ulcerative colitis	erythema nodosum; Sweet's disease; pyoderma gangrenosum

neck. The skin becomes velvety and papillomatous, and warty lesions develop. Rarely, the condition may present in childhood, an inherited form of the disorder not associated with malignancy. It can also occur in younger, obese adults suffering from insulin resistance. When it presents in older patients, a carcinoma, most commonly of the gastrointestinal tract, should be excluded.

Paget's disease of the nipple

A unilateral plaque-like lesion on the nipple areola usually indicates the spread of an intraductal carcinoma of the breast. An eruption resembling eczema around the perineum or axilla may be caused by intraepidermal malignant spread. With both presentations, a skin biopsy should be performed to confirm the diagnosis.

Erythema gyratum repens

This is an extremely rare disorder that is caused by malignancy, usually of the lung or breast. Scaly concentric erythematous rings resembling wood-grain develop, which rapidly change their pattern.

Necrolytic migratory erythema

This extremely rare eruption is characterized by burning, erythematous, annular plaques, which usually begin in the perineum. It is caused by a glucagonoma, a glucagon-secreting tumour of the pancreas. It is associated with weight loss, anaemia, diabetes and angular stomatitis.

Secondary tumour deposits in skin

Skin metastases often present late in cases of malignancy, and so carry a poor prognosis. They usually appear as firm, pink nodules and are found most commonly on the scalp, umbilicus and trunk. Tumour tissue may metastasize to the skin from the following primary sites:

- Breast
- Gastrointestinal tract
- Ovary
- Lung
- Melanoma (primary cutaneous or ocular)
- Lymphomas and leukaemias may also involve the skin.

Conditions occasionally associated with malignancy

Other skin manifestations that may be associated with underlying malignancy, but also with more benign diagnoses, include:

- Generalized pruritus (jaundice)
- Acquired ichthyosis (lymphoma)
- Hyperpigmentation
- Pyoderma gangrenosum (lymphoma, leukaemia, myeloma)
- Dermatomyositis (carcinoma of the lung, breast, GI and GU tract)
- Erythroderma (lymphoma, leukaemia)
- Hypertrichosis (carcinoma of the ovary).

A careful history and examination should be obtained from all patients who present with the above where there is no obvious underlying cause.

Skin changes in pregnancy

Pregnant women may be affected by:

- Increased pigmentation, especially of the nipples
- Proliferation of melanocytic naevi and skin tags
- Development of spider naevi, abdominal striae (stretchmarks) and midline pigmentation (linea nigra)
- Pruritus
- Telogen effluvium may also occur in the postpartum period.

DRUG-INDUCED SKIN DISORDERS

Cutaneous drug reactions are common. Beware of a patient who claims to be 'allergic' to a drug,

Fig. 7.50 Mechanisms that produce drug-induced disorders

Mechanism	Example
excessive therapeutic effect	an overdose of anticoagulants may lead to subcutaneous bleeding and purpura
pharmacological side effects	dry lips and mucosa resulting from use of isotretinoin; bone marrow suppression with use of cytotoxic drugs
hypersensitivity	true allergy; may occur via any of the four skin type reactions
skin deposition of drug or metabolites	gold
facilitative effect	use of a drug upsets biological balance; use of wide-spectrum antibiotics may result in Candida, etc.
idiosyncratic reaction	reaction peculiar to individual

Fig. 7.51 Important drug reactions

	Toxic erythema	Erythema multiforme	Toxic epidermal necrolysis	Psoriasiform and bullous eruptions
aetiology	caused by drugs, scarlet fever and infection	drugs, viral/bacterial/ fungal infection, pregnancy, malignancy; immune mediated	drug-induced epidermal necrosis	lithium and chloroquine exacerbate psoriasis; β-blockers, gold and methyldopa may precipitate an eruption
clinical features	eruption, which may be morbilliform or urticarial; may be accompanied by fever or followed by skin peeling; eruption affects trunk more than limbs	target lesions, dermal oedema, inflammatory infiltrate, vasodilatation	intraepidermal split in skin; skin red, swollen and separates as in scalding	psoriatic eruption
complications	erythroderma, dehydration, hypothermia	erythroderma, mucosal ulceration and scarring	problems in fluid and electrolyte balance; mortality around 25%	
management	stop precipitating drug; clears up within 1–2 weeks	treat underlying cause; systemic steroids	in-hospital management in intensive care unit	stop precipitating drug; emollients if necessary

as true allergies are less common and a mild eruption may be the cause of such a statement. As always, a thorough history should be taken and the features documented in the patient's notes.

Mechanisms of drug-induced skin disorders

There are several mechanisms that produce a drug-induced skin disorder (Fig. 7.50). The four most important drug reactions are listed in Figure 7.51.

CLINICAL ASSESSMENT

Common presentations of muscle, bone and skin diseases

8

Objectives

By the end of this chapter you should be able to:
- Understand the classifications of arthritis and be able to give some examples of each
- List the four classifications of back pain
- List the common causes of blistering
- Give some examples of causes of hyperpigmentation.

COMMON PRESENTING COMPLAINTS OF THE MUSCULOSKELETAL SYSTEM

Arthritis

Arthritis is classified as:

- Monoarticular
- Pauciarticular (up to four joints involved)
- Polyarticular (five or more joints involved).

Monoarticular arthritis

Monoarticular arthritis is a common presenting joint complaint (Fig. 8.1). It can be classified into acute and chronic forms.

Acute monoarticular arthritis

The more commoner causes of acute monoarticular arthritis include:

- Sepsis, e.g., from staphylococcal infection
- Crystal-induced, e.g., gout, pseudogout
- Psoriasis
- Trauma
- Reactive arthritis
- Haemarthrosis.

Chronic monoarticular arthritis

If monoarticular arthritis persists for more than 2 months it is referred to as chronic (Figs 8.2 and 8.3. Causes include those of both acute monoarticular arthritis and polyarticular arthritis. It can also occur because of:

- Rheumatoid arthritis
- Ankylosing spondylitis
- Chronic infection, e.g., TB
- Psoriasis.

> Diseases linked to HLA-B27 include ankylosing spondylitis, iritis and reactive arthritis. There is a weaker association with psoriasis and inflammatory bowel disease.

Polyarticular arthritis

Polyarticular arthritis is inflammation of five joints or more. It can be classified into acute or chronic forms. Where the condition lasts for more than 6–8 weeks it is described as chronic.

Causes of acute polyarthritis include:

- Rheumatoid arthritis
- The spondylarthritides, e.g. ankylosing spondylitis
- Viral arthritis (e.g. rubella and hepatitis B)
- Systemic lupus erythematosus
- Acute rheumatic fever
- Psoriasis.

Causes of chronic polyarthritis include:

- Osteoarthritis
- Rheumatoid arthritis
- Some of the spondylarthritides, such as psoriatic arthritis, Reiter's syndrome
- Sarcoid arthritis
- Systemic lupus erythematosus.

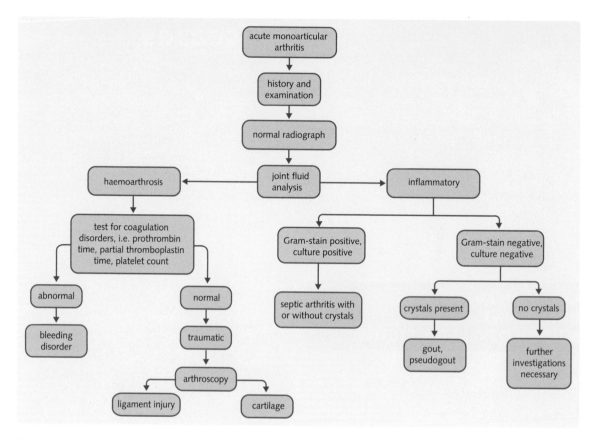

Fig. 8.1 Stages involved in determining a diagnosis of monoarticular arthritis.

Fig. 8.2 Stages involved in determining a diagnosis of chronic monoarticular arthritis with no joint effusion.

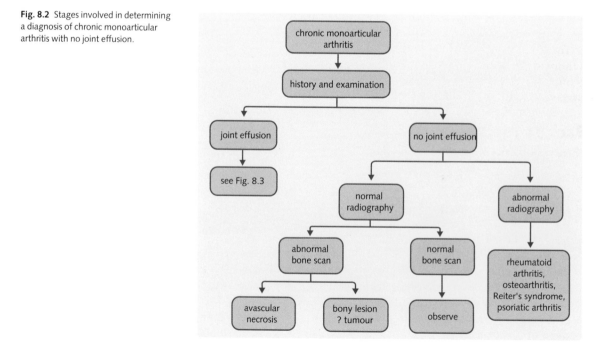

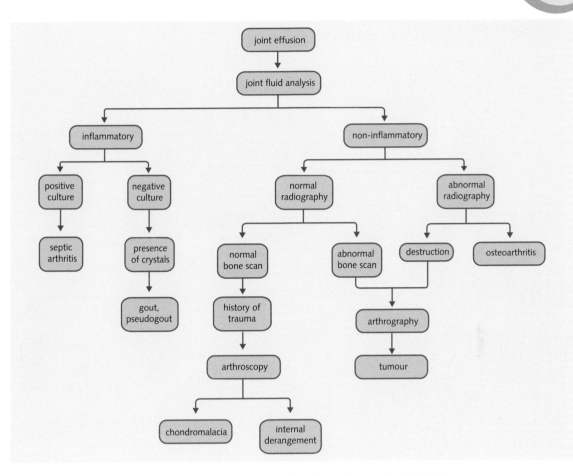

Fig. 8.3 Stages involved in determining a diagnosis of chronic monoarticular arthritis with an associated joint effusion.

The diagnosis of polyarticular arthritis is aided by a thorough systemic history, as this type of arthritis is often associated with extra-articular features that would indicate the most likely cause (Fig. 8.4).

Back pain

There are four common causes of back pain (Fig. 8.5):

- Inflammatory—stiffness and pain after inactivity, pain relieved by use
- Mechanical—pain that is aggravated by use. Can be associated with symptoms such as locking
- Neuropathic/referred—pain that is difficult to localize: it may be dermatomal, aggravated by moving the source of the referred pain, rather than the actual site of pain, and may be relieved by rubbing
- Destructive—progressive pain that may be worse at night. Destructive pain usually indicates serious pathology.

Metabolic—normal bone physiology is disrupted by metabolic conditions.

Inflammatory back pain is caused by:

- Rheumatoid arthritis
- Infective lesions of the spine.

Mechanical back pain is caused by:

- Trauma (damage to either ligaments or muscles)
- Poor posture
- Prolapsed intervertebral disc, lumbar spondylosis, spondylolisthesis
- The spondylarthritides
- Congenital hemivertebrae or sacralization
- Spinal stenosis (accompanied by non-referred pain down into the legs)
- Cauda equina syndrome (accompanied by sciatica to below knee).

Fig. 8.4 Systemic symptoms that may aid diagnosis of polyarthritis

System	Symptoms	Possible diagnoses
general	unexplained weight loss, fatiguability	systemic lupus erythematosus (SLE), rheumatoid arthritis, ankylosing spondylitis, Reiter's syndrome, sarcoidosis
eyes	dryness	Sjögren's syndrome
	pain	SLE, rheumatoid arthritis, ankylosing spondylitis, Reiter's syndrome, Behçet's syndrome, sarcoidosis
mucocutaneous	dry mouth	Sjögren's syndrome
	rash	SLE, dermatomyositis, psoriasis, Reiter's syndrome, Sjögren's syndrome
	nail pitting	psoriasis, Reiter's syndrome
	subcutaneous nodules	rheumatoid arthritis, SLE, gout, sarcoidosis
respiratory	shortness of breath, pleuritic pain	SLE, rheumatoid arthritis
gastrointestinal	symptoms of inflammatory bowel disease	enteropathic arthritis
genitourinary	dysuria	Reiter's syndrome
	painful intercourse	Sjögren's syndrome, Behçet's syndrome
musculoskeletal	muscle weakness	polymyositis, dermatomyositis, rheumatoid arthritis, SLE, sarcoidosis
	muscle tenderness, stiffness	rheumatoid arthritis, SLE
	joint symptoms	inflammatory arthritis
nervous	headaches and visual problems	SLE

It is estimated that seven out of 10 people will experience low back pain (or lumbago) at some point in their life. It is the commonest cause of sick leave from work, with an estimated loss of 52 million working days in Britain each year and an estimated cost to the NHS of over £500 million a year.

Neuropathic/referred back pain is caused by:

- Nerve root compression from a prolapsed intervertebral disc; tumour of a vertebra, nerve or fibro-osseous canal through which the nerve root leaves the spinal column; spondylosis, abscess or, less commonly, congenital diastematomyelia and tuberculosis
- Referred pain caused by an intracranial tumour, pelvic mass, osteoarthritis of the hip, retroperitoneal or urogenital pathology, aortic dissection.

Destructive back pain is caused by:
- Malignancy, primary and metastatic tumours of the bone
- Metabolic disturbance (i.e., osteoporosis, osteomalacia, Paget's disease)
- Sepsis
- Multiple myeloma.

The age of the patient can help to determine a list of differential diagnoses:

- 15–30 years
  - Trauma
  - Ankylosing spondylitis
  - Pregnancy
  - Slipped disc.
- 30–50 years
  - Slipped disc
  - Malignancy
  - Inflammatory joint disease, e.g., rheumatoid arthritis
  - Degenerative joint disease.

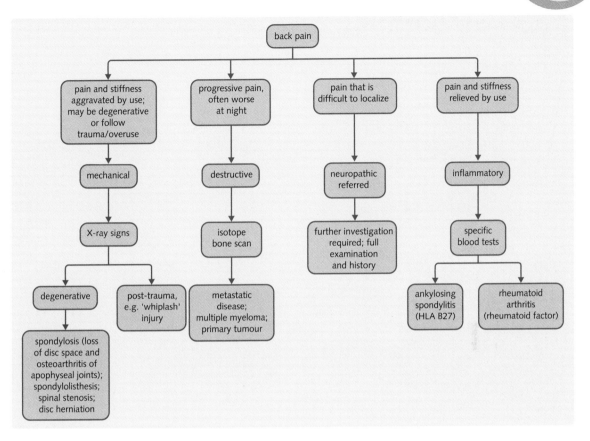

Fig. 8.5 Diagnostic features of mechanical, destructive, neurogenic/referred and inflammatory back pains.

- Over 50
  - Malignancy
  - Osteoarthritis
  - Degenerative joint disease
  - Myeloma
  - Paget's disease of bone.

Muscle weakness

Patients with muscle weakness can be divided into two categories: those with 'true' muscle weakness and those with normal muscle strength.

Muscle weakness may result from disorders anywhere along the motor cortex, the corticospinal tracts, anterior horn cells, peripheral nerves, neuromuscular junction and muscle. Only the last two will be considered here.

Diagnosis of muscle weakness is aided by considering the distribution of the weakness (Fig. 8.6).

Further investigations, involving electromyography and muscle biopsy, are required for the definitive diagnosis of muscular weakness.

COMMON PRESENTING COMPLAINTS OF THE SKIN

Eruptions

Eruptions are generally classified according to their site on the body. They can occur on or in the:

- Face
- Scalp
- Feet
- Hands
- Anogenital folds
- Axillae
- Glans penis.

Facial eruptions can be caused by:

- Acne vulgaris
- Rosacea
- Atopic dermatitis
- Contact dermatitis
- Systemic lupus erythematosus
- Perioral dermatitis.

191

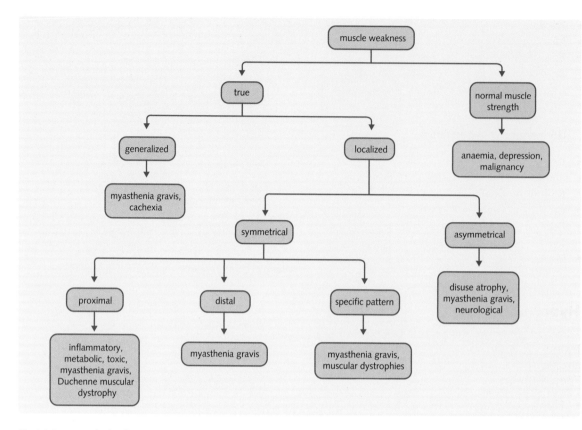

Fig. 8.6 Stages involved in determining a diagnosis of muscle weakness. Note that myasthenia gravis can potentially affect any part of the body (see Chapter 2, p. 39).

Scalp eruptions are caused by:

- Pityriasis capitis
- Seborrhoeic dermatitis
- Psoriasis
- Tinea capitis
- Discoid lupus erythematosus.

Eruptions of the hands and feet are caused by:

- Tinea
- Psoriasis
- Contact dermatitis
- Endogenous dermatitis.

Anogenital fold eruptions are caused by:

- Candidiasis
- Tinea
- Seborrhoeic dermatitis
- Psoriasis.

Eruptions in the axillae are caused by:

- Seborrhoeic dermatitis
- Psoriasis
- Contact dermatitis.

Eruptions of the glans penis are caused by:

- Candidiasis
- Psoriasis
- Lichen planus
- Scabies
- Intraepidermal carcinoma.

The most important factor in skin ageing is exposure to the UV rays of the sun, with ageing occurring faster in those who have spent more time out in the sun or using sunbeds. The longer-wavelength UVA rays destroy dermal collagen and elastin, resulting in reduced tensile strength and elasticity in the skin.

Blistering

Blistering can occur at several levels of cleavage in the skin. There are common and uncommon causes of blistering. Common causes include:

- Friction
- Insect bites and stings
- Burns
- Impetigo
- Contact dermatitis
- Drugs.

Uncommon causes include:

- Pemphigus vulgaris
- Pemphigus foliaceus
- Bullous pemphigoid
- Cicatricial pemphigoid
- Pemphigoid gestationis
- Dermatitis herpetiformis
- Linear IgA disease.

Hypopigmented lesions

These are classified into generalized and patchy hypopigmentation (with or without inflammation, atrophy or induration).
The causes of generalized hypopigmentation include:

- Phenylketonuria
- Hypopituitarism
- Albinism.

The causes of patchy hypopigmentation include:

- Vitiligo
- Achromic naevus
- Piebaldism
- Waardenburg's syndrome
- Ash-leaf macules
- Chemical induced.

The causes of patchy hypopigmentation with inflammation include:

- Tinea versicolor
- Leprosy
- Pityriasis alba.

The common causes of patchy hypopigmentation with atrophy or induration include:

- Radiodermatitis
- Morphoes
- Lichen sclerosus
- Burns.

Features that assist in the diagnosis of hypo-pigmentation can be found in Figure 8.7.

> Palmar erythema is redness caused by vasodilatation occurring over the thenar and hypothenar eminences of the palm. Although this can be present in normal healthy individuals, it can sometimes be a sign of liver disease.

Hyperpigmented lesions

Hyperpigmented lesions can be split into hyperpigmented naevi and all other causes.

A naevus consists of non-functional cells and may be defined as a congenitally determined tissue defect.
Hyperpigmented naevi include:

- Congenital melanocytic naevus
- Acquired melanocytic naevus
- Mongolian spot
- Acquired blue naevus
- Spitz naevus
- Halo naevus
- Pigmented hairy epidermal naevus
- Café-au-lait spots

Other causes of hyperpigmentation include:

- Tanning
- Postinflammatory pigmentation
- Hypoadrenalism
- Hyperoestrogenism
- Chloasma
- Metabolic causes (e.g., cirrhosis, haemochromatosis)
- Chemicals and drugs, e.g., oral contraceptives, chlorpromazine, busulfan, gold therapy
- Peutz–Jeghers syndrome

Fig. 8.7 Complications of some causes of hypopigmentation

Cause of hypopigmentation	Clinical signs
vitiligo	pernicious anaemia; Addison's disease; thyroid disease
albinism	white hair; lack of pigmentation in iris; poor sight; photophobia; nystagmus
phenylketonuria	if untreated, mental retardation; choreoathetosis

- Simple lentigo
- Actinic (solar) lentigo
- Pregnancy
- Malabsorption
- Chronic renal failure
- Addison's disease.

Peau d'orange is a characteristic skin appearance that commonly occurs in breast cancer, creating fine dimpling at the opening of hair follicles so that the skin resembles orange peel. It is due to infiltration and destruction of the lymphatic vessels of the area by the tumour, producing oedema and impaired lymphatic drainage. Skin can also tether to produce dimpling as a result of infiltration of the dermis by the tumour.

Skin ulcers

Ulcers are abnormal breaks in the epidermis and dermis. Causes are classified as:

- Specific, e.g. due to TB infection
- Non-specific, e.g. due to trauma
- Malignant.

They may originate from:

- Venous pathology
- Arterial pathology
- Neuropathy (Fig. 8.8).

Pubic hair is dark, coarse and curly hair that develops as a result of adrenal androgen production independent of gonadotrophin secretion. Patients with gonadotrophin deficiency can develop pubic hair without other signs of pubertal development.

Hair loss or gain

Hair loss (or alopecia) can be classified as diffuse localized scarring and localized non-scarring (Fig. 8.9).

Types of abnormal hair development include hirsutism [excessive female growth of terminal hair in a male (androgenic) pattern] and hypertrichosis (excessive growth of terminal hair in a non-androgenic pattern), in either a localized or a generalized distribution (Fig. 8.10). If menstruation is normal then testosterone production is usually normal. If menstruation is abnormal the cause is usually polycystic ovary syndrome (PCOS), associated with oversecretion of androgens. Another differential to exclude is late-onset congenital adrenal hyperplasia.

Causes of hirsutism are split into five categories:

- Pituitary
- Adrenal—late-onset congenital adrenal hyperplasia
- Ovarian—PCOS, ovarian tumours (rare)
- Iatrogenic—drug treatment e.g. minoxidil
- Idiopathic—benign.

Thinning of the outer third of the eyebrows has been noted to occur in hypothyroidism. However, it is also common in normal healthy people and so is of little diagnostic value.

Hypertrichosis can occur in a localized or generalized distribution.

Fig. 8.8 Stages involved in determining the cause of leg ulceration.

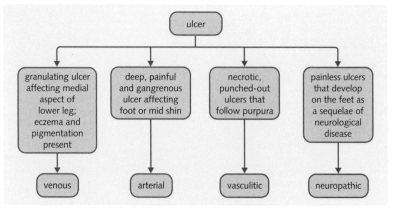

194

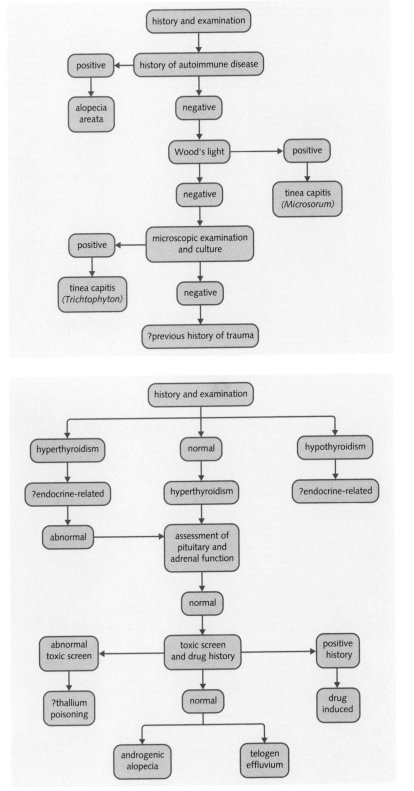

Fig. 8.9 (A) Stages involved in determining the cause of localized non-scarring alopecia. (B) Stages involved in determining a diagnosis of diffuse non-scarring alopecia.

Fig. 8.10 Stages involved in determining the cause of hirsutism/hypertrichosis and consideration of their possible causes.

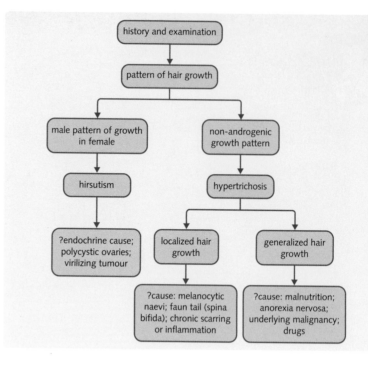

History and examination

TAKING A HISTORY

For a comprehensive guide to history taking, please refer to the Crash Course guide *History and examination*.

Things to remember when taking a history

First contact

When meeting a patient for the first time, you should:

- Always introduce yourself by name and status, e.g. medical student
- Mention the consultant's name, as this reassures the patient you are genuine and provides a common link between you. Obtain consent for the interview before you begin. Ask permission in a non-leading manner so that the patient can decline if he or she wishes
- Check that the patient is sitting/lying comfortably before you begin
- Try to put the patient at ease by sitting a reasonable distance away, and take the interview at a relaxed pace; do not worry about any silences between your questions. You should always aim to sit at the same level of the patient
- Dress appropriately, as many patients feel uncomfortable giving personal details to people who do not make an effort at personal presentation.

The patient's surroundings

Try to observe the patient walking into the consulting room, as any disabilities can be seen more easily during movement.

On the ward, look around the bedside for any clues to the patient's level of disability, or see what they bring to the consultation, e.g. an inhaler, oxygen, walking stick/frame, wheelchair, sputum pot, reading material, etc.

The patient's appearance and behaviour

Everyone subconsciously makes assumptions about people based on their appearance—you should try to be aware of someone's physical features and clothing.

Watch the patient's behaviour for clues while taking the history, e.g. is there agitation or distress; can you see any tremors, abnormal behaviour, or abnormal eye and body movements?

Taking a musculoskeletal history

Presenting complaint

When a patient presents with a muscular complaint, determine what symptom or symptoms brought him or her to seek medical attention, e.g. muscle weakness or stiffness. This should be recorded in the notes in the patient's own words, rather than medical jargon, quoting the patient where possible. If there is more than one presenting complaint, you should try and determine the patient's order of importance and enquire about each one separately.

History of presenting complaint

Nature of complaint
Determine the effect the complaint has on the patient's daily activities. Some important examples are presented below. A patient with proximal weakness, i.e. weakness involving the upper parts of the arms and legs, will describe difficulties in:

- Getting out of the bath
- Ascending stairs
- Getting up out of a chair
- Brushing the hair.

A patient with weakness of the hands may find it difficult to brush the hair.

Distal weakness in the limbs is suggested by:

- Difficulties in opening jars
- Footdrop in some cases
- Tripping over rugs.

Patients with myotonic dystrophy may present with an inability to let go upon shaking hands.

You should phrase your questions openly, giving the patient plenty of opportunity to tell his or her story before you begin to close in on aspects you have gathered from the history.

Onset of complaint
The time the patient first noticed the onset of a muscular complaint will depend on lifestyle and level of daily activity, e.g. athletes will notice a change in muscle strength at an early stage.

With muscular dystrophies, inflammatory myopathies and myasthenia gravis, the onset is usually gradual. However, the inflammatory myopathies, periodic paralyses and myasthenia gravis may also present suddenly.

The age of onset is also important. For instance, an underlying malignancy should be excluded in elderly patients presenting with myasthenic symptoms.

Pattern of symptoms
In the case of the inflammatory myopathies and muscular dystrophies, weakness is progressive as opposed to intermittent as in the periodic paralyses.

Precipitating or relieving factors
Some examples include:

- Exercise: an important precipitating factor, particularly in the metabolic myopathies, periodic paralyses and myasthenia gravis. The symptoms of Lambert–Eaton myasthenic syndrome improve with exercise
- Temperature: myotonia associated with Thomsen's disease and paramyotonia congenita is worse in the cold.

Other associated symptoms
Muscle pain may be a feature of viral myalgia (very common), metabolic myopathies and myopathy secondary to alcohol abuse. You should ask about dysphagia, dysarthria and respiratory symptoms, as these may be present, depending on the muscle groups involved.

Bone pain is suggestive of myopathy occurring secondary to osteomalacia. Bone pains must be enquired about in detail, in order to exclude bony metastases. Question the nature of the pain, any exacerbating or relieving factors, the time of the day it begins etc.

> SOCRATES is a very useful mnemonic, commonly used for remembering the questions you should ask to determine the characteristics of pain in a history. The letters stand for: Site; Onset (nature, circumstance, acute/chronic, etc.); Characteristics (sharp, dull, etc.); Radiation; Alleviating factors, associated symptoms; Timing (duration and frequency); Exacerbating factors; Severity.

Past medical history
A history of HIV infection should be excluded, as the infection itself, or its treatment (e.g. zidovudin), may be responsible for myopathy.

Drug history
Ask about medications the patient is taking, how long they have been taken, as well as any recent change in dose. Ask if the patient has recently stopped taking any medications.

A range of drugs, e.g. steroids, cholesterol-lowering agents, chloroquine and lithium, can result in proximal myopathy.

Family history
If other family members are affected by a muscular disorder, a family tree should be constructed. The gender of the patient and affected relatives should be noted.

Social history
Alcohol   When taking the social history, you should ask about alcohol consumption. How many units does the patient consume and how often?

Sexual practices You should try to establish if the patient is at risk of HIV infection. This requires a professional and diplomatic approach. Some ways in which to go about this include asking the patient if he or she is currently in a relationship, how long he or she has been in the relationship, and whether it is stable. Also ask about the current method of contraception used. You should ask how many sexual partners the patient has had in the last 2 years, explaining that this is a routine question asked of all patients. Explaining this often puts the patient at ease.

Exercise Ask the patient about exercise, as this can help exclude disuse atrophy. If a patient plays a sport or undertakes physical exercise, ask about levels of exercise, the type of activity and frequency of participation.

Systems review

A systems review is best approached systematically to ensure you give yourself the chance to ask all relevant questions, which can help in refining differential diagnoses, particularly of multisystem diseases. You should try to establish whether the patient has symptoms of other disorders, e.g. dark urine is suggestive of myoglobinuria and is associated with metabolic myopathies and acute alcoholic myopathy.

Does the patient have symptoms of endocrine disease, e.g. Cushing's syndrome or thyroid abnormalities?

Summary of patient's history

Always write a summary of a patient's history when clerking. When presenting the case, begin with a brief overview of the patient: 'Mr Jones is a 63-year-old man with rheumatoid arthritis who presents with exacerbation of his joint pain'. This helps the listener to focus on the relevant parts of the subsequent history.

Joints
Presenting complaint

Presenting complaints of joint disorders are usually:

- Pain
- Swelling
- Stiffness
- Deformity
- Loss of function
- Numbness or paraesthesia.

History of presenting complaint

For each complaint the patient reports, ask about specific details such as when and where the symptom started, if anything makes it better or worse, and how daily life is affected. Where more than one is reported, ask about each one separately and in turn.

Past medical history

Enquire about any previous injuries or diagnosed conditions, as some may predispose to new disorders.

Family history

Genetic disorders should be considered in joint complaints. Has anything similar affected anyone in the family—parents, siblings, relatives? Do any other conditions run in the family, e.g. diabetes mellitus?

Social history

Information about the patient's social life, e.g. occupation, exercise and hobbies, can help to assist in a diagnosis, as well as in understanding the impact of the complaint on the patient's lifestyle.

The 'red flags' of musculoskeletal history include:

- Pain that wakes the patient at night
- Severe, progressive pain that is unremitting
- Pain accompanied by weight loss.

These features point to a diagnosis of malignancy or sepsis; both must be excluded.

Taking a skin history
Presenting complaint

Presenting complaints of skin disorders are usually:

- Rash
- Itching
- Psychological distress (severe acne, extensive psoriasi, etc.).

History of presenting complaint

For each of these, ask when and where the symptom started, whether anything makes it better or worse (e.g. sunlight) and how daily life is affected. With lesions, ask how and where the problem started, how it first looked, and if it has changed in appearance or spread. Bear in mind that having a skin disease can be very stressful for patients, who frequently devalue their own body image and thus suffer psychological distress. However minor the problem may seem to you, it may genuinely cause the patient intense distress and psychosocial impairment. This should be noted in the history.

Past medical history

Enquire about any previous skin disease or atopic syndromes such as hay fever, asthma or eczema. Coexisting medical conditions may also involve the skin.

Drug history

Skin eruptions are one of the common side effects of many prescribed drugs, so take a full drug history. Also enquire about over-the-counter drugs and alternative medicines (such as herbal remedies), as they may have been used inappropriately and may cause irritant or allergic reactions. Ask whether the patient is allergic to any drugs and, if so, what happened when he or she took them. This should also be recorded in brackets in the notes as not all drug reactions are true allergic reactions, and this may be important in certain circumstances.

Family history

There may be a genetic component to skin disorders (tuberous sclerosis, psoriasis, etc.). Also, disorders caused by infestation and infection may also have affected family members recently. It is therefore important to ask who lives at home and whether they have been affected recently.

Social history

Occupational factors often lead to skin complaints, e.g. chemical engineers with contact dermatitis, health workers with latex allergies, etc. Enquire about recent foreign travel, as this may elicit the cause of an infection, as well as point towards a reaction to strong sunlight. A sexual history and contact tracing may be necessary in some disorders such as HIV, genital warts, syphilis.

GENERAL EXAMINATION OF JOINTS AND THE MUSCULOSKELETAL SYSTEM

Clinical examination

The clinical examination of a patient should be performed in a systematic way so that important signs are not missed. All findings should be recorded and

summarized. First and foremost, you should make sure the patient feels at ease and explain instructions clearly. Remember to watch the patient's face when eliciting signs, and explain your findings at the end of the examination.

When examining limbs or joints, you should start by examining the normal or trouble-free joint/limb before the troubled one, as this allows the two to be compared.

Joints should be examined from the front, back and sides.

> Learning examination sequences and specific tests for each joint can seem a daunting task. However, it need not be: if you remember that each sequence is based around LOOK, FEEL, MOVE, you will automatically have a systematic structure to your examination and will find it easier to remember what to do next.

General examination of joints

The routine for examination of joints can be remembered as:

- Look
- Feel
- Move.

The joint should be carefully inspected before you touch the patient. The joint should then be palpated before movement and stability are assessed. It is advisable to examine painful areas last.

This routine can often be followed by X-rays.

Inspection

The area for examination should be adequately exposed and viewed in good light. You should look at:

- The alignment of the bones—look for any obvious deformities, shortening or subluxation
- The position of the joint and limbs at rest—is there any unusual posture? Valgus or varus? (see Chapter 5)
- The joint contour—any effusions or other abnormalities, and general or localized swellings?
- Scars or sinuses—from operations (linear scar), injury (irregular scar) or suppurations (broad, adherent puckered scar)? Ask about the origin of any scars
- Any skin changes
- Muscle wasting.

Palpation

Preferably with warm hands, initially feel gently and then more firmly while simultaneously watching the patient's face for any signs of pain or apprehension. You should consider:

- Skin temperature changes by noting any warmth (inflammation, rapidly growing tumour) or coldness in local areas. Using the back of the hand, start on the contralateral (normal) joint
- Swellings—are they bony abnormalities or diffuse joint swellings?
- Areas of tenderness—these should be precisely located so as to relate them to anatomical structures
- Pain.

Measurements

Measurements of limb length and width are carried out to determine any discrepancies between the two sides. Length is especially important in the lower limbs, and width provides information on muscle wasting, soft tissue swellings or bone thickenings. Measurements should be made from fixed points so that findings are reproducible.

Sensation

Where a patient's symptoms could be caused by neurological pathology, sensation should be tested, e.g. nerve impingement such as sciatica, slipped disc or spinal cord compression.

Movement

Both active and passive ranges of movement must be recorded for the directional planes of each joint. These should be equal. Passive movement exceeds active when there is muscle paralysis, myopathy or weakness affecting voluntary control, or torn or slack tendons.

A goniometer—a hinged rod with a protractor in the centre—is the instrument used to measure the range of joint movements. Measurements usually begin with the joint in extension, and movement is expressed as degrees of flexion from this point. Measuring and recording these allow you to quantify and accurately assess the degree of disability and give a clinical picture from which you can make comparisons in future joint examinations.

In order to make an adequate clinical assessment, the normal ranges of joint movement need to be fully understood. Both sides should be measured and recorded. Restricted movements in all directions are suggestive of arthritis, whereas restrictive movements in some directions and free movements in others suggest a mechanical disorder or damage to particular structures.

As you elicit passive movements, place your hand over the moving joint to detect any crepitus on movement. Pain and crepitations must be noted. Joint crepitations are coarse and diffuse.

> Hypermobile joints can move beyond the normal range of movement, the most commonly affected joints being the elbows, wrists, fingers and knees. The differential diagnoses of hypermobile joints include Marfan's syndrome, Ehlers–Danlos syndrome, Down syndrome and benign familial hypermobility.

Stressing

Straining of the ligaments supporting certain joints provides information about joint stability, most notably the knee joint. When assessing ligaments, the muscles moving the joint must be relaxed as contraction can conceal unstable ligaments.

Pain is usually present in ligaments that have been recently injured, whereas those that are torn or stretched produce an increased range of movements.

Power

The strength of a particular muscle or muscle group can be tested by asking the patient to move a joint against the resistance of the examiner. Muscle weakness is easily detectable and an important sign of motor impairment.

Muscle power (or strength) is graded according to the Medical Research Council (MRC) scale as:

- 0—no power
- 1—a flicker of contraction
- 2—slight power to move a joint with gravity eliminated: this is when the joint is supported, usually by the edge of a bed or manually by the observer
- 3—sufficient power to move a joint against gravity
- 4—power to move a joint against gravity plus added resistance
- 5—normal muscle power.

The power of each muscle or muscle group should be recorded in the notes using this scale, for example 4/5, 5/5 etc.

X-rays

Anteroposterior and lateral views of a joint are routinely taken during an X-ray examination, except for certain joints such as the hands and feet. They can also allow bones, joints and soft tissues to be examined.

Bones

It is important to observe the general outline of bones: are there areas of increased density (e.g. osteopetrosis) or reduced density (e.g. osteoporosis)? Where present, is reduced density generalized, suggesting osteoporosis, or periarticular only, suggestive of rheumatoid arthritis?

Joints

When assessing joints you should check for:

- Narrowing of the joint space, indicating loss of cartilage thickness
- Joint margin erosion, typical of rheumatoid arthritis
- New bone-forming osteophytes, typical of osteoarthritis
- Flattening or thickening of bone
- Bone erosion, sclerosis or cavitation.

Soft tissues

Areas of calcification, foreign bodies and increased density (suggestive of fluid) should all be noted.

REGIONAL EXAMINATION OF JOINTS AND THE MUSCULOSKELETAL SYSTEM

The principles of general examination are applied to local areas in different ways. This section focuses on specific features that should be noted and manoeuvres that should be performed on different structures.

Examination of the back

Although the spinal examination is often described according to the vertebral segment, in practice the entire spine is examined.

Cervical spine

Inspection

Inspect from the front, both sides and from behind the patient.

During inspection of the cervical spine you should note any deformities, such as:

- Torticollis (wry neck)
- Hyperextension.

Palpation

Palpate the bony contour, checking for midline tenderness in the spine and adjacent muscles, e.g. trapezius and paraspinal muscles, e.g. from a sprain or whiplash injury.

Movement

Movements of the cervical spine include flexion, extension, lateral rotation and lateral flexion. These movements are best seen from the side or front, and are expressed as a fraction of the usual range (Fig. 9.1). Restriction of movement occurs in arthritis and nerve compression. Ask the patient to look left and right (rotation), tilt the head to the left and right (lateral flexion), and to flex and extend the neck.

Neurological examination

A neurological examination of the upper limbs should be performed.

Thoracic spine

Inspection

During inspection of the thoracic spine you should note any scoliosis (lateral fixed curvature) or kyphosis (anterior-facing concave curvature, the so-called 'dowager's hump'), which may be rounded or angular, owing to collapsed vertebrae. In addition, you may observe pectus carinatum (pigeon chest), pectus excavatum (funnel chest), scoliosis and 'gibbus' (a sharp angular deformity caused by collapsed vertebrae from infection).

Palpation

Palpate the bony contour. Any tenderness of the thoracic spine can be due to collapse of T12 or L1 vertebrae, e.g. osteoporosis or trauma. Where there is no local tenderness, gently percuss the spine with a fist.

Movement

Movement of the thoracic spine is mainly rotational, but there is a small amount of flexion, extension and lateral flexion (Fig. 9.2). Observe the range of movement (ROM) from behind the patient. Ask the patient to perform movements to elicit rotation, flexion and extension. Observe whether any apparent scoliosis is corrected by spinal flexion.

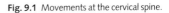

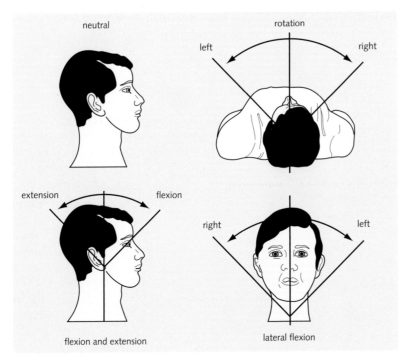

Fig. 9.1 Movements at the cervical spine.

Stressing
Stressing is not useful at the thoracic spine.

Lumbosacral spine

Inspection
Inspect the spine from behind and observe whether it is straight or if any scoliosis is apparent. Inspect from the sides for the presence of the physiological lordosis (posterior-facing concave curvature) or scoliosis. You may also observe other signs, e.g. vestigial ribs on the upper lumbar vertebrae.

Palpation
Palpate the bony contours and lightly percuss along the spinous processes with the side of a fist. During palpation, note any tenderness of the lumbosacral spine.

Movement
Movement of the lumbosacral spine includes flexion, extension, lateral rotation and lateral flexion (see Fig. 9.2). Restriction follows different patterns, i.e. general restriction in osteoarthritis, asymmetrical flexion in disc prolapse or scoliosis, and painful 'catch' on extension in muscle strain.

There is a range of clinical tests to determine whether there is nerve root pathology. Some important ones include straight-leg raising and the femoral nerve stretch test.

Straight-leg raising
The supine patient raises each leg as far as it will go, keeping it as straight as possible. It is normal to manage 70–120°. Painful restriction below this usually indicates a prolapsed disc.

> Intervertebral disc prolapse commonly occurs at the L4/5 and L5/S1 levels, causing compression of the L5 and S1 nerve roots. Straight-leg raising applies tension to these nerve roots, so hip flexion will be reduced and pain be felt in the lumbar region as well as the leg.

Femoral nerve stretch test
In this test the patient lies prone and the examiner attempts to flex the knee. This stretches the nerve roots of the femoral nerve, L2–L4, which are sometimes also affected by prolapse.

Schober's test
With the patient standing straight, the examiner locates the dimples of Venus at the base of the spine, and a mark is made 10 cm above and 5 cm below this level using a non-permanent marker. The patient is then asked to bend forwards. Using a tape measure, the distance that the upper mark has moved in relation

Fig. 9.2 Movements at the thoracic and lumbar spine.

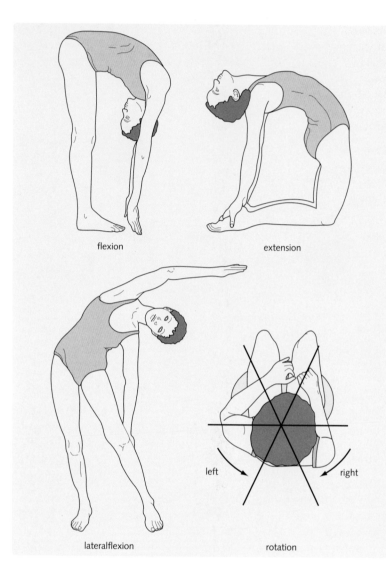

flexion

extension

lateralflexion

rotation

left

right

to the lower one is measured. It should normally be 5 cm or more. Where it is less it is indicative of lumbar spinal pathology, e.g. ankylosing spondylitis.

Stressing

Stressing is not useful at the lumbosacral spine. Stressing of the sacroiliac joints is not reliable, as signs of sacroiliac pathology are not readily demonstrable clinically, and sacroiliac pain also radiates to the buttocks and back of the thigh.

Examination of the upper limb

Shoulder

Inspection

You should inspect both shoulders simultaneously from the front, back and side. Note their contour ('squaring off' in dislocation), any swellings caused by effusion (synovitis in the subacromial bursa and glenohumeral joint), deltoid muscle wasting, winging of the scapulae (congenital or muscular dystrophies), alignment of the clavicle and acromion, and the way in which the arms are held (chronic conditions and pain may affect this).

Palpation

In the rotator cuff disorders, tenderness and pain may be localized to different areas during palpation of the shoulder. This may be caused by glenohumeral or acromioclavicular arthritis, other arthropathies, or referred pain from other parts of the body. Palpate over the front aspect and the point of the shoulder, the acromioclavicular and sternoclavicular joints.

Movement

Glenohumeral (abduction, adduction, flexion, extension, medial and lateral rotation) and scapular movements (elevation, retraction and rotation) (Fig. 9.3) are possible at the shoulder.

You can quickly assess overall ROM by asking the patient to:

- Place the hands behind the head, elbows pointing out sideways
- Slide each hand down the back between the shoulder blades.

If there is pain, limited range of movement or swelling you should then examine the glenohumeral joint and rotator cuff individually to determine the site of pathology.

In order to assess glenohumeral joint function, you should eliminate scapular movement by pressing the scapula down at the top and asking the patient to move the shoulder.

The patient should flex the shoulder (normally 90°) and abduct the arm (90°).

Check the power of deltoid (abduct the arm), serratus anterior (abnormality causes scapular 'winging' when both hands push firmly on a wall), and pectoralis major (push hands into waist). The range of internal and external rotation of the shoulder can be tested with the patient's arm by the side, the elbow flexed 90°.

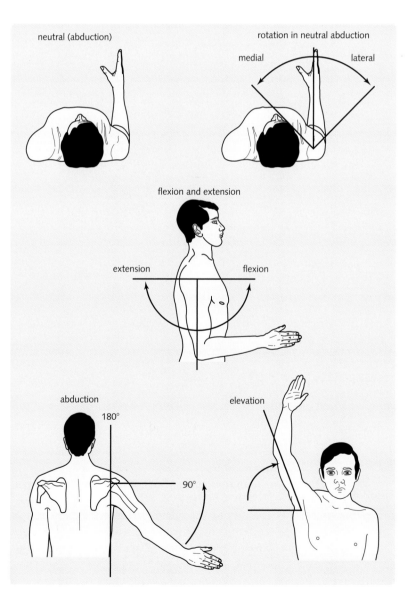

Fig. 9.3 Movements at the shoulder joint.

Painful arc syndrome is caused by pathology affecting the supraspinatus muscle and rotator cuff, such as degeneration and tendonitis, producing impingement pain between 60° and 120° of abduction. Impingement produces pain on abduction as the tendon becomes compressed under the acromion. Inflammatory and degenerative conditions of the rotator cuff produce tenderness over the sites of insertion of the rotator cuff and bicipital tendons.

The rotator cuff consists of four muscles: subscapularis, supraspinatus, infraspinatus and teres minor. The patient should stand with the arm by the side and attempt to abduct the arm against resistance. If the patient cannot start abducting the arm from the side, there may be rupture of the rotator cuff. The patient may also be seen to shrug the shoulder in the attempt to abduct it. The examiner should then passively abduct the arm to 45° and ask the patient to continue to abduct.

Impingement is caused by pinching of the rotator cuff tendons as they pass under the acromion and causes pain in the mid-arc of abduction or adduction. The examiner can test for this by assisting the patient to elevate the arm fully, and then asking for the arm to be lowered slowly. Where this produces pain it is called painful arc syndrome.

Stressing
Stressing is useful at the shoulder in checking for capsular lesions and osteoarthritis.

Elbow
Inspection
During inspection of the elbow you should look for 'gunstock' deformity (malunion of a previous supracondylar fracture), joint effusion swellings (usually in the posterolateral position), soft lumps posteriorly (olecranon bursitis), and pebbly osteophytes (osteoarthritis).

Palpation
During palpation of the elbow you should note any tenderness of the lateral epicondyle ('tennis elbow'), medial epicondyle ('golfer's elbow') and radial head (rheumatoid arthritis).

Movement
Flexion and extension movements are seen in the humeroulnar joint. Examine for active flexion and extension, noting any flexion deformity. With the arms by the sides, elbows flexed to 90°, the patient should be asked to supinate and pronate (turn the palms up to the ceiling and down to the floor; Fig. 9.4). Feeling over the joint during movement can detect crepitus. You should also test the median, radial and ulnar nerves.

To test for epicondylitis, the patient should extend the elbow and grip the examiner's hand. Where the epicondyles are inflamed this produces pain, which is relieved by flexion of the elbow.

Stressing
Stressing is not useful at the elbow.

Hands
Inspection
During inspection of the hands you should look for deformities of the fingers, thumb and joints, notably:

- Mallet finger
- Trigger finger
- Dropped finger
- Swan-neck or Boutonnière deformities
- A Z-deformity of the thumb
- Ulnar deviation of the fingers (rheumatoid arthritis)
- Heberden's nodes at the distal interphalangeal joint
- Bouchard's nodes at the proximal interphalangeal joints (osteoarthritis)
- Ganglia and thickening of the palmar aponeurosis (Dupuytren's contracture).

When examining for dilated capillaries and vasculitic changes on the hands, a magnifying glass should be used to ensure nothing is missed.

Palpation
During palpation of the hands you should note any tenderness over the joints, which in rheumatoid arthritis is commonly symmetrical. The joints of the hands and wrist should be palpated. Palpating over the flexor tendons in the palm can detect crepitus, such as that occurring at the carpometacarpophalangeal joint in osteoarthritis. The examiner places the index finger over the volar side of the patient's extended fingers, then asks the patient to open and close the fingers. Gently palpate any swelling over the joints to determine whether it is hard or boggy, and whether it is warm or appears inflamed. Note the distribution of any swelling. Metacarpophalangeal and proximal interphalangeal

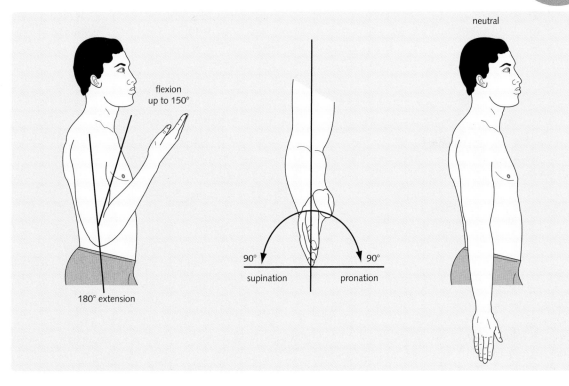

Fig. 9.4 Movements at the elbow joint.

joints are commonly affected in rheumatoid arthritis, whereas the distal interphalangeal joints are affected by osteoarthritis and psoriatic arthritis.

> When examining swelling of the joints, you should look for a pattern of joint involvement. In rheumatoid arthritis the metacarpophalangeal and proximal interphalangeal joints are commonly affected symmetrically, whereas in osteoarthritis and psoriatic arthritis the distal interphalangeal joints are affected.

Movement
Flexion, extension, adduction and abduction movements can be seen at the metacarpophalangeal joints. There is also opposition of the thumb and little finger (Fig. 9.5). The interphalangeal joints show only flexion and extension. Test fine pinch by asking the patient to bring the tip of the thumb to meet the tip of the index, middle, ring and little fingers in succession. Grip strength should be assessed by asking the patient to grip your fingers as hard as possible.

To assess the interosseus muscles, the patient splays the fingers apart and resists the examiner's attempts to squeeze them together.

Assess the range of wrist flexion and dorsiflexion.

Stressing
Stressing is useful at the hands—applying pressure on the fingers along their axis tests the mechanical stability of the metacarpals and phalanges.

Wrist
Inspection
During inspection of the wrist you should note any deformities or swellings of the tendon sheaths or joint capsule.

Palpation
During palpation of the wrist you should note any tenderness over the radial area (scaphoid fracture, de Quervain's tenosynovitis, osteoarthritis) or the ulnar area (tenosynovitis of extensors).

Movement
Flexion, extension, adduction and abduction movements may be seen at the radiocarpal joint, and

Fig. 9.5 Movements at (A) the finger joint, and (B) the thumb joint.

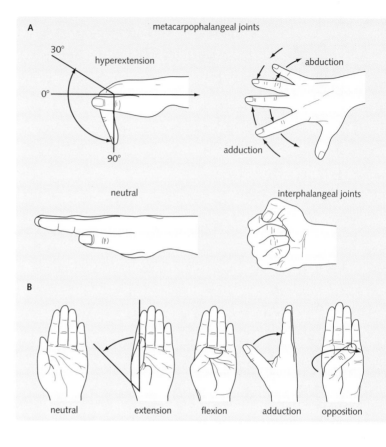

supination and pronation at the inferior radioulnar joints (Fig. 9.6).

Stressing
Stressing is not useful at the wrist.

Examination of the lower limb

Hip

Inspection
It is important to assess the hip visually when the patient is standing and walking, with the hips adequately exposed, and observe for any abnormalities of the gait, looking for any tilting or scoliosis. The Trendelenburg test is important to assess stabilization of the hip by the gluteal muscles. The patient stands on one leg, then on the other. Weak gluteals cause pelvic tilt.

With the patient supine the hip can be inspected for fixed flexion deformities, swellings, asymmetry or muscle wasting.

Palpation
During palpation you should note any pain at the front of the hip and the skin over the greater trochanter. You should measure the limbs to find:

- The true length (from the anterior superior iliac spine to the medial malleolus, with the angle between the pelvis and limbs equal on both sides)
- The apparent length (from the xiphisternum to the medial malleolus, with the limbs lying parallel to the trunk).

> True limb shortening is caused by a loss of bone or cartilage, for example arthritis, fracture or dislocation, missed congenital dislocation of the hip, or displacement of the femur, which can occur in Perthes' disease, slipped femoral epiphysis and avascular necrosis. Apparent shortening is caused by an adduction deformity causing elevation of the pelvis, which can occur in arthritis.

Movement
Flexion, extension, abduction, adduction, medial (internal) rotation and lateral (external) rotation are possible at the hip (Fig. 9.7). By immobilizing the other hip by pressing down on the iliac crest of that side, abduction and adduction can be assessed

Fig. 9.6 Movements at the wrist joint.

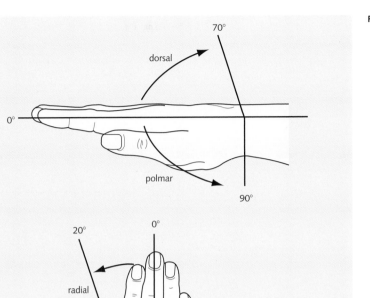

passively. You should note any fixed deformities, which may be flexed, abducted or adducted. Fixed flexion can be confirmed by performing Thomas's test. Lie the patient flat on the back and place a hand under the lumbar spine. Flex the hip and knee of the leg on the unaffected side, and flex the hip up to and beyond its limit so the normal lordosis disappears. If the other leg also flexes, this demonstrates fixed flexion of the hip on that side and Thomas's test is positive. Straight-leg raising test will allow the detection of nerve impingement caused by slipped disc, as well as a quadriceps lag.

Stressing
Stressing is not very useful at the hip.

Knee

Inspection
The knee should be inspected with the patient both standing and supine. During inspection you should look for genu valgum or genu varum, wasting of the quadriceps femoris, and swelling around the knee (thickened bone or synovium, fluid within the joint, bursitis). Assess the gait.

> You should always perform a thorough examination of the hip as well as the knee in any patient presenting with knee pain, as hip pathology can cause referred pain at the knee.

Palpation
During palpation of the knee you should note any tenderness over the joint or joint line caused by torn menisci, synovitis or osteoarthritis. Loose bodies may be felt in the suprapatellar region. An effusion can be elicited by one of two tests: the patellar tap and the sweep test:

Fig. 9.7 Movements at the hip joint.

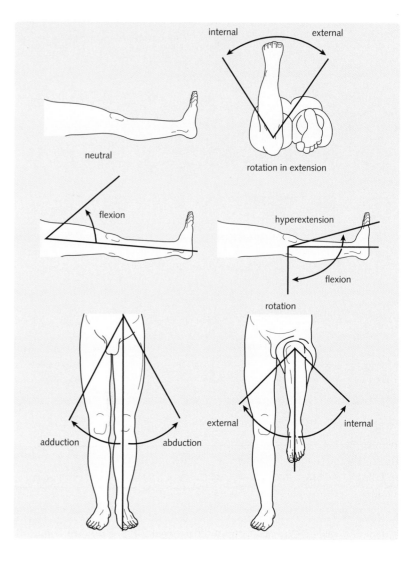

- Patellar tap: the examiner applies pressure to the suprapatellar region to drain any fluid, so the kneecap will float off of the femoral condyle. The other hand presses down on the kneecap, noting any fluctuation or 'tap'
- Sweep test: the examiner strokes the medial side of the knee so that any fluid there is stroked into the lateral compartment. A brisk stroke to the lateral compartment will create a transient bulge on the medial side of the knee as the fluid moves back to the medial compartment.

A small effusion may be found in athletic and sporting persons, and is not abnormal.

Movement

Flexion and extension movements are possible at the knee (Fig. 9.8). Many of these movements can be hyperextended. Measure any apparent degrees of genu valgum and varum with a measuring tape, and document it.

Stressing

During stressing of the knee you should check the collateral ligaments in full extension. Place the patient's ankle between your elbow and your side, and use both hands to try and abduct/adduct the tibia, looking and feeling for any laxity of these ligaments. The cruciate ligaments are assessed with the knee flexed at a right-angle. Sit on the patient's foot and, using your hands, attempt to draw the

Fig. 9.8 Movements at the knee joint.

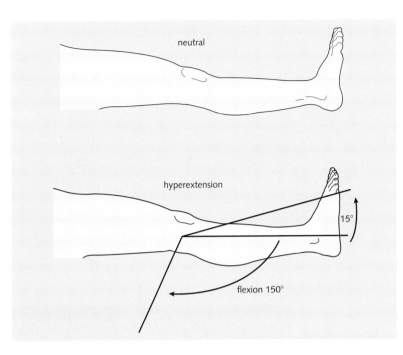

tibia back and forth, looking and feeling for any laxity.

Feet

Inspection

The feet should be inspected while the patient is standing and during walking. You should assess the condition of the skin and structural abnormalities such as:

- Congenital club foot
- Flat or hollow feet (pes planus and pes cavus)
- Claw toes
- Hammer toes (hallux valgus)
- Hallux rigidus
- Bunions
- Calluses
- Toenail lesions
- Hindfoot lesions.

> Inspection of the footwear should be a routine part of the examination of the foot and ankle, to look for signs of abnormal wear.

Palpation

During palpation of the feet you should check for a hot, swollen, first metatarsophalangeal joint, which can be apparent in gout. You should also check the metatarsal heads for prominence and pain. The fore, mid and hindfoot should be palpated, squeezing the forefoot to determine whether there is any tenderness in those joints. The calf muscles and Achilles tendon can also be palpated for tenderness.

> Nail growth is slowed by acute illness and ischaemia. It is increased in psoriasis. Spoon-shaped nails (or koilonychias) can indicate chronic iron-deficiency anaemia.

Movement

Flexion and extension movements occur in the toes; inversion and eversion of the foot occur at the midtarsal joint (Fig. 9.9). To prevent subtalar inversion when examining the ROM of the foot, the heel should be immobilized in one hand while the other rotates the forefoot.

Stressing

During stressing of the feet, longitudinal pressure will enable you to determine the integrity of the toes.

Ankle

Inspection

During inspection of the ankle you should check for swelling.

Fig. 9.9 Movements at the foot.

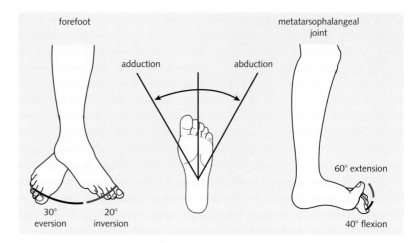

forefoot

metatarsophalangeal joint

adduction   abduction

60° extension

30° eversion   20° inversion

40° flexion

Palpation

During palpation of the ankle you should note any swelling near the joints that may indicate tenosynovitis.

Movement

Plantarflexion and dorsiflexion movements at the ankle are possible (Fig. 9.10). Inversion and eversion also occur at the subtalar joint.

Stressing

Stressing of the ankle will enable the integrity of the ligaments to be checked.

Systemic examination

The systemic examination should be tailored to different systems in order to elicit any signs that are suggested in the history, or that you expect to find clinically (Fig. 9.11).

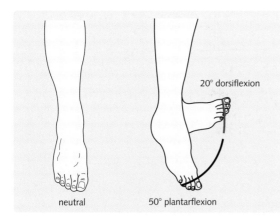

20° dorsiflexion

neutral   50° plantarflexion

Fig. 9.10 Movements at the ankle joint.

EXAMINATION OF THE SKIN

Inspection

Ideally, the skin should be examined in natural daylight, with full exposure for atypical or widespread lesions. Inspection involves noting the distribution and morphology of lesions.

Distribution

Specific skin disorders commonly show different patterns of lesion distribution (see Chapter 7). It is important to determine whether the eruptions are:

- Symmetrical or asymmetrical
- Central or peripheral
- Localized or widespread
- On flexor or extensor surfaces.

Some disorders may show specific patterns: shingles erupts in a dermatomal pattern, rosacea occurs on the face, contact dermatitis usually affects the hands or face, etc.

Morphology

It is important to note whether the lesions are:

- Grouped
- Linear
- Annular
- Show the Koebner phenomenon.

Fig. 9.11 Systemic features of disease

System	Sign	Association
abdomen	splenomegaly	Felty's syndrome
	enlarged inguinal nodes	rheumatoid arthritis metastatic spread
	renal enlargement	ankylosing spondylitis
eyes	redness, dryness	Sjögren's syndrome
	nodular scleritis, thin blue sclera	rheumatoid arthritis
	iritis	ankylosing spondylitis
	conjunctivitis	Reiter's syndrome
	uveitis	Behçet's syndrome
	difficulty in closing eyes	scleroderma
mouth	dry mouth, dental caries	Sjögren's syndrome
	ulcers	rheumatoid arthritis, SLE, Reiter's syndrome
skin	butterfly rash	SLE
	skin tethering and pigmentation	scleroderma

Skin-derived structures

Examination of the skin should also involve inspection of the hair, scalp, nails and mucous membranes for associated physical signs.

Palpation

Palpation of skin lesions (a task often feared and hence avoided by medical students) is necessary to assess the consistency, depth and texture of a lesion.

Palpation of lymph nodes is essential in patients with suspected skin malignancy.

Pulses must be assessed in patients with leg ulcers.

Skin examination includes the essential basic morphology of skin lesions, including their shape, size, colour, margins and surfaces.

Further investigations

10

Objectives

By the end of this chapter you should be able to:
* Understand the techniques available to determine bone density
* Understand the uses and limitations of the EMG technique
* Describe the technique of muscle biopsy
* List the important blood tests in investigating the musculoskeletal system
* Describe the characteristics of synovial fluid found in osteoarthritis, rheumatoid arthritis and septic arthritis
* Understand different ways of measuring bone density
* Describe the diseases in which rheumatoid factor can be detected
* List some methods of assessing muscle function
* Interpret normal radiographs of the skeleton
* Differentiate between prick tests and patch tests
* List the techniques used for taking skin biopsies.

INVESTIGATION OF MUSCULOSKELETAL FUNCTION

Bone

X-rays can identify gross abnormalities of bone that can be characteristic of certain conditions, for example chronic osteomyelitis. However, there are more sensitive investigations that can be used depending on individual factors, such as the suspected pathology, the time of presentation, etc. They do not detect abnormal bone density.

Magnetic resonance imaging

In magnetic resonance imaging (MRI) the region under investigation is put into a magnetic field. Hydrogen nuclei (protons) are lined up in the direction of this magnetic field, assuming a new orientation when the electromagnetic radiation is altered. When the radiation is stopped the protons return to their original position and emit radiofrequency signals as they do so. It is these signals that can be analysed and converted into a two-dimensional image.

MRI scanning can detect variations in the density of tissues. It provides a means of scanning without the use of X-rays, and gives detailed images of subchondral areas, as well as other areas of bone.

Radioisotope scanning

During routine investigations using radioisotope scanning, an intravenous injection of radiolabelled technetium is administered. Rays emitted from the technetium can be measured with a gamma camera or rectilinear scanner.

As the isotope diffuses from bone matrix to blood, its increased uptake provides a measure of hyperaemia of bone and increased osteogenic activity.

> The choice of imaging used in back pain depends on the information given in the patient's history. Generally, plain X-rays are used for suspected sacroiliitis. MRI is used for suspected tumours, spinal cord compression and spinal stenosis, and disc prolapse. Vertebral fractures can be imaged by plain X-ray, radionuclide bone scan or MRI.

Bone densitometry

Bone mineral density can be assessed using:

* DEXA scans
* CT scans
* Ultrasound of the calcaneum.

DEXA scan

Dual-energy X-ray absorptiometry (DEXA) measures the amount of mineral per surface area, and is usually performed on the lumbar vertebrae and proximal femur. It is a clinical gold standard as it produces minimal radiation while also producing an accurate picture.

X-ray computed tomography

X-ray computed tomography (CT) involves X-ray scanning of part of the body from several angles with oscillators that detect the X-rays. Cross-sectional images are then compared and reconstructed by computer. These images can show variations in density between bone and surrounding tissue.

This test can distinguish cortical from trabecular bone, thus allowing assessment of the volume of bone rather than mineral content. Despite this, it has not been shown to be superior to other methods of assessment. It also exposes the patient to higher doses of radiation and is more expensive.

Ultrasound of the calcaneum

The results of this test are not easily reproducible, and so it is not often used.

Muscle

Electromyography

Electromyography is a technique used to record the electrical activity in muscle both at rest and during contraction.

Method

During electromyography, a needle electrode is inserted into muscle. Electrical activity in the muscle is displayed on a cathode ray oscilloscope and heard on a speaker.

Electromyography is used:

- To determine whether a disorder is caused by disease of the muscle or abnormalities of innervation
- If there is an abnormality of innervation: this may be localized to the central nervous system, peripheral nerves or neuromuscular junction
- To aid in the diagnosis of myopathy, myotonia and myasthenia
- To obtain information about the distribution of a disorder so that a biopsy specimen can be taken from the appropriate site
- To obtain information on the characteristics of motor units.

Assessment of muscle function

Normal muscle   Normal muscle at rest is electrically silent. The insertion of an electrode results in insertional activity because the muscle fibres are mechanically stimulated or damaged. If there is disease, the extent of this spontaneous activity may increase or decrease.

When insertional activity subsides, further activity may be seen only if the electrode is moved or the muscle contracts (Fig. 10.1).

Denervated muscle   Abnormal spontaneous activity of muscle at rest is termed fibrillation potentials. However, diseases of the neuromuscular junction and myopathies may also result in this pattern.

Myasthenia gravis   Single-fibre electromyography is used in the diagnosis of myasthenia gravis. This technique records the time interval between the potentials of two fibres belonging to the same motor unit. In normal muscle this interval is 10–50 s, but in myasthenia gravis it is increased.

Myopathic muscle   In myopathic muscle the number of active muscle fibres in a motor unit is reduced (see Fig. 10.1). This results in a reduced amplitude and a shorter action potential.

Reinnervated muscle   Muscle fibres are often reinnervated as a result of axonal sprouting of adjacent nerves (see Fig. 10.1). This results in a larger motor unit and hence an increased amplitude of the recorded potential. In addition, there is an unusual arrangement of fibres in the same unit, which may now lie next to each other.

Limitations   Electromyography does not provide a specific diagnosis, as certain types of recording may occur in more than one disorder. It is therefore always important to confirm a diagnosis with clinical findings and laboratory results.

Muscle biopsy

Method

Muscle samples are usually taken by needle biopsy, a procedure that requires local anaesthesia.

An open biopsy may be needed to diagnose focal abnormalities such as myositis.

Evaluation

A muscle biopsy can be assessed in one or more ways, including:

- Histology
- Histochemistry
- Electron microscopy
- Assays of enzyme activities.

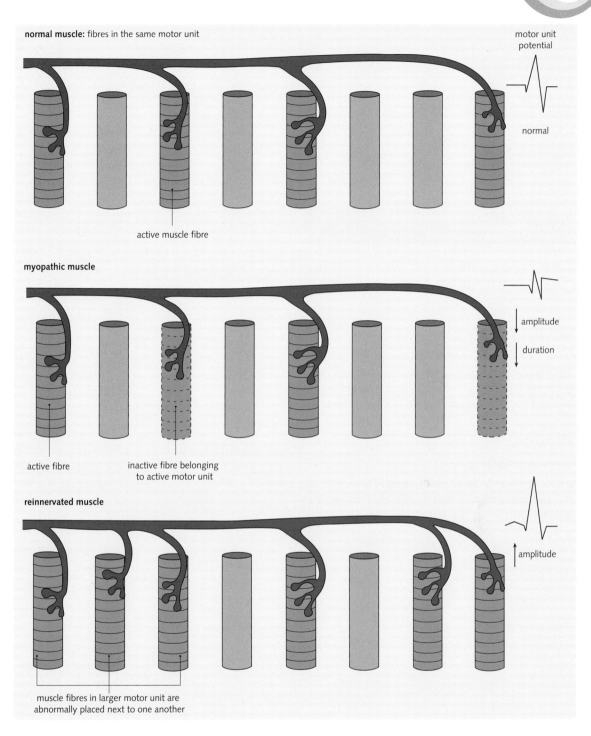

Fig. 10.1 Comparison of the motor unit action potentials recorded in normal muscle, myopathic muscle and reinnervated muscle.

With these techniques it is possible to assess muscle fibre types, the presence of inflammation or degeneration, the presence of abnormal mitochondria and enzyme abnormalities.

Indications
Muscle biopsy differentiates between neuropathic and myopathic disorders. It is used to aid in the diagnosis of a range of inflammatory, dystrophic and metabolic myopathies.

INVESTIGATIONS OF SKIN DISORDERS

Surgical biopsies
Biopsies are classified as follows: excisional, incisional, punch, shave or curettage.

Excisional biopsy
Excisional biopsy is used not only to facilitate histological diagnosis of the lesion, but also as a therapeutic procedure. The lesion is removed along with a defined margin of skin, which depends on the lesion. Benign and malignant skin lesions can both be biopsied in this way.

Incisional biopsy
This is similar to excisional biopsy but is used for diagnostic sampling rather than complete removal of a lesion.

Punch biopsy
A biopsy in which a small (3–6 mm) punch tool is used to remove a cylindrical section of skin for histological examination.

Shave biopsy
The lesion is shaved off parallel to the skin surface, with any resultant bleeding treated by cauterization. This is only used for benign lesions, as some of the lesion remains after the procedure; it is usually used for intradermal naevi and seborrhoeic warts.

Curettage
The lesion is removed using a curette spoon, with bleeding points being cauterized. This method is used to remove seborrhoeic warts, pyogenic granulomas and viral warts.

Whichever biopsy method is used, the tissue removed should always be sent for histopathological examination to confirm the suspected diagnosis.

Immunological tests
Prick tests
Prick tests are used to detect immediate (type I) hypersensitivity reactions, and involve injecting tiny amounts of antigen solutions into the skin of the forearm. After 15 minutes the skin is inspected and a wheal of 5 mm or larger is regarded as a positive result. The test can be useful to detect allergies, such as those to foods or house-dust mites, but it is important that antihistamines are stopped 48 hours before the test.

Patch testing
This detects cell-mediated (type IV) hypersensitivity reactions by applying a range of test substances to aluminium discs, which are then taped to the skin of the back. The patches are left on for 2 days, after which erythematous patches are correlated to specific test substances. The skin is re-examined after 4 days, as some reactions take longer to develop. Patch testing is used in the investigation of contact dermatitis.

Immunofluorescence
Used to diagnose the primary blistering disorders, this process targets specific immunoglobulins or complement fractions using an antibody labelled with fluorescein (a marker). The marker then shows up on fluorescence microscopy.

An indirect method of immunofluorescence is also used in which an animal substrate is used to reveal certain human serum antibodies tagged with antihuman immunoglobulin antibody.

Wood's lamp
This light emits ultraviolet (UV) radiation, which causes certain fungal infections to fluoresce on skin, and especially hair. It can also be used to detect hypopigmentation, such as that seen in vitiligo.

Microscopy
Skin scrapings treated with potassium hydroxide solution can be viewed under a light microscope to confirm the presence of fungal hyphae. Microscopy is also used in the diagnosis of scabies: the mite can be extracted from its burrow with a needle and viewed.

ROUTINE INVESTIGATIONS IN MUSCULOSKELETAL AND SKIN DISORDERS

Haematology

Erythrocyte sedimentation rate

The erythrocyte sedimentation rate (ESR) is the rate at which red blood cells settle out of suspension in blood plasma in anticoagulated blood. A standard ESR tube is used and the amount of clear plasma at the top of the settled blood cells is measured at 1 hour. The normal rate is <10 mm/h.

The ESR is raised in inflammatory conditions such as rheumatoid arthritis, systemic lupus erythematosus (SLE) and inflammatory myopathy.

C-reactive protein

C-reactive protein (CRP) is normally present in small amounts in serum, and is synthesized in greater amounts by the liver in response to a variety of insults, including infection.

CRP is raised in inflammatory conditions. It is a more sensitive indicator than ESR, but the results are not available as quickly.

Haemoglobin

Anaemia—usually normochromic or normocytic—occurs in inflammatory conditions such as rheumatoid arthritis and SLE.

White blood cell count

The numbers of white blood cells are raised in infections such as septic arthritis.

Thyroid function

The thyroid function test is able to exclude myopathy caused by thyroid dysfunction; parathyroid hormone levels exclude myopathy associated with osteomalacia.

Blood biochemistry

Uric acid

Uric acid levels need be checked only if gout is suspected.

Muscle enzymes

Creatine kinase, a muscle enzyme, may be raised in inflammatory myopathy, muscular dystrophy, alcohol myopathy and metabolic myopathy.

Bone enzymes

Alkaline phosphatase, a bone enzyme, is raised in Paget's disease, osteomalacia and rickets, but not in osteoporosis.

Immunopathology

Autoantibodies

Autoantibodies that can be measured in musculoskeletal disorders include:

- Rheumatoid factor in rheumatoid arthritis, Sjögren's syndrome, SLE, polymyositis and dermatomyositis
- Antinuclear antibodies (ANA) in SLE (anti-Ro), Sjögren's syndrome, Still's disease, polymyositis (anti-Jo) and dermatomyositis
- Anti-acetylcholine receptors in myasthenia gravis
- Anti-cyclic citrullinated peptide antibodies are very specific for rheumatoid arthritis.

Synovial fluid analysis

Synovial fluid should be analysed for appearance, the presence of white blood cells and the presence of crystals, and should also be cultured for infections (Fig. 10.2).

Joint crystals found in gout are negatively birefringent, whereas in pseudogout they are positively birefringent.

IMAGING OF THE MUSCULOSKELETAL SYSTEM

The radiograph, or plain X-ray, is the imaging technique most commonly used to diagnose musculoskeletal disorders. It is simple, quick, and relatively cheap. However, in some instances, radiographs may not yield sufficient information;

Fig. 10.2 Synovial fluid changes in some rheumatic diseases

Disease state	Appearance	White blood cells ($\times 10^6$/L)	Crystals	Culture
normal	clear viscous fluid	<200 mononuclear	none	sterile
osteoarthritis	increased volume; normal viscosity	3000 mononuclear	5% have pyrophosphate	sterile
rheumatoid arthritis	may be turbidly yellow or green; low viscosity	30 000 neutrophils	none	sterile
septic arthritis	turbid; low viscosity	50 000–100 000 neutrophils	none	positive
gout	clear; low viscosity	10 000 neutrophils	needle-shaped; negative birefringence	sterile
pyrophosphate arthropathy (pseudogout)	clear; low viscosity	10 000 neutrophils	brick-shaped; positive birefringence	sterile

Adapted with permission from Kumar P, Clark M. Clinical medicine, 3rd edn. London: Baillière Tindall, 1994.

then, other imaging techniques, such as MRI, CT or radioisotope imaging, need to be employed.

Normal anatomy

The normal appearance of the musculoskeletal system during imaging is depicted in Figures 10.3–10.10. These include the:

- Skull (Fig. 10.3)
- Shoulder (Fig. 10.4)
- Elbow (Fig. 10.5)
- Hand (Fig. 10.6)
- Female pelvis (Fig. 10.7)
- Knee and leg (Fig. 10.8)
- Ankle (Fig. 10.9)
- Cervical spine (Fig. 10.10).

Bone disorders

Radiography can detect conditions of various aetiologies, including the following.

Hereditary disorders

Hereditary bone disorders include:

- Congenital scoliosis (Fig. 10.11).

Infections and trauma

Bone is prone to infection, called osteomyelitis (see Fig. 4.18D), and trauma.

Metabolic disease

Metabolic bone disorders include:

- Hyperparathyroidism (see Fig. 4.23B)
- Vitamin D deficiency (Fig. 10.12)
- Periarticular osteoporosis.

Tumours

Hereditary bone tumours include:
- Osteosarcoma (Fig. 10.13).

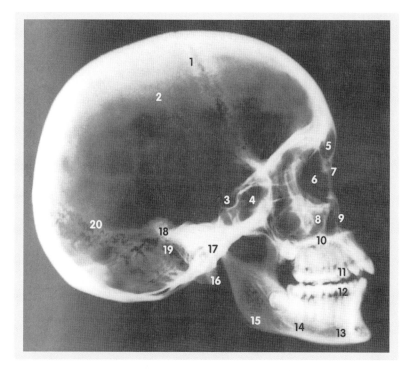

Fig. 10.3 Lateral radiograph of skull. (Courtesy of Dr B Berkovitz and Dr B Moxham.)
1 Coronal suture
2 Grooves for meningeal vessels
3 Pituitary fossa
4 Sphenoidal sinus
5 Frontal sinus
6 Orbit
7 Nasal bones
8 Maxillary sinus
9 Anterior nasal spine
10 Hard palate
11 Caxilla and teeth
12 Mandible and teeth
13 Mental foramen
14 Mandibular canal
15 Angle of mandible
16 Mastoid process
17 External acoustic meatus
18 Petrous ridge
19 Groove for sigmoid sinus
20 Lambdoid suture

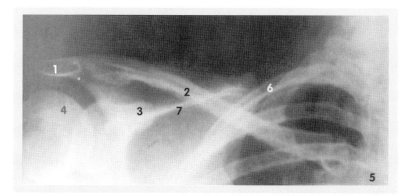

Fig. 10.4 Radiograph of the right shoulder. (Courtesy of Dr J Calder and Dr G Chessell.)
1 Acromion process of scapula
2 Clavicle
3 Coracoid process of scapula
4 Head of humerus
5 Manubrium
6 Ribs
7 Spine of scapula

Fig 10.5 Anteroposterior radiograph of the right elbow. (Courtesy of Dr J Calder and Dr G Chessell.)
1 Capitulum of humerus
2 Trochlea of humerus
3 Medial epicondyle of humerus
4 Olecranon fossa of humerus
5 Lateral epicondyle of humerus
6 Olecranon process of ulna
7 Coronoid process of ulna
8 Head of radius
9 Radial tuberosity

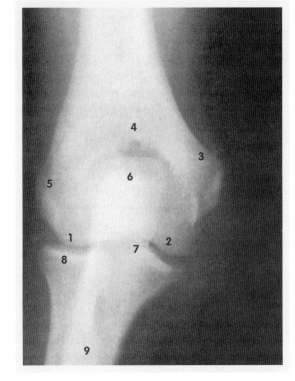

Fig. 10.6 Radiograph of an adult hand. (Courtesy of Drs J Gosling, P Harris, J Humpherson, I Whitmore and P Willan.)
1 Distal phalanx
2 Middle phalanx
3 Proximal phalanx
4 Second metacarpal
5 Sesamoid bone
6 Trapezoid
7 Trapezium
8 Scaphoid
9 Lunate
10 Triquetral
11 Pisiform
12 Hamate
13 Capitate
14 Styloid process of ulna
15 Styloid process of radius

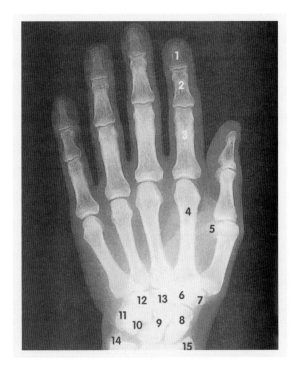

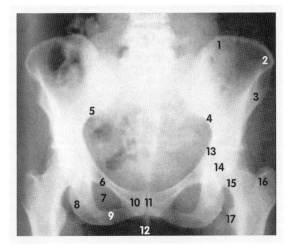

Fig. 10.7 Anteroposterior radiograph of the female pelvis.
(Courtesy of Dr J Calder and Dr G Chessell.)
 1 Iliac crest
 2 Anterior superior iliac spine
 3 Anterior inferior iliac spine
 4 Pelvic brim
 5 Sacroiliac joint
 6 Superior pubic ramus
 7 Obturator foramen
 8 Inferior ischial ramus
 9 Inferior pubic ramus
10 Body of pubis
11 Pubic symphysis
12 Subpubic arch
13 Acetabulum
14 Head of femur
15 Neck of femur
16 Greater trochanter of femur
17 Lesser trochanter of femur

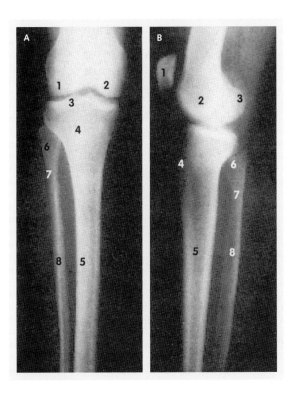

Fig. 10.8 (A) Anteroposterior radiograph of the right tibia
and fibula; (B) lateral radiograph of the right tibia and fibula.
(Courtesy of Dr J Calder and Dr G Chessell.)

A
1 Lateral femoral condyle
2 Medial femoral condyle
3 Tibial spine
4 Tibial tuberosity
5 Shaft of tibia
6 Head of fibula
7 Neck of fibula
8 Shaft of fibula

B
1 Patella
2 Medial femoral condyle
3 Lateral femoral condyle
4 Tibial tuberosity
5 Shaft of tibia
6 Head of fibula
7 Neck of fibula
8 Shaft of fibula

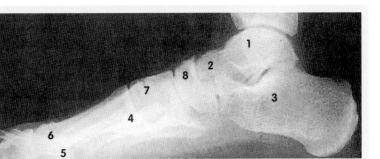

Fig. 10.9 Radiograph of the right foot
and ankle showing longitudinal arches.
(Courtesy of Drs J Gosling, P Harris, J
Humpherson, I Whitmore and P Willan.)
1 Medial malleolus
2 Head of talus
3 Calcaneus
4 Base of first metatarsal
5 Sesamoid bone
6 Head of first metatarsal
7 Cuneiforms
8 Navicular

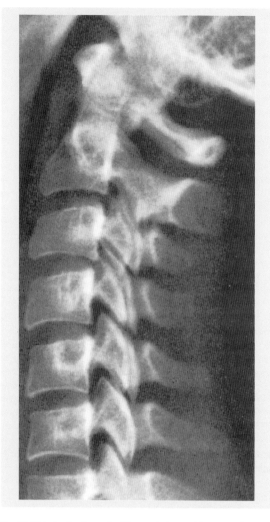

Fig. 10.10 Lateral radiograph of the cervical spine. (Courtesy of Dr A Greenspan and Dr P Montesano.)

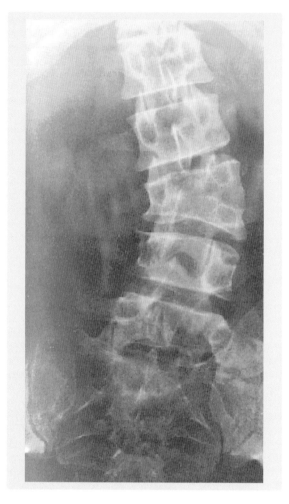

Fig. 10.11 Congenital scoliosis. This case in a 22-year-old man was due to hemivertebrae, a complete unilateral failure of formation. (Courtesy of Dr A Greenspan.)

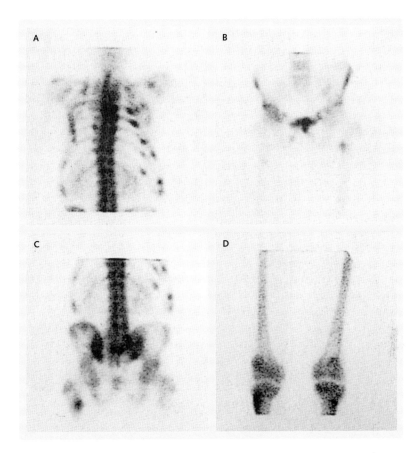

Fig. 10.12 Radioisotope bone scan demonstrating a generalized increase in technetium uptake with multiple hot spots due to small fractures in the thoracic spine. The patient had metabolic bone disease caused by vitamin D deficiency. The darker areas indicate increased uptake of technetium, representing altered cell growth. (Courtesy of Dr PM Bouloux.)

Fig. 10.13 Osteosarcoma in a child. The radiograph shows an infiltrative, poorly demarcated tumour in the metaphyseal region of the tibia. (Courtesy of Dr S Taylor.)

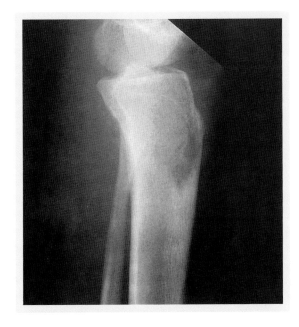

SELF ASSESSMENT

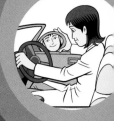

Multiple-choice questions (MCQs)

Skeletal muscle

1. **Skeletal muscle contraction:**
   (a) Is under voluntary and reflex control.
   (b) The greater the length of the muscle fibre, the less range of movement it can produce.
   (c) Synergistic muscles oppose the movement of a muscle.
   (d) A functional muscle can belong to more than one group.
   (e) Skeletal muscle contraction is under the control of the autonomic nervous system.

2. **Regarding skeletal muscle attachment:**
   (a) Muscle attaches to bone through tendons made of closely compacted cartilage fibres.
   (b) All skeletal muscle attaches to bone.
   (c) Multiple muscles can insert into one site through an aponeurosis.
   (d) It can attach at epiphyses of long bones.
   (e) Tendon fibres insert into the periosteum of the bone.

3. **Regarding skeletal muscle fibres:**
   (a) They are arranged in bundles called fasciculi.
   (b) Their nerve and blood supply runs throughout the epimysium that surrounds them.
   (c) The greater the size of a fasciculus, the finer the movement that muscle performs.
   (d) Satellite cells replace damaged muscle fibres with scar tissue.
   (e) Damage to the basal lamina results in scar tissue formation.

4. **Resting membrane potential (RMP):**
   (a) The RMP of skeletal muscles is around −70 mV.
   (b) The main ion responsible for maintaining the RMP is Na^+.
   (c) The charge is predominantly positive on the outside and negative on the inside.
   (d) The membrane is mainly permeable to K^+.
   (e) The Na^+/K^+-ATPase pump makes no contribution to the RMP.

5. **Action potentials in skeletal muscles:**
   (a) Are only initiated at synaptic clefts.
   (b) Occur at greater force when a greater threshold is reached.
   (c) Can occur in both directions from a stimulus.
   (d) Saltatory conduction results in greater conduction velocity.
   (e) Conduction velocity is increased in increased temperatures of up to 50°C.

6. **Regarding synapses:**
   (a) Synapses can be chemical or electrical.
   (b) Action potentials occur at electrical synapses but not at chemical synapses.
   (c) At a chemical synapse, neurotransmitters are released by exocytosis.
   (d) Unlike chemical synapses, electrical synapses are not mediated by receptors.
   (e) Depolarization is produced by electrochemical changes in the target membrane.

7. **Comparing the action potentials of skeletal muscle and nerve fibres:**
   (a) The resting membrane potentials in both skeletal muscle and nerve remain fairly constant.
   (b) Action potentials of skeletal muscles last between 1 and 5 ms.
   (c) The conduction velocity of a nerve fibre is more variable than that of skeletal muscle.
   (d) The ionic basis of the action potential in muscle differs from that of nerve in that it is mainly due to calcium ions.
   (e) Action potentials in muscle and nerve both travel along the membranes of the adjacent cell.

8. **The nicotinic acetylcholine receptor:**
   (a) Is activated by the binding of one acetylcholine molecule.
   (b) Activation produces Na^+ influx.
   (c) Acetylcholine is produced in the nerve terminal from acetic acid and choline.
   (d) End-plate potentials produce depolarization.
   (e) Receptor stimulation ceases when acetylcholine is broken down enzymatically in the cleft.

9. **Drugs at the neuromuscular junction:**
   (a) Botulinum toxin acts by binding to and blocking the nicotinic acetylcholine receptor.
   (b) Edrophonium acts by binding irreversibly to acetylcholinesterase.
   (c) Tubocurarine is an example of a depolarizing drug that desensitizes nicotinic acetylcholine receptors.
   (d) Neuromuscular blocking agents bind competitively to acetylcholine receptors.
   (e) The effect of neuromuscular blockers can be reversed with anticholinesterases.

10. **Regarding muscle contraction:**
    (a) Contraction occurs as a result of the interaction of thick filaments called actin with thin filaments called myosin.
    (b) Interaction is prevented by tropomyosin–protein complexes.
    (c) Binding of sodium to tropomyosin is required for actin–myosin interaction and contraction to occur.

(d) Contraction results from actin 'walking along' the myosin molecule.
(e) Actin–myosin interaction is dependent on the ATPase activity of the actin molecule.

11. **Regarding motor units:**
(a) The greater the number of muscle fibres a motor neuron supplies, the larger the motor unit.
(b) Slow muscle fibres are innervated by larger motor neurons than fast muscle fibres.
(c) Denervation of a motor unit can result in the muscle fibre becoming insensitive to acetylcholine.
(d) Denervation of a motor unit results in the manifestation of lower motor neuron signs.
(e) On excitation, fast fatiguable units are activated before slow units.

12. **Regarding muscle tension:**
(a) The greater the stimulus applied to a muscle, the greater the tension produced.
(b) The greater the sarcoplasmic calcium concentration, the greater the force produced.
(c) The more muscle fibres stimulated, the greater the tension produced.
(d) Tetany occurs when there is no muscular relaxation between stimuli applied to a muscle fibre, resulting in a smooth, sustained contraction.
(e) During sustained contraction of a muscle, its motor units are activated together in synchrony.

13. **Myasthenia gravis:**
(a) Is an autoimmune condition.
(b) Produces symptoms and signs only when nicotinic acetylcholine receptors are reduced by 50%.
(c) Follows a progressive course.
(d) Also affects cardiac and smooth muscle nicotinic acetylcholine receptors.
(e) Is diagnosed by EMG.

14. **Myotonic dystrophy:**
(a) Commonly presents in the 40s and 50s.
(b) Is inherited in an autosomal recessive fashion.
(c) Can display the genetic phenomenon of anticipation.
(d) Does not affect cognitive function.
(e) Death can be caused by cardiomyopathy.

15. **Duchenne muscular dystrophy:**
(a) Is an autosomal dominant condition.
(b) Genetic mutation results in muscles susceptible to tearing on contraction due to dystrophy of the muscle fibre attachment to the extracellular matrix.
(c) Death usually occurs by 25 years of age.
(d) Almost all sufferers are affected by intellectual impairment.
(e) Pseudohypertrophy is a sign of established disease.

16. **Polymyositis:**
(a) Is the most common inflammatory myopathy seen.
(b) Inflammation of type I and II muscle fibres is mediated by a cytotoxic T-cell response.

(c) Rheumatoid factor can be found in sufferers.
(d) Muscle weakness is asymmetrical and progresses to involve the entire body.
(e) Can be associated with underlying malignancy.

17. **True or false:**
(a) Muscles involved in fine movements have smaller motor units.
(b) Dermatomyositis is clinically diverse from polymyositis.
(c) Gower's sign is a feature of myotonic dystrophy.
(d) The *treppe* effect commonly occurs in cardiac contraction.
(e) Thymus disease should be excluded in myasthenia gravis.

Cardiac muscle

18. **Regarding the structure of the heart:**
(a) The inner layer of the heart is called the endocardium.
(b) The myocardium is thickest in the atria.
(c) The parietal pericardium is in close contact with the myocardium.
(d) The parietal cavity separates the epicardium and the pericardium.
(e) Endocardial epithelial cells are irresponsive to circulatory substances.

19. **Cardiac action potentials:**
(a) Atrial and ventricular action potentials share the same characteristics.
(b) The action potential is initiated in the atrioventricular node.
(c) Myocardial gap junctions stop the action potential from deviating from its course.
(d) Left and right bundle branches branch from the bundle of His.
(e) The ventricles contract after the atria due to slowed conduction at the AV node.

20. **Regarding the action potential:**
(a) The plateau phase is caused by Ca^{2+}/K^+ channels.
(b) Purkinje cells have a stable resting membrane potential.
(c) Pacemaker function is determined by those cells that produce stronger action potentials than cells elsewhere in the heart.
(d) Tissue in the Purkinje fibres and the bundles of His can act as latent pacemakers.
(e) The action potential threshold in SA and AV nodes is lower than that of ventricular myocytes.

21. **Cardiac contraction:**
(a) The sarcoplasmic reticulum is arranged into dyads around the T-tubules in a less organized fashion than in skeletal muscle.
(b) Cardiac T-tubules are narrower than those of skeletal muscle.
(c) Action potential causes calcium influx through the sarcolemma to initiate the contractile apparatus.

(d) Cardiac sarcoplasmic reticulum stores more calcium than that of skeletal muscle.
(e) Increased frequency of action potentials leads to increased force of successive contractions.

22. Factors affecting contractility:
(a) Chronotropes affect the force of contraction.
(b) Positive inotropes increases calcium concentration by blocking the Na$^+$/K$^+$-ATPase pump.
(c) Acetylcholine has a positive inotropic effect on the heart.
(d) Glucagon has a negative inotropic effect.
(e) β-Blockers have a negative inotropic effect.

23. The autonomic nervous system:
(a) Vagal innervation slows the heart rate.
(b) Norepinephrine (noradrenaline) is only released from the adrenal medulla.
(c) Epinephrine (adrenaline) opens calcium channels to produce increased force of contraction by stabilizing the plateau.
(d) Parasympathetic innervation is mediated through nicotinic acetylcholine receptors.
(e) Parasympathetic effects are mediated at SA and AV nodes.

24. Regarding cardiac contraction:
(a) Force of contraction is inversely proportional to the initial length of the cardiac muscle fibre.
(b) Excessive stretching of the muscle fibres reduces contractile ability.
(c) Action potentials last longer in the conducting system than in the contractile system.
(d) Ventricles contract from the apex up to the base.
(e) Potassium efflux in the SA node is reduced, producing a state of self-excitability.

25. Hypertrophic obstructive cardiomyopathy:
(a) Can be autosomal dominantly inherited.
(b) Usually causes right ventricular hypertrophy.
(c) Is the cause of sudden death in over 75% of adolescents.
(d) ECG is diagnostic.
(e) The prognosis is variable.

26. In dilated cardiomyopathy:
(a) There is cardiomegaly.
(b) Presentation is usually with congestive heart failure.
(c) A significant complication is atherosclerosis.
(d) Prognosis is good if the disease is diagnosed early enough.
(e) It can cause sudden death.

27. True or false:
(a) Thyroid hormones act as positive inotropes.
(b) Repolarization is mediated by opening of K$^+$ channels.
(c) Intercalated discs do not anchor actin filaments to each end of the cell.
(d) Cardiac myocytes are multinucleated.
(e) Cardiac myocytes are small, at only 10 μm long.

28. Smooth muscle in the respiratory tract:
(a) Alters resistance to airflow.
(b) Is not under sympathetic control.
(c) Is arranged longitudinally.
(d) Is sensitive to aspirin.
(e) Is the target of first-line treatment of asthma attacks.

29. Smooth muscle:
(a) The intestine is composed of three muscle layers.
(b) The bladder consists of three layers of circular muscle.
(c) The stomach has a middle oblique layer of muscle.
(d) The lower third of the oesophagus consists of smooth muscle.
(e) Smooth muscle layers in the blood vessels are arranged circumferentially.

30. Smooth muscle contractile apparatus:
(a) Dense bodies in smooth muscle cells are a pathological sign.
(b) Synchronous contraction of smooth muscle cells depends on the electrical activity of the cells.
(c) Actin and myosin are the main contractile proteins.
(d) The contractile apparatus is structured similar to that of skeletal muscle, giving it a striated appearance.
(e) Desmin is the product of myosin breakdown in smooth muscle.

31. Regarding the nerve supply to smooth muscle:
(a) Varicosities are tumours that grow on nerve fibres that innervate smooth muscle.
(b) The nerve fibres are in direct contact with smooth muscle cells.
(c) Norepinephrine is a sympathetic neurotransmitter.
(d) Sympathetic and parasympathetic innervation is possible in the same tissue.
(e) Where there are multiple layers of smooth muscle only the inner layer is usually innervated.

32. True or false:
(a) H$^+$ is a local tissue factor that affects smooth muscle tone.
(b) Smooth muscle cells communicate electrically via gap (nexus) junctions.
(c) Organic nitrates increase smooth muscle tone.
(d) Muscle spindles are present in smooth muscle.
(e) Smooth muscle facilitates peristalsis.

33. Smooth muscle:
(a) Na$^+$ is responsible for the action potential.
(b) The resting membrane potential is more negative than that of skeletal muscle.
(c) Calmodulin is a component of the thin filament.
(d) Auerbach's plexus has an inhibitory effect on peristalsis.
(e) Serotonin has no effect on smooth muscle.

34. **In smooth muscle contraction:**
    (a) Three calcium ions bind to calmodulin.
    (b) Action potential characteristics are unlike those of skeletal muscle in that they are spiked.
    (c) Myosin light chain phosphorylation is required in order for myosin to interact with actin.
    (d) Myosin kinase is only active when it is part of the calmodulin complex.
    (e) Caveolae are equivalent to the T-tubules of skeletal muscle.

35. **In contrast to skeletal muscle, in smooth muscle contraction:**
    (a) Troponin molecules are larger than those found in skeletal muscle.
    (b) Myosin kinase phosphorylation is the cause of low conduction velocities in smooth muscle.
    (c) Cross-bridge formation is ATP independent.
    (d) Is resistant to fatigue.
    (e) Is prolonged.

Bone

36. **Cartilage:**
    (a) Is composed of collagen and oligosaccharides.
    (b) Is produced by chondrocytes.
    (c) Is derived from mesenchyme.
    (d) Is mainly produced by appositional growth.
    (e) Is a very vascular tissue.

37. **Regarding cartilage:**
    (a) Hyaline cartilage consists of predominantly type I collagen fibres.
    (b) Fibrocartilage is a major component of articular joints.
    (c) Perichondrium contains support cells for growth.
    (d) Chondroblasts eventually turn into chondroclasts.
    (e) Proteoglycans are formed from glycosaminoglycans linked to aggrecan molecules.

38. **Regarding long bones:**
    (a) The epiphysis is the shaft of the bone.
    (b) Cancellous bone lines the inside of compact bone-forming trabeculae.
    (c) Active bone marrow is mostly confined to the distal epiphyses of larger long bones.
    (d) The epiphyses consist mainly of compact bone.
    (e) The metaphysis is the epiphyseal end of the diaphysis.

39. **True or false:**
    (a) Lacunae are small cavities within the bone matrix.
    (b) Blood supply enters the bone through the epiphyseal plate.
    (c) The inorganic component consists of calcium and magnesium.
    (d) Osteoclasts are derived from macrophages.
    (e) Periosteum lymph drains to regional lymph nodes.

40. **True or false:**
    (a) Fracture repair leads to immature bone formation.
    (b) Osteoporosis mostly affects compact bone.
    (c) There is no cancellous bone in flat bone.
    (d) Haversian canals are lined by osteoblasts.
    (e) Sesamoid bones are of no functional significance.

41. **Bone production:**
    (a) Most commonly occurs by endochondral ossification.
    (b) Compact bone is produced solely by endochondral ossification.
    (c) The skull is produced by endochondral ossification.
    (d) Endochondral ossification occurs during fetal development and is complete 1 week before birth.
    (e) Bone remodelling does not have a significant role in bone production.

42. **Concerning bone growth:**
    (a) Endochondral growth leads to an increase in the width of bone.
    (b) Vitamin C has no role in bone growth.
    (c) Endochondral ossification continues throughout life but at a much slower rate.
    (d) Growth plates fuse at around 25 years of age.
    (e) Alkaline phosphatase induces matrix calcification.

43. **Regarding calcium:**
    (a) The skeleton maintains an optimal blood calcium level.
    (b) Parathyroid hormone decreases high blood calcium.
    (c) Calcitonin decreases renal reabsorption of calcium and phosphate.
    (d) Gastrointestinal absorption is controlled by vitamin C.
    (e) Vitamin D is required for osteoblast synthesis of the collagen of the bone matrix.

44. **Concerning hormonal influence on bone:**
    (a) Growth hormone stimulates chondrocyte production.
    (b) Precocious puberty causes early epiphyseal growth.
    (c) Testosterone is required for growth hormone production.
    (d) Thyroid hormone deficiency can cause gigantism.
    (e) Acromegaly causes disfiguring of the bone as the bone lengthens irregularly.

45. **Regarding the bone:**
    (a) Physical stress on a bone stimulates remodelling.
    (b) Physical stress reduces calcitonin production to inhibit bone resorption.
    (c) Bone density is reduced in osteoporosis but not in osteomalacia.
    (d) Bone destruction is associated with lowered plasma alkaline phosphatase.
    (e) Epiphyses are all present at birth.

46. **Regarding bony metastases, some characteristic features are:**
    (a) Bone destruction alongside bone formation.
    (b) Pathological fractures.
    (c) Lowered plasma alkaline phosphatase.
    (d) Red marrow involvement more than yellow marrow.
    (e) Increased immature red blood cell levels in peripheral blood.

47. **Metastatic tumours of the skeleton:**
    (a) Are more common than primary tumours.
    (b) Lytic metastases arise from the breast, kidney, thyroid and lung.
    (c) Can be detected by isotope bone scanning.
    (d) Red-flag symptoms include progressive pain that is worse in the mornings.
    (e) If suspected, a full history and examination of all systems should be undertaken.

48. **True or false:**
    (a) Osteogenesis imperfecta is caused by abnormal synthesis of type II collagen.
    (b) Osteopenia means bone pain.
    (c) Osteopetrosis occurs when there is irregular osteoclast activity.
    (d) Achondroplasia is an autosomal recessive condition.
    (e) Bone marrow transplant can cure osteopetrosis.

49. **Regarding osteomyelitis:**
    (a) Commonly occurs in the distal humerus.
    (b) Spreads locally but not haematogenously.
    (c) Usually affects cancellous bone.
    (d) Complications include the development of Brodie's abscesses.
    (e) Pathological changes are visible on X-ray within 3 days of onset.

50. **Regarding fractures:**
    (a) Fractures involving joints require closed reduction.
    (b) Healing begins with the development of a callus.
    (c) Systemic complications include DVT (deep vein thrombosis) and PE (pulmonary embolism).
    (d) Greenstick fractures are pathological.
    (e) Subluxed fractures require external fixation.

51. **True or false:**
    (a) Avascular necrosis is an autosomal dominant condition.
    (b) Avascular necrosis spares the marrow.
    (c) Osteoporosis of the spine can cause nerve root compression.
    (d) Osteomalacia is caused by excessive vitamin D or phosphate.
    (e) Patients with bony metastases rarely present initially with fractures.

52. **Osteoporosis:**
    (a) Has a female to male ratio of 1:1.
    (b) Can occur secondary to neoplasia.
    (c) An isotope bone scan is the gold standard for diagnosis.
    (d) Has an association with oestrogen deficiency.
    (e) Bisphosphonates work by stimulating osteoblast activity.

53. **Hyperparathyroidism:**
    (a) Leads to a raised calcitonin level, which causes increased osteoclastic activity and increased absorption.
    (b) Clinical features arise due to low calcium levels.
    (c) Bone damage due to the condition is irreversible.
    (d) Is a complication of renal disease.
    (e) Plasma phosphate levels are low.

54. **Regarding Paget's disease of bone:**
    (a) It affects women more than men.
    (b) In 85% of cases it affects one bone only.
    (c) Is caused by an initial increase in osteoblast activity.
    (d) Serum calcium levels are markedly raised.
    (e) Complications include high-output heart failure.

55. **True or false:**
    (a) Chondromas are malignant and progressive.
    (b) Osteosarcomas can occur as a complication of Paget's disease of bone.
    (c) Paget's disease of bone presents most commonly during the third decade of life.
    (d) Avascular necrosis occurs secondary to infection.
    (e) Renal osteodystrophy occurs as a consequence of congenital dystrophic kidneys.

56. **Possible differential diagnoses of an acute monoarthritis include:**
    (a) Gout.
    (b) Septic arthritis.
    (c) Haemophilia.
    (d) Trauma.
    (e) Systemic lupus erythematosus.

57. **True or false:**
    (a) C-reactive protein is produced by the kidneys.
    (b) True limb shortening can occur with a fractured femur.
    (c) Chest pain can be referred to the lateral side of the upper arm.
    (d) Cancellous bone is less metabolically active than compact bone.
    (e) Carpal tunnel syndrome commonly occurs in the first trimester of pregnancy.

58. **Kyphosis can be caused by:**
    (a) Ankylosing spondylitis.
    (b) Hemivertebrae.
    (c) Sciatica.
    (d) Fractured vertebrae.
    (e) Spinal tumours.

59. **Extra-articular features of rheumatoid arthritis include:**
    (a) Peripheral neuropathy.
    (b) Aortic regurgitation.
    (c) Carpal tunnel syndrome.
    (d) Dry mouth.
    (e) Spider naevi.

Joints

60. HLA B27 may be associated with:
(a) Rheumatoid arthritis.
(b) Osteoarthritis.
(c) Reiter's syndrome.
(d) Behçet's syndrome
(e) Ankylosing spondylitis.

61. Reactive arthritis:
(a) Occurs after genital infection with *Trichomonas vaginalis*.
(b) Occurs after gastrointestinal infection with *Escherichia coli*.
(c) Is associated with HLA B27.
(d) Reiter's syndrome is an example of reactive arthritis.
(e) May lead to severe spondylitis.

62. Developmental dysplasia of the hip:
(a) Occurs in girls more than boys.
(b) Requires surgical correction in the first instance.
(c) Occurs more commonly following breech delivery.
(d) May cause delayed walking and abnormal gait.
(e) Is routinely examined for on the neonatal check.

63. Slipped upper femoral epiphysis:
(a) Is more prevalent in overweight patients.
(b) Is a pathological complication of osteoarthritis.
(c) Can be complicated by avascular necrosis.
(d) Management is conservative in the first instance.
(e) Affects males more than females.

64. True or false:
(a) Chondromalacia patellae most commonly affects adolescent girls.
(b) Meniscal cysts require excision.
(c) Adhesive capsulitis causes restriction of abduction only.
(d) Painful arc syndrome is caused by biceps rupture.
(e) Patellar dislocation usually occurs medially.

65. Carpal tunnel syndrome:
(a) Can wake the patient at night.
(b) Causes paraesthesia of the ulnar nerve.
(c) Can occur in myxoedema.
(d) Is caused by nerve compression from the flexor retinaculum.
(e) Can be treated by hydrocortisone injections.

66. Concerning gout:
(a) Gout is caused by urate crystals.
(b) Crystals are needle-shaped.
(c) Is associated with hyperuricaemia.
(d) Can occur due to chronic thiazide diuretic therapy.
(e) Is associated with abstinence from alcohol.

67. True or false:
(a) Medications can cause myopathy.
(b) Muscle weakness gets worse on exertion in Lambert–Eaton myasthenic syndrome.

(c) Straight-leg raising test is positive where there is a prolapsed disc.
(d) Trendelenburg test reveals pathology of the neck of femur.
(e) Uveitis is associated with scleroderma.

68. Regarding joint pathology:
(a) The urate crystals of gout are negatively birefringent.
(b) Transient synovitis commonly affects those in their 20s.
(c) A bunion is a protective bursa.
(d) Swan-neck deformity is caused by a flexed PIP joint and a hyperextended DIP joint with an extended MCP joint.
(e) Sjögren's syndrome can affect the exocrine glands.

69. Regarding the elbow joint:
(a) Olecranon bursitis causes pain in all directions of movement of the elbow joint.
(b) Cubitus valgus can be associated with Klinefelter's syndrome.
(c) The paraesthesia arising from ulnar neuritis is felt over the thumb, index, middle and lateral ring fingers.
(d) Tennis elbow can be caused by hitting a tennis ball awkwardly during a backstroke.
(e) The ulnar nerve runs in a groove behind the lateral epicondyle.

70. Regarding the hands and wrists:
(a) Ganglia are diagnosed by excision and biopsy of the swelling.
(b) In trigger finger the affected finger locks or snaps on forced extension.
(c) In mallet finger there is damage to the insertion of the flexor tendon with loss of full flexion.
(d) Tenosynovitis is caused by overuse of the affected tendons.
(e) Dropped finger can occur as a complication of rheumatoid arthritis.

71. Regarding septic arthritis:
(a) It should always be excluded where there is an acutely painful, hot, swollen joint.
(b) Neutropenia is seen on joint aspiration.
(c) Plain radiographs are diagnostic.
(d) In patients taking immunosuppressant therapy the signs of systemic sepsis may be exacerbated.
(e) Predisposing factors to septic arthritis include rheumatoid arthritis.

72. Regarding Perthes' disease:
(a) It affects girls five times more than boys.
(b) It occurs bilaterally in 60% of cases.
(c) It predisposes to arthritis of the affected joint in later life.
(d) It requires surgical debridement.
(e) It usually affects adolescents between 10 and 15 years of age.

73. Regarding systemic lupus erythematosus:
(a) It commonly causes a migrating symmetrical arthralgia.
(b) Rheumatological features resemble those of rheumatoid arthritis.
(c) Affected joints commonly develop effusions.
(d) Patients commonly develop Raynaud's phenomenon.
(e) Complement C3 and C4 levels are raised in active disease.

Skin

74. Regarding the epidermis:
(a) It is avascular.
(b) It forms three layers, through which keratinocytes mature.
(c) The prickle cell layer projects into the underlying dermis to form rete ridges.
(d) Melanocytes are mainly located in the horny cell layer.
(e) It is derived from endoderm.

75. Regarding the dermis:
(a) The papillary layer contains many capillaries and nerves.
(b) It contains mast cells.
(c) It contains many adipose cells.
(d) It is thicker in areas that undergo repeated trauma, such as the palms and soles.
(e) Sweat glands originate from this layer.

76. Regarding keratinocytes:
(a) They contain the low molecular weight keratin molecule.
(b) They take 28 days to mature through the layers of the epidermis.
(c) Turnover rate is reduced in psoriasis.
(d) Desquamation occurs within 14 days after maturation is achieved.
(e) Keratin molecules are stronger in hair than skin.

77. Regarding nails:
(a) They consist of a plate of collagen.
(b) The hyponychium contains the dividing keratinocytes.
(c) Fingernails grow slower than toenails.
(d) Clubbing causes a marked increase in the angle between the base of the nail and the nail fold.
(e) Beau's lines are longitudinal grooves in the nail caused by systemic illness disrupting the growth of the nail matrix.

78. Causes of clubbing include:
(a) Empyema.
(b) Lung cancer.
(c) Subacute infective endocarditis.
(d) Rheumatoid arthritis.
(e) Ulcerative colitis.

79. Sebaceous glands:
(a) Communicate indirectly with hair follicles.
(b) Become active at puberty.
(c) The sebum they produce is bactericidal.
(d) Are derived from epidermal cells.
(e) Are important in maintaining a waterproof skin barrier.

80. Eccrine sweat glands:
(a) Are under sympathetic adrenergic control.
(b) Become active at puberty.
(c) Are modified sexual scent glands.
(d) Are found in abundance on the palms and soles.
(e) Secrete a protein-rich secretion.

81. Regarding the cutaneous blood vessels:
(a) Branches of the skin's plexuses directly penetrate all layers of the epidermis.
(b) Arteriovenous anastomoses are formed in the basal layer of the epidermis.
(c) Arteriovenous anastomoses control direct heat loss through dilatation or constriction.
(d) Arteriovenous anastomoses are under parasympathetic and sympathetic control.
(e) The skin does not have a lymphatic drainage system.

82. Regarding melanin:
(a) It is produced by melanosomes.
(b) It shields keratinocytes from the effects of UV radiation.
(c) Skin colour is genetically determined by the number of melanocytes present.
(d) Phaeomelanin pigments the skin brown–black.
(e) It scavenges free radicals.

83. Side effects of topical steroid therapy can include:
(a) Infection.
(b) Pruritus.
(c) Skin atrophy.
(d) Telangiectasia.
(e) Allergic contact dermatitis.

84. Atopic eczema:
(a) Has no associations or known aetiology.
(b) 10% of those likely to present with it do so in the first year of life.
(c) Half remit by the age of 15.
(d) Affects the flexures in the older child.
(e) Affects both the dermis and the epidermis.

85. Predisposing factors for *Candida albicans* infection include:
(a) HIV infection.
(b) Good hygiene.
(c) Corticosteroid treatment.
(d) Pregnancy.
(e) Diabetes mellitus.

86. Concerning scabies:
(a) It is caused by a bacterium.
(b) Most commonly involves the finger webs.
(c) Norwegian scabies is the variant of scabies that occurs in Norway.

(d) Skin rash occurs within 2 weeks of contracting the infestation.
(e) It causes a great deal of itching.

87. Regarding tumours of the skin:
(a) Seborrhoeic warts are caused by overproliferation of melanocytes.
(b) Epidermal cysts are filled with keratin.
(c) Keloid scars occur most common in Caucasian individuals.
(d) Melanocytic naevi develop exclusively in the epidermis.
(e) Melanocytic naevi can transform into malignant melanoma.

88. Regarding vascular naevi:
(a) Port-wine naevi resolve spontaneously by 7 years of age.
(b) Salmon patch commonly occurs on the neck at birth.
(c) Strawberry naevi can cause parents great anxiety.
(d) Strawberry naevi require surgical excision.
(e) Epidermal naevi can recur after excision.

89. Regarding malignant melanoma:
(a) It is thought to be associated with sunbathing.
(b) Almost all occur on the site of a pre-existing melanocytic naevus.
(c) It occurs twice as often in men than in women.
(d) Prognosis is related to the depth of invasion.
(e) Lentigo maligna melanoma follows a slower course.

90. Regarding skin tumours:
(a) Squamous cell carcinoma is usually a pigmented tumour.
(b) Basal cell carcinoma is the rarest form of skin tumour.
(c) Kaposi's sarcoma occurs more commonly in immunocompromised patients.
(d) Keratoacanthoma is a malignant, rapidly growing tumour that occurs on sun-exposed areas.
(e) Basal cell carcinoma commonly arises on the face.

91. Regarding acne:
(a) There is colonization with *Staphylococcus aureus*.
(b) Comedones may leave 'ice-pick' scars.
(c) Affects both sexes equally.
(d) Clinical features arise from chronic inflammation of the stratum corneum.
(e) There is a sebum deficiency.

92. Hirsutism can be caused by:
(a) Polycystic ovaries.
(b) Gigantism.
(c) Congenital adrenal hyperplasia.
(d) Cushing's syndrome.
(e) Porphyria cutanea tarda.

93. Hypopigmentation is a feature of:
(a) Hyperoestrogenism.
(b) Phenylketonuria.

(c) Lichen sclerosus.
(d) Peutz–Jeghers syndrome.
(e) Albinism.

94. Causes of hyperpigmentation include:
(a) Chloasma.
(b) Burns.
(c) Cirrhosis.
(d) Vitiligo.
(e) Hypoadrenalism.

95. True or false:
(a) Pacinian corpuscles detect touch.
(b) Lanugo hairs are formed at 12 weeks' gestation.
(c) Mature keratinocytes become corneocytes.
(d) The stratum corneum is no longer pliable if its water content falls below 30%.
(e) Skin melanin scavenges free radicals.

96. Regarding disorders of pigmentation:
(a) Vitiligo is associated with pernicious anaemia, thyroid disease and Addison's disease.
(b) Albinism has a prevalence of 1 in 5000.
(c) Phenylketonuria leads to increased melanin synthesis.
(d) Chloasma may be induced by puberty.
(e) Amiodarone may cause pigmentation.

97. Regarding cutaneous bacterial infections:
(a) Erythrasma eruptions will not fluoresce under a Wood's lamp.
(b) Trichomycosis axillaris affects the hair.
(c) Impetigo is highly contagious.
(d) Ecthyma leads to ulcer development.
(e) Scalded skin syndrome is caused by a streptococcal infection.

98. Viral infections:
(a) Viral warts are caused by infection with herpes virus.
(b) Molluscum contagiosum mainly affects children and adolescents.
(c) Herpes simplex type I primary infection is genital.
(d) Herpes zoster occurs in a dermatomal distribution.
(e) Neonatal infection with herpes simplex is commonly fatal.

99. True or false:
(a) Skin-prick tests are used to detect type II hypersensitivity.
(b) Wood's lamp detects fungal infection.
(c) ESR is decreased in SLE.
(d) Serum uric acid is raised in gout.
(e) Patch skin testing is used to detect type I hypersensitivity reactions.

100. The normal skin flora include:
(a) Staphylococci.
(b) Streptococci.
(c) *Escherichia*.
(d) *Corynebacteria*.
(e) *Propionebacteria*.

Short-answer questions (SAQs)

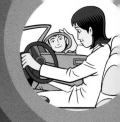

1. Discuss the pathological features of type I hypersensitivity reactions against those of type IV hypersensitivity reactions, and give examples of conditions in which they occur.

2. Draw the structure of a simple hair follicle.

3. Compare the pathophysiologies of pemphigus and pemphigoid.

4. List some of the characteristic features of arterial, venous and neuropathic ulcers.

5. Discuss the differences between the cardiac action potentials that occur in sinoatrial cells and those cells of the conducting system, and the relevance of these features to cardiac function.

6. Make brief notes on the processes involved in fracture repair.

7. List the characteristic features of basal cell carcinoma and compare these to the features of squamous cell carcinoma.

8. Discuss the sinister features of back pain and produce a list of possible causes. What initial investigations are usually required?

9. List the features of compact and cancellous bone, in particular with relation to their location, structure and function.

10. Make brief notes on vitamin D production and list some causes of vitamin D deficiency.

11. Make brief notes on the roles of parathyroid hormone and calcitonin in calcium homoeostasis.

12. Draw a normal synovial joint and list examples of factors that can affect it, with examples.

13. Make notes on cartilage production.

14. List the pathological joint changes that occur with rheumatoid arthritis and osteoarthritis.

15. Define the following and give examples of clinical conditions in which they occur: macule; wheal; blister; plaque; papule; purpura.

16. A 78-year-old woman fell onto the left side of her hip and presented with severe pain in her left lower leg, which was externally rotated and shortened. What is the diagnosis and treatment for this woman, and what is the most severe complication?

17. A 24-year-old man presents with a 5-month history of lower back pain. The pain is worse upon rest and his back is particularly stiff in the mornings. His lumbar spine movement is reduced in all planes. What is the likely diagnosis, what blood tests should be taken, and what changes may be apparent on X-ray?

18. A 35-year-old blonde woman presents with a mole that has become increasingly itchy and darker over the past month. She is concerned she might have skin cancer. What features would suggest malignant change of the lesion, and what investigations would be required?

19. List some of the skin changes that occur with diabetes mellitus.

20. List some skin conditions that can be associated with malignancy.

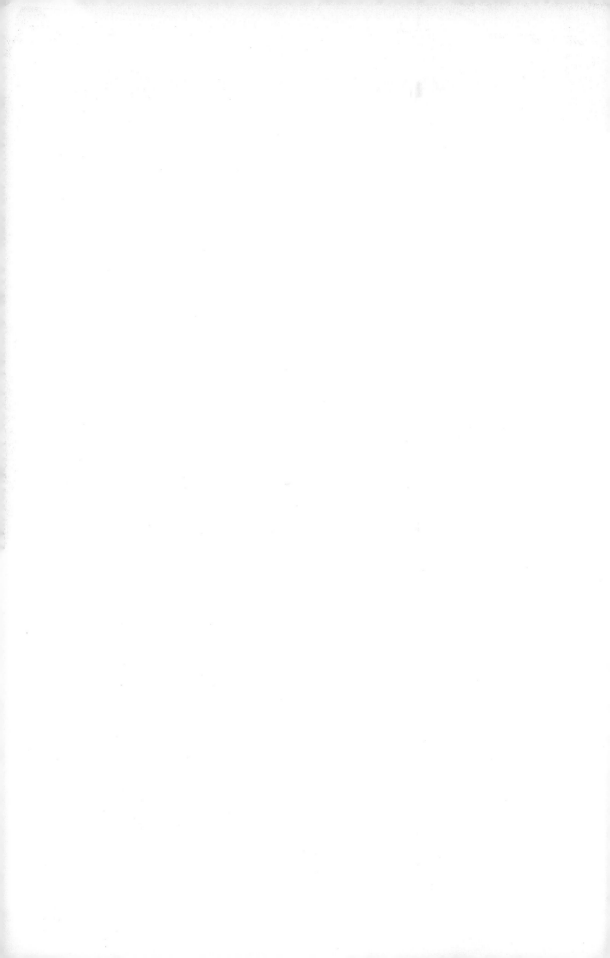

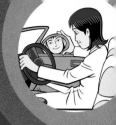
1. Fractures

A. Comminuted
B. Simple
C. Compound
D. Stress
E. Greenstick
F. Avulsion fracture

1. Partial fracture on radiograph in a young child
2. Fracture of the second metatarsal in a young woman who developed symptoms on a sponsored 20-mile walk
3. A fracture producing three bony fragments
4. One clean break, e.g. humerus
5. A traumatic tibial fracture, a fragment protruding through the skin
6. A fragment of bone detached by the force applied through a tendon on traction force

2. Cutaneous sensation

A. Free nerve endings
B. Meissner's corpuscles
C. Pacinian corpuscle
D. Merkel cells
E. Substance P
F. Corpuscular receptors

1. Receptors located within the dermis, detecting pressure and vibration
2. Within the dermis and epidermis, detect pain, itch and temperature
3. Mechanoreceptors, also containing neurotransmitters
4. Within dermal papillae of hands and feet, sensitive to touch

3. Match the terms

A. Urticaria
B. Angio-oedema
C. Contact dermatitis
D. Nodule
E. Papule
F. Vesicle
G. Plaque

1. Skin blister filled with fluid less than 5 mm across
2. Eczema precipitated by an exogenous substance, e.g. chemicals
3. Palpable lesion of less than 5 mm elevation but measuring more than 2 cm in diameter
4. Transient, pruritic wheals caused by extravascular plasma leakage into dermis
5. Solid or oedematous lesion elevated no more than 5 mm

6. Widespread collection of extravascular fluid involving the dermis and subcutis
7. Solid elevation of skin less than 5 mm in diameter

4. Match the disease with the organism

A. *Staphylococcus aureus*
B. *Streptococcus pyogenes*
C. Human papillomavirus
D. *Corynebacterium*
E. *Mycobacterium tuberculosis*

1. Viral warts
2. Lupus vulgaris
3. Folliculitis
4. Erysipelas
5. Trichomycosis axillaris

5. Match signs and syndromes

A. Sjögren's syndrome
B. Systemic lupus erythematosus
C. Felty's syndrome
D. Scleroderma
E. Ankylosing spondylitis
F. Rheumatoid arthritis

1. Skin tethering
2. Mouth ulcers
3. Butterfly rash
4. Splenomegaly
5. Iritis
6. Difficulty in closing eyes
7. Dry mouth

6. Joint pain

A. Gout
B. Transient synovitis
C. Septic arthritis
D. Enteropathic arthritis
E. Rheumatoid arthritis
F. Tennis elbow
G. Osteoarthritis

1. A 32-year-old man with ulcerative colitis presents with a 2-week of history of pain, swelling and reduced mobility of the left hip joint, with one previous episode at the same joint in the previous year lasting for 4 weeks. No other joints have been affected. No features are evident on a plain radiograph of the joint.
2. A 68-year-old former professional footballer presenting for the first time with progressive pain, stiffness, and reduced mobility of the left knee

joint. He complains of stiffness in early mornings, and the pain is worse on exertion.

3. A 5-year-old apyrexial girl presenting to A&E in distress with a painful, hot right hip joint that she woke up with the previous day. She is reluctant and apprehensive about weightbearing on the right leg, and her mobility is reduced. No swelling is apparent. Plain radiograph is normal.

4. An 82-year-old woman presenting with a hot, swollen and exquisitely tender left metatarsophalangeal joint. No other joints have been affected. Her past medical history includes hypertension.

5. A 38-year-old woman with an 8-week history of intermittent stiffness in the joints of both hands that is worse in the mornings, which has recently become more regular and painful. She also complains of feeling increasingly tired, and her partner remarks that she has lost weight.

7. Skin lesions

A. Lichen planus
B. Urticaria
C. Allergic dermatitis
D. Plaque psoriasis
E. Pityriasis rosacea
F. Atopic eczema
G. Parapsoriasis

1. A 28-year-old man with raised, scaly, silvery lesions on both elbows.

2. An 8-month-old girl with reddened, scaly patches that have developed on the face and ears, with weeping lesions that are causing her to scratch.

3. A 20-year-old domestic worker with erythematous, itchy lesions on the hands and flexor surface of the left wrist.

4. A student presenting with unusual transient itchy, red wheals developing on the arms that disappear after a few hours.

5. A man presenting with flat, itchy, red lesions on the flexor surfaces of the wrists that have developed a fine white lacework surface. He has also developed a few ulcers and lesions around the mouth.

8. Skin infections

A. Scabies
B. Impetigo
C. Viral warts
D. Cellulitis
E. Folliculitis
F. Candidiasis
G. Ringworm

1. A 68-year-old pyrexial woman presenting 5 days after orthopaedic surgery to the left ankle with an acute onset of erythema of the lower left leg that has become increasingly swollen and painful, and is progressing up the limb.

2. A 12-year-old girl with lesions spreading over the chin that are weeping and developing yellow crusts.

3. A 15-year-old schoolgirl with red papules over the wrists and finger webs that are extremely itchy, especially at night.

4. A 2-month-old baby girl with erythematous, ragged patches down the flexor creases of both hips, with small white pustules.

5. A 14-year-old girl with two roughened, raised, rounded and itchy lesions that have developed on the palms.

9. Skin conditions: match the causative organism with the clinical features it causes

A. Molluscum contagiosum
B. Staphylococcus aureus
C. Propionibacterium acnes
D. Phthirus pubis
E. Varicella zoster virus
F. Tinea capitis
G. Streptococcus pyogenes

1. An 11-year-old girl with some hair loss associated with itchy, round, scaly patches on the scalp, with pustules.

2. A 17-year-old boy with very greasy skin and red, inflamed spots over the face and chest, who has recently begun to develop red, sore cysts in these areas.

3. A 21-year-old man who presents with itching and excoriation of the pubic region, with itching most intense at night.

4. An 80-year-old woman with painful, vesicular eruptions developing down the right side of the face, preceded by pins and needles of the area.

5. A 9-year-old girl with crops of pearly-pink papules with a central punctum, which are expressible.

10. Muscle disorders

A. Myocarditis
B. Gastro-oesophageal reflux disease
C. Irritable bowel disease
D. Hypertrophic obstructive cardiomyopathy
E. Myocardial infarction
F. Leiomyoma
G. Ischaemic heart disease

1. A 24-year-old woman with chest pain and shortness of breath associated with feeling faint, and a family history of sudden death.

2. A 42-year-old man with an acute presentation of fever, dyspnoea and malaise following a recent chest infection. He presents with the features of cardiac failure.

3. A 78-year-old man presenting with intermittent chest pain, worse on exertion and alleviated by rest. He has been treated by his GP for hypertension for the past 10 years.

4. A 38-year-old woman presenting to gynaecology outpatients with an 8-month history of abnormally heavy menstrual bleeding associated with increasing period pain and recent onset of urinary frequency.

5. A 32-year-old athletic man who complains of a 10-month history of progressive intermittent chest pain and a troublesome cough brought on by spicy foods and aggravated by bending.

11. Hypersensitivity reactions

A. Type III hypersensitivity reactions
B. Type I hypersensitivity reaction
C. Type IV hypersensitivity reaction
D. Type II hypersensitivity reaction

1. Infective endocarditis
2. Pemphigus
3. Penicillin allergic reaction
4. Contact dermatitis
5. Systemic lupus erythematosus

Skeletal muscle

1. Skeletal muscle contraction:
   (a) True
   (b) False   the longer the muscle fibre, the more range of movement it can produce
   (c) False   synergistic muscles help with the movement of a muscle
   (d) True
   (e) False   it is under somatic or voluntary control

2. Regarding skeletal muscle attachment:
   (a) False   tendons are made of closely compacted collagen fibres
   (b) False   not always, e.g. sphincters
   (c) True
   (d) False
   (e) True

3. Regarding skeletal muscle fibres:
   (a) True
   (b) False   they run through the surrounding perimysium
   c) False   the smaller a fasciculus, the finer the movement that muscle performs
   (d) False   satellite cells form myoblasts as part of the repair process
   (e) True

4. Resting membrane potential:
   (a) False $-90\,mV$
   (b) False K^+ is the main ion responsible for maintaining the RMP
   (c) True
   (d) True
   (e) False   the Na^+/K^+-ATPase pump contributes to the RMP

5. Action potentials in skeletal muscles:
   (a) False   they are initiated from the hila of the axons that supply the neuromuscular junctions
   (b) False   action potentials occur according to an all-or-none principle
   (c) True
   (d) True
   (e) False   conduction velocity is increased in increased temperatures up to 40°C

6. Regarding synapses:
   (a) True
   (b) False   action potentials can occur at chemical synapses as well as electrical ones
   (c) True
   (d) True
   (e) True

7. Comparing action potentials of skeletal muscle and nerve fibres:
   (a) False   they are not constant
   (b) True
   (c) True
   (d) False   it is mainly due to Na^+ ions
   (e) False   in muscle action potentials run along T-tubules

8. The nicotinic acetylcholine receptor:
   (a) False   it is activated by two acetylcholine molecules
   (b) True
   (c) False   it is produced from acetyl CoA and choline
   (d) True
   (e) True

9. Drugs at the neuromuscular junction:
   (a) False   it binds and blocks presynaptic acetylcholine release
   (b) False   it binds reversibly
   (c) False   tubocurarine is a non-depolarizing drug that competitively binds and blocks the nicotinic acetylcholine receptor
   (d) True
   (e) True

10. Regarding muscle contraction:
   (a) False   muscle contraction occurs as a result of the interaction of thin filaments called actin and thick filaments called myosin
   (b) True
   (c) False   calcium binding to tropomyosin is required for actin–myosin interaction and contraction to occur
   (d) False   the myosin molecule head 'walks along' the actin filament
   (e) False   it is dependent on the ATPase activity of the myosin molecule, as well as calcium being bound to tropomyosin

11. Regarding motor units:
(a) True
(b) False
(c) False
(d) True
(e) False

12. Regarding muscle tension:
(a) False the more frequently the muscle is stimulated, the greater the tension produced
(b) False an action potential results in sufficient Ca^{2+} to produce the maximal response. This principle only applies to cardiac muscle
(c) True
(d) False that is tetanus
(e) True

13. Myasthenia gravis:
(a) True
(b) False it produces signs and symptoms only when nicotinic acetylcholine receptors are reduced to 30%
(c) False intermittent remission and relapse
(d) False they have a different antigenicity from those of skeletal muscle
(e) False It is diagnosed by the Tensilon (edrophonium) test

14. Myotonic dystrophy:
(a) False it commonly presents in the 20s to 30s
(b) False it is inherited in an autosomal dominant fashion
(c) True
(d) False it can affect cognitive function
(e) True

15. Duchenne muscular dystrophy:
(a) False it is an X-linked recessive condition
(b) False mutated dystrophin protein means impaired anchorage of muscle to the extracellular matrix, causing susceptibility to tearing on repeated contraction
(c) True
(d) False 30% of sufferers are affected by intellectual impairment
(e) True

16. Poliomyelitis:
(a) True
(b) True
(c) True
(d) False the proximal myopathy is symmetrical
(e) True

17. True or false:
(a) True
(b) False
(c) False Gower's sign is a feature of Duchenne muscular dystrophy
(d) False it does not occur in cardiac muscle, otherwise the heart would be unable to beat
(e) True

18. Regarding the structure of the heart:
(a) True
(b) False thickest in the ventricles, particularly the left
(c) False visceral pericardium is in close contact with the myocardium
(d) False the visceral and parietal pericardium separates the myocardium and the pericardium
(e) False endocardial epithelial cells are responsive to circulatory substances

19. Cardiac action potentials:
(a) False atrial and ventricular action potentials have different characteristics
(b) False the action potential is initiated at the sinoatrial node
(c) False the cardiac action potential travels through muscle tissue through gap junctions which are electrical in nature
(d) True
(e) True

20. Regarding the action potential:
(a) False the plateau phase is caused by Ca^{2+}/Na^+ channels
(b) False Purkinje cells are unstable and self-excitable
(c) False pacemaker function is determined by those cells that generate a greater number of action potentials. An action potential is an all-or-nothing phenomenon, and therefore cannot be stronger than other action potentials
(d) True
(e) True

21. Cardiac contraction:
(a) True
(b) False cardiac T-tubules are wider than those of skeletal muscle
(c) False calcium is released from the sarcoplasmic reticulum
(d) False it stores less
(e) True known as the *treppe* effect

22. Factors affecting contractility:
(a) False   chronotropes affect the rate of contraction
(b) True
(c) False
(d) False
(e) True

23. The autonomic nervous system:
(a) True
(b) False   also from sympathetic postganglionic nerve fibres
(c) True
(d) False   parasympathetic innervation is mediated through muscarinic acetylcholine receptors
(e) True

24. Regarding cardiac contraction:
(a) False   force of contraction is proportional to the initial length of the cardiac muscle fibre
(b) True
(c) False   action potentials in the conducting and contractile systems are the same length
(d) True
(e) True

25. Hypertrophic obstructive cardiomyopathy:
(a) True   in 50% of cases
(b) False   usually left ventricular hypertrophy
(c) False   it is the cause of sudden death in 6% of adolescents
(d) False   echocardiography is diagnostic
(e) True   but most stay stable for years

26. In dilated cardiomyopathy:
(a) True
(b) True
(c) False   atherosclerosis is not a complication
(d) False   prognosis is poor
(e) True

27. True or false:
(a) True
(b) True
(c) False   intercalated discs anchor actin filaments to each end of the cell
(d) False   cardiac myocytes are uninucleated
(e) False   they are 100 µm long

28. Smooth muscle in the respiratory tract:
(a) True
(b) False   it is under sympathetic control
(c) False   it is arranged circumferentially
(d) True
(e) True

29. Smooth muscle:
(a) False   the intestine is composed of two muscle layers
(b) False   the bladder consists of inner and outer longitudinal layers, and a middle circular layer
(c) False   the stomach has an inner oblique layer
(d) False   the lower two-thirds
(e) True

30. Smooth muscle contractile apparatus:
(a) False   they anchor thin filaments to the cell membrane
(b) False   it occurs when the force of contraction is transmitted through the dense bodies to which the cell fibres attach
(c) True
(d) False   it does not appear striated
(e) False   desmin is an intermediate filament in the smooth muscle contractile apparatus

31. Regarding the nerve supply to smooth muscle:
(a) False   varicosities are swellings from which neurotransmitters are released to act on smooth muscle
(b) False   nerve fibres release neurotransmitters that act on receptors on the smooth muscle
(c) True
(d) True
(e) False   the outer layer is usually innervated

32. True or false:
(a) True
(b) True
(c) False   organic nitrates decrease smooth muscle tone
(d) False   muscle spindles are not present in smooth muscle
(e) True

33. Smooth muscle:
(a) False Ca^{2+} is responsible for the action potential
(b) False   the RMP is less negative, around −50 to −60 mV
(c) False   calmodulin is a component of the thick filament
(d) False   along with Meissner's plexus, Auerbach's plexus coordinates peristalsis
(e) False   serotonin influences smooth muscle contraction

34. In smooth muscle contraction:
(a) False   four calcium ions bind to calmodulin
(b) False   action potentials can be plateau-like as well as spiked
(c) True
(d) True
(e) True

35. In contrast to skeletal muscle, in smooth muscle contraction:

(a) False   troponin is not present in smooth muscle

(b) True

(c) False   cross-bridge formation is ATP dependent

(d) True

(e) True

Bone

36. Cartilage:

(a) False   composed of collagen and glycosaminoglycans

(b) False   chondroblasts

(c) True

(d) False   mainly derived from interstitial growth, from the centre outwards

(e) False   it is avascular

37. Regarding cartilage:

(a) False   type II

(b) False   hyaline cartilage is a major component of articular joints

(c) True

(d) False   chondroblasts eventually turn into chondrocytes

(e) True

38. Regarding long bones:

(a) False   the diaphysis is the shaft of the bone

(b) True

(c) False   proximal epiphyses

(d) False   cancellous bone

(e) True

39. True or false:

(a) True

(b) False   it enters by penetrating the periosteum

(c) False   calcium and phosphate

(d) False   monocytes

(e) True

40. True or false:

(a) True

(b) False   cancellous bone

(c) False   it lies between two layers of compact bone and is called diploe

(d) False   Haversian canals are lined by osteocytes

(e) False   sesamoid bones lie within tendons that protect them from rubbing on the underlying bones

41. Bone production:

(a) True

(b) False   it can be produced by either intra-membranous or endochondral ossification

(c) False   intramembranous ossification

(d) False   it forms a cartilaginous model in which secondary ossification centres convert it to bone

(e) False   bone remodelling does have a significant role in bone production

42. Concerning bone growth:

(a) False   endochondral growth leads to an increase in length

(b) False

(c) False   it ceases when the epiphyseal growth plates fuse

(d) True

(e) True

43. Regarding calcium:

(a) True

(b) False   parathyroid hormone increases low blood calcium levels

(c) True

(d) False   gastrointestinal absorption is controlled by vitamin D

(e) False   vitamin C

44. Concerning hormonal influence on bone:

(a) True

(b) True

(c) False   thyroid hormones are required for growth hormone production

(d) False   thyroid hormone deficiency can cause dwarfism

(e) False   bones in acromegaly increase in width because the epiphyseal plates have fused

45. Regarding the bone:

(a) True

(b) False

(c) False   it is reduced in both

(d) False   it is raised

(e) False   not all of them

46. Regarding bony metastases, some characteristic features are:

(a) True

(b) True

(c) False   raised alkaline phosphatase

(d) True

(e) True

47. Metastatic tumours of the skeleton:
- (a) True
- (b) True
- (c) True
- (d) False   pain worse at night, keeping the patient awake
- (e) True

48. True or false:
- (a) False   type I collagen
- (b) False   it is defined as bone thinning
- (c) False   osteopetrosis occurs where there is a lack of osteoclastic bone resorption
- (d) False   autosomal dominant
- (e) True

49. Regarding osteomyelitis:
- (a) False   commonly occurs in the distal femur and proximal tibia
- (b) False   both can occur
- (c) True
- (d) True
- (e) False   7–10 days

50. Regarding fractures:
- (a) False   open reduction and internal fixation
- (b) True
- (c) True
- (d) False
- (e) False   comminuted fractures do

51. True or false:
- (a) False   it is caused by poor blood supply
- (b) False   it affects marrow
- (c) True
- (d) False   it is caused by vitamin D and phosphate deficiency
- (e) False   it is a common mode of presentation

52. Osteoporosis:
- (a) False   the female to male ratio is 4:1
- (b) True
- (c) False   dual emission X-ray absorptiometry (DEXA) scanning is the gold standard
- (d) True
- (e) False   bisphosphonates inhibit osteoclastic activity

53. Hyperparathyroidism:
- (a) False   it leads to a raised parathyroid hormone level
- (b) False   clinical features arise from raised calcium levels

- (c) False   reversible with treatment
- (d) True
- (e) True

54. Regarding Paget's disease of bone:
- (a) False   it affects men more than women
- (b) False   in 85% of cases it affects several bones
- (c) False   it is caused by an initial increase in osteoclastic activity
- (d) False   serum calcium levels are usually normal
- (e) True

55. True or false:
- (a) False
- (b) True
- (c) False   later life
- (d) False
- (e) False   renal osteodystrophy occurs secondary to chronic renal disease

56. Possible differential diagnoses of an acute monoarthritis include:
- (a) True
- (b) True
- (c) True
- (d) True
- (e) False   causes acute polyarthritis

57. True or false:
- (a) False   C-reactive protein is produced by the liver
- (b) True
- (c) False   chest pain can be referred to the medial side of the upper arm
- (d) False   cancellous bone is more metabolically active than compact bone
- (e) False   it commonly occurs in the third trimester of pregnancy

58. Kyphosis can be caused by:
- (a) True
- (b) False   this can cause scoliosis
- (c) False   this can cause scoliosis
- (d) True
- (e) True

59. Extra-articular features of rheumatoid arthritis include:
- (a) True
- (b) False   it does not cause aortic regurgitation
- (c) True
- (d) True   as part of a triad known as secondary Sjögren's syndrome, with dry eyes and arthritis
- (e) False   it does not cause spider naevi

Joints

60. HLA B27 may be associated with:
(a) False
(b) False
(c) True
(d) False
(e) True

61. Reactive arthritis:
(a) False   occurs after genital infection with *Chlamydia*
(b) False   occurs after gastrointestinal infection with *Salmonella*, *Campylobacter* or *Shigella*
(c) True
(d) True   it forms a triad with arthritis, urethritis/cervicitis and conjunctivitis
(e) True

62. Developmental dysplasia of the hip:
(a) True
(b) False
(c) True
(d) True   if not detected early and it does not resolve spontaneously
(e) True

63. Slipped upper femoral epiphysis:
(a) True
(b) False   it occurs in adolescents
(c) True
(d) False   surgical pinning or osteotomy is required
(e) True

64. True or false:
(a) True
(b) True
(c) False   it affects movement in all planes
(d) False   painful arc syndrome is caused by rotator cuff pathology
(e) False   patellar dislocation commonly occurs laterally

65. Carpal tunnel syndrome:
(a) True
(b) False   it affects the median nerve
(c) True
(d) True
(e) True   although this is not first-line treatment

66. Concerning gout:
(a) True
(b) True
(c) True

(d) True
(e) False   it is associated with excessive alcohol intake

67. True or false:
(a) True
(b) False
(c) True
(d) False   it reveals gluteal pathology
(e) False   scleroderma is associated with difficulty in closing the eyes and a tight, beaked mouth

68. Regarding joint pathology:
(a) True
(b) False   it commonly affects children
(c) True   it arises where the shoe rubs
(d) False   this is a Boutonnière deformity. Swan-neck deformity has a flexed DIP joint and a hyperextended PIP joint. Both deformities occur in rheumatoid arthritis
(e) True

69. Regarding the elbow joint:
(a) False   movement is not usually painful: pain is produced on pressure
(b) False   it can be associated with Turner's syndrome
(c) False   it is felt over the little finger and medial ring finger
(d) False   caused by inflammation or trauma of the common extensor attachment at the lateral epicondyle
(e) False   it runs in a groove behind the medial epicondyle

70. Regarding the hands and wrists:
(a) False
(b) True
(c) False   it affects the extensor tendon, with loss of full extension
(d) True
(e) True

71. Regarding septic arthritis:
(a) True
(b) False   neutrophilia is seen on joint aspiration
(c) False   radiographs can exclude trauma but are not diagnostic of acute infection
(d) False   the signs may be absent
(e) True

72. Regarding Perthes' disease:
(a) False   it affects boys five times more than girls
(b) False   it occurs bilaterally in 10–20% of cases
(c) True

(d) False   management requires bed rest and traction

(e) False   it affects children between 5 and 10 years of age

73. Systemic lupus erythematosus:

(a) False   it commonly causes a migrating asymmetrical arthralgia

(b) True

(c) False   they are rare

(d) True

(e) False   they are low

Skin

74. Regarding the epidermis:

(a) True

(b) False   it is formed of four layers

(c) False   the basal cell layer projects into the underlying dermis to form rete ridges

(d) False   melanocytes are mainly located in the basal cell layer

(e) False   it is derived from ectoderm

75. Regarding the dermis:

(a) True

(b) True

(c) False

(d) True

(e) True

76. Regarding keratinocytes:

(a) False   keratin is high molecular weight, at 67 kDa

(b) False   14 days

(c) False   turnover rate is accelerated

(d) True

(e) True

77. Regarding nails:

(a) False   they consist of a plate of keratin

(b) False   the hyponychium is the free margin of the nail at the proximal end; dividing keratinocytes originate from the nail matrix

(c) False   toenails grow slower than fingernails

(d) False   there is a loss of the angle between the base of the nail and the nail fold

(e) False   Beau's lines are transverse, not longitudinal

78. Causes of clubbing include:

(a) True

(b) True

(c) True

(d) False

(e) True

79. Sebaceous glands:

(a) False   they communicate directly as they release sebum into the follicles

(b) True   they are androgen sensitive

(c) True

(d) True

(e) True

80. Eccrine sweat glands:

(a) False   they are under wrong cholinergic control

(b) False   apocrine glands become active at puberty

(c) False   apocrine sweat glands are modified sexual scent glands

(d) True

(e) False   they produce a watery fluid containing fatty acids, lipids, urea, glycoproteins and mucopolysaccharides

81. True or false:

(a) False   they do not

(b) False   they are formed in the papillary dermis

(c) True

(d) False   arteriovenous anastomoses are under sympathetic control

(e) False   lymphatic drainage occurs through lymphatic meshes that originate in the papillae, ultimately draining into regional lymph nodes

82. Regarding melanin:

(a) False   it is produced by melanocytes

(b) True

(c) False   it is determined by the level of activity of the melanocytes present

(d) False   that is eumelanin

(e) True

83. Side effects of topical steroid therapy can include:

(a) True

(b) False

(c) True

(d) True

(e) True

84. Atopic eczema:

(a) False   has a strong association with a positive family history of atopic disorders

(b) False   60% of those likely to present do so within the first year of life

(c) True

(d) True

(e) True

85. Predisposing factors for *Candida albicans* infection include:
(a) True
(b) False   poor hygiene is a predisposing factor
(c) True
(d) True
(e) True

86. Concerning scabies:
(a) False   it is caused by a mite, *Sarcoptes scabei*
(b) True   it also commonly involves the wrist, ankle, nipples and genitalia
(c) False   Norwegian lesions are large, encrusted eruptions that occur in the immunocompromised
(d) False   infestation occurs within 4–6 weeks
(e) True   rash

87. Regarding tumours of the skin:
(a) False   seborrhoeic warts are caused by overproliferation of keratinocytes
(b) True
(c) False   Afro-Caribbeans
(d) False   junctional naevi develop at the dermoepithelial junction, intradermal naevi develop in the dermis, and compound naevi occur in both
(e) True

88. Regarding vascular naevi:
(a) False   strawberry naevi resolve spontaneously by 7 years of age. Port wine naevi do not
(b) True
(c) True
(d) False   they resolve by 7 years of age
(e) True

89. Regarding malignant melanoma:
(a) True
(b) False   30% occur on the site of a pre-existing naevus
(c) False   it is twice as common in women than men
(d) True
(e) True

90. Regarding skin tumours:
(a) False
(b) False   basal cell carcinoma is the most common type of skin tumour
(c) True
(d) False   keratoacanthoma is benign
(e) True

91. Regarding acne:
(a) False   there is colonization with *Propiobacterium acnes*
(b) False   ice-pick scars are left by cysts
(c) True
(d) False   clinical features occur as a result of chronic inflammation of the pilosebaceous gland
(e) False   there is excessive production of sebum

92. Hirsutism can be caused by:
(a) True
(b) False
(c) True
(d) True
(e) True

93. Hypopigmentation is a feature of:
(a) False   hyperoestrogenism is a cause of hyperpigmentation
(b) True
(c) True
(d) False   Peutz–Jeghers syndrome can cause hyperpigmentation
(e) True

94. Causes of hyperpigmentation include:
(a) True
(b) False   burns cause patchy hypopigmentation
(c) True
(d) False   vitiligo causes patchy hypopigmentation
(e) True

95. Components of the dermis include:
(a) False   Pacinian corpuscles detect vibration and pressure
(b) False   lanugo hairs are formed at 20 weeks' gestation
(c) True
(d) False   the stratum corneum is no longer pliable if its water content falls below 10%
(e) True

96. Regarding disorders of pigmentation:
(a) True
(b) False   it has a prevalence of 1 in 20 000
(c) False   phenylketonuria leads to decreased melanin synthesis
(d) False   chloasma may be induced by pregnancy or the oral contraceptive pill
(e) True

97. Regarding cutaneous bacterial infection:
(a) False   lesions do fluoresce under a Wood's lamp
(b) True
(c) True

(d) True

(e) False   scalded skin syndrome is caused by a staphylococcal infection

98. Viral infections:

(a) False   human papilloma virus

(b) True

(c) False   perioral

(d) True

(e) True

99. True or false:

(a) False   skin-prick tests are used to detect type I hypersensitivity

(b) True

(c) False   ESR is raised in SLE

(d) True

(e) False   patch skin testing is used to detect type IV hypersensitivity reactions

100. The normal skin flora include:

(a) True

(b) False

(c) False

(d) True

(e) True

1. In a type I hypersensitivity reaction, an antigen causes the surface IgE of mast cells to cross-link, stimulating the production of inflammatory mediators such as histamine, prostaglandins and leukotrienes, producing urticaria and anaphylaxis. It can occur as a reaction to allergens such as bee stings and foods, and is an immediate to intermediate reaction. In type IV hypersensitivity reactions, antigen-presenting cells present presensitized T cells with an antigen, stimulating cytokine release, which activates other T cells and macrophages. The reaction is cell mediated and tissue damage is relatively delayed, occurring after 48–72 hours. Examples: allergic contact dermatitis, tuberculosis, leprosy.

2. Refer to Figure 6.10.

3. Autoantibodies are produced in both conditions against proteins in desmosomal structures that have a role in holding cells together – desmoglein 3 in pemphigus and BP-1 in pemphigoid. In pemphigus, autoantibodies are deposited in the intracellular matrix, inducing the release of proteolytic enzyme from keratinocytes, which produces fragile intraepidermal blisters that rupture easily. In pemphigoid, autoantibodies are deposited at the basement membrane, producing subepidermal splitting and blisters that are relatively more robust and less easily ruptured than those of pemphigus.

4. Venous ulcers are due to valvular incompetence in veins. Resulting venous hypertension produces increased venous permeability, allowing fibrin to leak through the walls and deposit next to capillaries, impeding oxygen and nutrient transfer and leaving them prone to ulceration. Skin discoloration, pain, venous eczema and lipodermatosclerosis can occur. They are initially exudative and become granulative, taking weeks to months to heal. Arterial ulcers occur secondary to ischaemia due to arterial disease. They are well demarcated and appear 'punched out'. The limb is often cold and numb due to arterial disease, with weak or absent pulses and hair loss from the limb. Neuropathic ulcers occur on areas subjected to repeated minor trauma on limbs with damaged nerve supply, especially diabetics with peripheral neuropathy.

5. Sinoatrial node cells have a drifting resting membrane potential because of their leakiness to Na^+, which allows slow Na^+ influx, so the potential drifts to threshold. This allows automatic rhythmicity, with the cell producing its own action potential. Depolarization produces Ca^{2+} influx and repolarization is produced by K^+ efflux. The membranes of myocytes of the conducting system are brought to threshold by opening of fast Na^+ channels, with a fast Na^+ influx. These channels are rapidly inactivated and repolarization occurs, with passive Cl^- influx. Slow Ca^{2+}/Na^+ channels open producing a plateau, with the Ca^{2+} producing contraction. Late repolarization occurs when these Ca^{2+}/Na^+ channels close and K^+ channels open, producing an efflux until the RMP is restored to normal. It does not drift as it does in the SA nodal cells.

6. With fracture repair, a haematoma initially forms at the fracture site. This becomes a procallus, which is converted into a fibrocartilaginous callus. This becomes an osseous callus, remodelled to form trabecular lamellar bone.

7. BCC and SCC commonly occur in areas exposed to excessive sun, such as the face and chest. They arise from keratinocytes. Common in middle to late life, BCC are composed of basophilic cells, grow slowly over years, and bud downwards to invade the dermis in a lobular manner. Telangiectatic papules or nodules that ulcerate. Almost never metastasize. SCC are composed of keratinocytes growing in disorderly manner, with nuclear abnormalities, beginning as small plaques that can progress to keratotic nodules or plaques and ulcerate and crust. They metastasize if untreated.

8. The 'red flags' of back pain include pain that wakes the patient at night; severe, unremitting pain that is progressive in nature and associated weight loss. Also bilateral leg pain or neurological involvement. Age less than 20 or over 55. Previous diagnosis of cancer. Altered perianal sensation. Thoracic or non-mechanical pain. Features can suggest cord compression, (cauda equina syndrome), metastases, infection, fracture. Investigations include FBC, ESR, CRP, calcium, alkaline phosphatase, spinal X-ray, bone scan, urgent MRI if cord compression suspected.

9. Compact bone forms circumferential layers around the outside of a long bone, in between which run Haversian canals, canals lined by osteocytes through which run neurovascular branches that supply the bone. They protect the bone from external forces. Cancellous bone forms lattices of lamellae called trabeculae, orientated in lines of stress, which act as scaffolding to the bone. It is more metabolically active than compact bone and hence more affected by metabolic conditions such as osteoporosis.

10. Small amounts of vitamin D are taken in the diet, e.g. fish. Most produced in epidermis from 7-dehydrocholesterol via photolysis by UV rays in sunlight. Two hydroxylation steps activate it, first in the liver and then in the kidney to form 1, 25-dihydroxyvitamin D_3 (calcitriol). Vitamin D deficiency can occur as a result of lack of sun exposure and poor dietary intake of foods containing vitamin D.

11. Parathyroid hormone stimulated by low calcium levels. Acts to restore calcium levels to normal by stimulating osteoclastic activity, subsequent bone resorption causing calcium and phosphate release; increases renal calcium reabsorption; directly stimulates vitamin D hydroxylation/activation at the kidney, and vitamin D stimulates intestinal absorption of calcium. Calcitonin is stimulated by high calcium levels. It inhibits osteoclasts, opposing the effects of PTH. It decreases calcium and phosphate renal reabsorption (refer to Figure 4.11).

12. It can be affected by inflammatory conditions, e.g. rheumatoid arthritis; infection, e.g. septic arthritis; fractures or mechanical injury, e.g. sport, trauma; metabolic conditions, e.g. gout; vascular abnormalities, e.g. avascular necrosis; degeneration, e.g. osteoarthritis (refer to Figure 5.4).

13. Cartilage is produced from mesenchyme. Mesenchymal differentiation produces chondroblasts, which secrete cartilage matrix. Deposition of matrix traps chondroblasts within the matrix, where they transform into chondrocytes, forming lacunae which they inhabit. They remain metabolically active, maintaining the integrity of the matrix for up to eight more divisions. This way cartilage is produced from the inside out.

14. Rheumatoid arthritis: joint pain with prolonged early morning stiffness and gelling after activity. In the joint there is synovial inflammation and thickening with lymphocytic and macrophage infiltration, cartilage destruction, juxta-articular osteoporosis, joint deformities. Osteoarthritis: intermittent, chronic pain worsens on exertion, early morning stiffness and pain lasting a few minutes, joint tenderness and instability, loss of function and deformity. Signs include swelling and effusion, crepitus on movement and osteophytes (bony swellings). Loss of joint space and cartilage destruction can appear on X-ray; also subchondral bone cysts arising due to repeated trauma.

15. Macule: flat, circumscribed lesion of colour change, e.g. vitiligo, freckles, capillary haemangioma; wheal– itchy, raised, discoloured, oedematous papules or plaques, e.g. urticaria and angio-odema; blister: lesion filled with clear fluid that occurs as a result of epidermal cleavage, e.g. due to trauma, pemphigus, pemphigoid; plaque extended, flat-topped lesion no more than 5 mm in elevation, up to 2 cm wide, e.g. psoriasis; papule solid, circumscribed, palpable elevation less than 5 mm wide, e.g. lichen planus (flat-topped); purpura rash caused by cutaneous capillary haemorrhage, e.g. septicaemia, thrombocytopenia.

16. Complete fracture of the neck of femur. At this age this would require a total hip replacement or, if the patient is not medically fit for surgery due to comorbidity, it would require pinning. The main complication is death, with a 50% mortality rate within 12 months. Another complication occurring in intracapsular fracture is avascular necrosis due to disruption of the joint's blood supply.

17. Most likely diagnosis is ankylosing spondylitis. Test for presence of HLA B27 antibody. An X-ray may show squaring of the vertebral bodies, syndesmophyte formation, ossification of anterior longitudinal and interspinous ligaments creating a bamboo-spine appearance, and calcification of the intervertebral discs.

18. Features suggestive of malignant change are asymmetry of the lesion and an irregular border, dark and irregular colour, diameter greater than 6 mm, elevation, itching, bleeding. Wide local excision of the lesion and histological examination are required.

19. Cutaneous candidal or bacterial infections, ulcers due to arterial or neuropathic disease (commonly at the feet), eruptive xanthomas due to hyperlipidaemia. Specific complications include diabetic dermopathy, necrobiosis lipoidica on the shins, granuloma annulare on the hands and feet.

20. Nodular skin metastases from primaries, including breast, GI tract, ovary, lung and melanoma. Pruritus (jaundice), acquired ichythyoses (lymphoma) , hyperpigmentation, pyoderma gangrenosum (leukaemia, lymphoma, myeloma), dermatomyositis (breast, lung, GI or GU carcinomas), erythroderma (lymphoma, leukaemia), hypertrichosis (ovarian carcinoma). Less commonly acanthosis nigricans (GI carcinoma), Paget's disease of the nipple (breast carcinoma).

1. 1E; 2D; 3A; 4B; 5B; 6F
2. 1C; 2A; 3D; 4B
3. 1F; 2C; 3G; 4A; 5D; 6B; 7E
4. 1C; 2E; 3A; 4B; 5D
5. 1D; 2F; 3B; 4C; 5E; 6D; 7A
6. 1D; 2G; 3B; 4A; 5E

7. 1D; 2F; 3C; 4B; 5A
8. 1D; 2B; 3A; 4F; 5C
9. 1F; 2C; 3D; 4E; 5A
10. 1D; 2A; 3G; 4F; 5B
11. 1A; 2D; 3B; 4C; 5A

Index

A

A band 18, 19
abscesses, Brodie's 83, 84
acantholysis 142
acanthosis 142
acanthosis nigricans 181–2
acetyl CoA 26, 27
acetylcholine (ACh)
  neuromuscular junction 26, 27
  receptors see nicotinic acetylcholine receptors
  smooth muscle 55, 56
acetylcholinesterase 26, 27
  inhibitors 28
Achilles tendonitis 14
achondroplasia 81–2
aciclovir 149, 156–7
acitretin 147
acne vulgaris 166–7
acral lentiginous melanoma 164
acrodermatitis of Hallopeau 144
acromegaly 78
actin 29–30
  filaments 17, 18, 19, 29–30
  function during contraction 30–1
  smooth muscle 56
actinic dermatitis, chronic 153
actinic prurigo 153
α-actinin 30
action potential (AP)
  cardiac 47–9, 50
  nerve 22–4
  neuromuscular transmission 26–7
  skeletal muscle 27, 28–9
  smooth muscle 56
active zones 26
Addison's disease 176
adenoma sebaceum 178
adenosine triphosphate (ATP) 30, 31, 57
adhesive capsulitis 116
adrenaline (epinephrine) 25, 53, 56
adrenocorticotrophic hormone (ACTH) 136
afferent neurons 5
ageing 7, 137, 192
airway smooth muscle 53–4
Albers–Schönberg disease 79–81
albinism 175, 193
alcohol abuse, myopathy 46
alcohol consumption 198
alkaline phosphatase 219

all-or-none principle 23, 34
allergy 134–5, 136
  contact dermatitis 139, 149
  drug 182–3, 200
allopurinol 112
alopecia 168, 169, 194
  diffuse non-scarring 195
  localized non-scarring 195
alopecia areata 168, 170
α-actinin 30
aminoglycoside antibiotics 27
amiodarone 58
anaerobic glycolysis 31
anagen effluvium 138
anal sphincters 55
androgenetic alopecia 168, 169
androgens 136
angioedema 150–1
angiotensin 56
ankle
  disorders 122–3
  examination 211–12
ankylosing spondylitis 108–9
anogenital fold eruptions 192
anorexia nervosa 169
antagonistic muscle groups 14, 16
anthrax 155–6
anti-acetylcholine receptor antibodies 39, 219
anti-androgens 167
anti-cyclic citrullinated peptide antibodies 219
antibiotics
  acne 167
  eczema 149
  pyogenic osteomyelitis 83–4
  septic arthritis 113
  skin infections 154, 155
anticholinesterases 28, 40
anticipation, genetic 43
antifungal agents 157, 158, 171
antihistamines 149
antinuclear antibodies (ANAs) 103, 106–7, 110, 219
antiseptics 149
antiviral agents 149, 156–7
apocrine sweat glands 140
aponeuroses 4–5, 15
appearance, patient's 197
appositional growth 66, 73
arrectores pilorum 137
arterial leg ulcers 173–4